# A Manual of Paedodontics

Train up a child in the way he should go: and when he
is old, he will not depart from it.

*Proverbs xxii 6*

# A Manual of Paedodontics

**R. J. Andlaw**
Senior Lecturer in Children's Dentistry,
University of Bristol Dental School

**W. P. Rock**
Senior Lecturer in Children's Dentistry and Orthodontics,
University of Birmingham Dental School

With illustrations by
**G. C. Van Beek** B. D. S.

SECOND EDITION

CHURCHILL LIVINGSTONE
EDINBURGH LONDON MELBOURNE AND NEW YORK 1987

CHURCHILL LIVINGSTONE
Medical Division of Longman Group UK Limited

Distributed in the United States of America by Churchill
Livingstone Inc., 1560 Broadway, New York, N.Y. 10036,
and by associated companies, branches and representatives
throughout the world.

First Edition 1982
Second Edition 1987
  Reprinted 1989

ISBN  0-443-03602-0

**British Library Cataloguing in Publication Data**
Andlaw, R.J.
   A manual of paedodontics.—2nd ed.
   1. Pedodontics
   I. Title II. Rock, W.P.
617.6'45      RK55.C5

**Library of Congress Cataloging-in-Publication Data**
Andlaw, R.J.
   A manual of paedodontics.
   Includes bibliographies and index.
   1. Pedodontics—Handbooks, manuals, etc.
I. Rock, W.P. II. Title. [DNLM: 1. Pedodontics—
handbooks. WU 39 A552m]
RK55.C5A53    1987      617.6'45      86-33374

Produced by Longman Singapore Publishers (Pte) Ltd.
Printed in Singapore.

# Preface to the Second Edition

We were extremely gratified by the favourable reaction to the first edition of this book. We are grateful for the constructive criticisms made by colleagues who reviewed the book, and we have taken these into account in preparing this second edition.

The aim of the book has not been changed: the book is essentially a practical manual of clinical techniques, not a comprehensive textbook. However, by including references to relevant literature and by making suggestions for further reading, we aim to help the reader who wishes to pursue the subject more deeply.

Almost every chapter has been modified to some extent but the greatest changes have been made to the chapters on fluoride (Chapter 4), the treatment of hypoplastic teeth (Chapter 13) and the immediate treatment of traumatised teeth (Chapter 27). An additional chapter has been in-cluded on the treatment of intrinsic staining of teeth (Chapter 16) and the section on periodontal disease in children has been expanded into a separate chapter (Chapter 23). New sections have been added to several chapters, for example on intraligamentary local analgesia (Chapter 6), on composite resin and glass ionomer restorations of primary teeth (Chapter 8), on porcelain veneers for hypoplastic or discoloured teeth (Chapter 13) and on root fractures (Chapter 27). The presentation of techniques in tabular form proved popular and has been retained.

We gratefully acknowledge the helpful suggestions of Herschel Horowitz and Stanley Heifetz on fluorides, of Don Glenwright on periodontal disease and of Crispian Scully on soft tissue lesions; and also the help given by Glyn Duggan in reading, correcting and improving several sections of the manuscript.

Bristol, 1987

RJA
WPR

# Preface to the First Edition

This book has been written primarily for undergraduate dental students but we hope it will also be of interest and value to practising dentists. Our aim has been to write a practical manual, not a comprehensive textbook. Thus, treatment aspects have been considered in detail but other aspects, such as aetiology, clinical features and histopathology, have been excluded or considered only briefly. We have included most of the common forms of treatment in paedodontics, but there are some omissions; for example, we have not described the extraction of teeth or other surgical procedures.

We would greatly value constructive criticisms from our colleagues, which would be most helpful in preparing further editions. The book is strongly influenced by current ideas and practices in the United Kingdom and, inevitably, it is orientated towards the British reader; for this we beg the indulgence of our overseas readers.

The tabular format chosen for describing many of the clinical techniques is a modification of that used by Dr Milton Houpt in *Task Analyses of Procedures in Paedodontics* (U.W. Public Helath Service, 1975). To avoid disrupting the continuity of the tables, illustrations are placed at the end of each table. We hope students will find this format instructive and easy to follow.

We wish to record our gratitude to the following colleagues who read sections of the drafts and made helpful suggestions: Tom Dowell, Glyn Duggan, Don Glenwright, Hugh Edmondson, Stephen Kneebone and Roger Smith. We also thank Mrs Elaine Collings, who typed the manuscript, and all those at Churchill Livingstone who helped in the publication of this book.

Bristol, 1982

RJA
WPR

# Contents

# The child patient

# 1

# The first appointment

The practice of paedodontics, as indeed of all branches of dentistry, should be governed by a simple but fundamental philosophy: treat the patient not the tooth. Implicit in this philosophy is a commitment to consider the child's feelings, to gain the child's confidence and cooperation, to perform treatment in a kind, sympathetic manner, and to be concerned not only with providing the treatment currently required but also with promoting the child's future dental health by stimulating positive attitudes and behaviour regarding dental care.

The first appointment should be used to establish a sound basis for achieving these aims. The appointment should be conducted in such a way that it is an enjoyable experience for the child, and should be regarded primarily as a mutual assessment session during which the dentist assesses the child, and the child assesses the dentist and his environment. It is recognised that sometimes, for example when the child attends in acute pain, the ideal procedure may have to be modified, but the fundamental aims of the first visit should never be abandoned.

## PREPARATION FOR THE FIRST APPOINTMENT

Parents usually try in some way to prepare their child for the dental appointment. Some parents, through their own fears or ignorance, do more harm than good in this attempt. It is therefore sensible to advise parents on how to prepare their child, and a letter that has been prepared for this purpose is presented below.

Dear parents,
    I enclose an appointment card for your child. I hope the following notes will be helpful to you.
*Preparation for the visit*
    Most people (adults included) are rather nervous at the prospect of visiting a dentist. Parents sometimes try to prepare their children for the visit by saying that the dentist 'will not hurt', or by bribing them to be good with the promise of a toy (or even a sweet!). I suggest that it is better to be as casual as possible. Simply inform the child (either on the morning of the appointment or on the day before) that you are taking him to visit the dentist, and that the dentist will look at his teeth and help to look after them. Avoid conversation in the home that might include unfavourable references to dentistry.
*What will be done at the first visit?*
    It has been said that a child's first dental appointment is the most important in his life. The main objective of the first appointment is that he should enjoy his visit and be happy to come again.
    I will first ask you and your child certain questions to obtain essential background information about, for example, medical condition, any past dental experience, etc.
    Your child's mouth will then be examined, and you will be informed of the nature of any treatment required and approximately how long it will take to complete.
    Your child's teeth will be brushed and possibly X-rayed.
    If your child has toothache or any other dental problem, this will be attended to, but treatment is not usually done at the first visit.
*Further visits*
    I hope that your child will continue to enjoy coming to see me. Treatment is started once the child's confidence and cooperation have been obtained. This is usually at the second visit, but for some children further introductory appointments are required.
    Following the first appointment you will usually be asked to remain in the Waiting Room, unless your child needs your continued moral support at the chairside.

Yours sincerely,

The aims of the first appointment are as follows:

1. To establish good communication with the child and parent.
2. To obtain important background information (i.e. the patient's history).
3. To examine the child, and to obtain radiographs if required.
4. To perform a simple operative procedure.
5. To explain treatment aims to the child and parent.

## COMMUNICATION WITH CHILD AND PARENT

Most patients have some anxiety about visiting a dentist for the first time, and it should therefore be an important objective for the dentist and his staff to allay this anxiety. The receptionist should greet the child in a friendly and cheerful manner, and the waiting room should contain evidence that children are welcome (e.g. children's posters, periodicals, books and toys). Thus, the whole environment of reception and waiting areas should communicate a warm sense of friendship and welcome.

On meeting the child and parent, the dentist should establish friendly communication with them while at the same time obtaining the information that constitutes the patient's history. Ideally, this meeting should not take place in the surgery, but in another room (Swallow, Jones and Morgan, 1975); if in the surgery, it is preferable to offer the child a chair other than the dental chair. This approach allows the dentist time to assess and, if necessary, to allay the child's anxiety before placing the child in a more stressful situation.

It is desirable to meet the parent with the child mainly to obtain a full history, important details of which may not be provided by the child. Moreover, very young or apprehensive children usually need the moral support of a parent in the surgery, at least at their first visit. At subsequent appointments, the dentist must decide whether to separate child and parent by asking the parent to remain in the waiting room. Some dentists invariably insist on working with the child alone; others are more flexible and base their decisions on the age and behaviour of the child, and on the character of the parent. However, it is always important to gain the parent's interest and cooperation, so that effective home care is encouraged.

Some dentists find communicating with children easy, others find it difficult. An essential ingredient in successful communication is to show interest in the child, and this can readily be achieved by asking simple questions about the home, school and favourite leisure activities. The dentist should also communicate visually by appearing relaxed, friendly and cheerful, and should use opportunities that may arise to communicate physically, for example by shaking hands or patting the child on the shoulder, or by stroking a girl's 'beautiful hair' or tickling a young child; there are many opportunities depending on the child's age and sex. Especially with the very young child, and with the mentally handicapped, this visual and physical communication is most important.

## HISTORY

The information that constitutes the patient's history is divided into three parts: the social, dental and medical histories. History-taking provides essential information on which treatment planning is based. A suggested outline for history taking is given on pages 6 and 7.

## EXAMINATION

### Clinical examination

*Extra-oral examination*

Any obvious extra-oral abnormalities noted during history-taking may be examined more closely. An outline of points to note is given in Table 1.1.

*Intra-oral examination*

It is hoped that any anxiety that the child may have felt on arrival will have been reduced or eliminated during the period of history-taking. He should then be happy to sit on the dental chair.

**Table 1.1** An outline for clinical examination.

*Extra-oral*
General appearance — size and weight.
Gait
Skin, complexion.
Eyes, lips.
Facial symmetry
Lymph glands

*Intra-oral*
Soft tissues
  cheeks
  lips
  tongue
  tonsils
  hard and soft palate
  gingiva
Teeth
  oral cleanliness
  teeth present
  position of teeth — crowding, spacing, drifting.
  occlusion
    first permanent molars and canines
    incisors — overjet, overbite.
  mobility — exfoliating primary tooth, abscess, periodontitis.
  colour — non-vital tooth, intrinsic staining, caries.
  structure — hypoplasia, hypomineralisation.
  caries

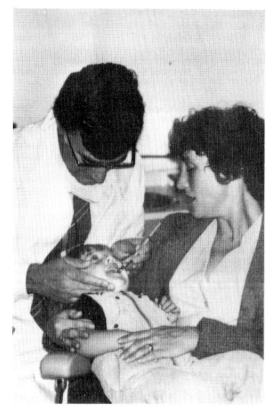

**Fig. 1.1** Position for examination of an uncooperative young child.

With a very young child, a good approach is for the dentist to ask 'how many teeth do you have?' and to suggest 'let's count your teeth'; this is probably less threatening to a child than to say 'I want to look at your teeth'. If the child is still unwilling to sit on the chair, the parent should be asked to do so and the child should be placed across the parent's lap, with the head supported on the parent's right arm (Fig. 1.1). In this position the child feels some sense of security, the parent may help in restraining undesirable movements if necessary, and the dentist has excellent access for oral examination. If the child should cry, access for the examination is improved; the dentist should ignore the cries while 'counting' the teeth aloud, after which the child is allowed to sit up again. He will have learned that there was nothing traumatic about the examination and that crying did not disturb the dentist. With these lessons learned, introduction to treatment may proceed in the normal manner.

An initial examination carried out under these conditions need not be very detailed. If a probe is used it should be remembered that the sight of any sharp, pointed instrument may cause anxiety, and that careless use of a probe may cause pain. Simple treatment may be started with the child lying on the parent's lap but, as the child's confidence grows, he should soon be happy to sit alone.

The approach outlined above clearly is not practicable with the older child who is too large to lie on a parent's lap. If such a child remains uncooperative after the history-taking period and is unwilling to sit on the dental chair, it may be preferable to postpone oral examination and to start the process of behaviour shaping (Ch. 2) at a different point, for example with oral hygiene instruction. Although this situation does not frequently arise, it is not uncommon with mentally handicapped children. Clearly, if the child was brought because of a specific problem that may require urgent treatment, some means must be

## Suggested outline for history-taking

|  | Information | Rationale | Notes |
|---|---|---|---|
| Social history | Name (including any abbreviated name or nickname). Address. School. | The dentist should address the child by the name he prefers. | |
| | Brothers and sisters. | Simple questioning about home and school is the most natural way of communicating with a child. In addition, the answers provide an insight into the child's interests and home environment. Recording these details provides the dentist with topics of conversation at subsequent meetings. | The type of response to questioning immediately gives some indication of the child's character and state of mind. He may respond in an easy, friendly manner, indicating that he is happy and relaxed, or he may refuse to respond at all, indicating that he is shy, very anxious or frankly antagonistic. |
| | Pets. Favourite activites at home, at school. | | |
| | Mother's occupation — any difficulties in bringing the child for further appointments? | Most commonly it is the mother who brings the child to his first dental appointment. Any difficulty in attending would have to be considered in treatment planning, especially if a long course of treatment is required. | |
| | Father's occupation. | Classifying the family by social class, based on the father's occupation, allows some prediction to be made of the family's attitudes towards dentistry (Beal, 1983). | Often, the father's occupation emerges while establishing the mother's occupation. Sometimes, however, it may seem inappropriate to question on this point, in which case the information may be obtained at a subsequent meeting, perhaps after asking the child 'what do you want to be when you grow up?' |
| Dental history | C/o — Complaining of: Is the patient attending because of a specific complaint? If not, what is the reason for attendance? e.g. routine check-up, referred following dental inspection at school. | It is important to establish the reason for the patient's attendance. | |
| | HPC — History of present complaint: If complaint is toothache, obtain the following information: location of pain, when did it start? is it intermittent or continuous? if intermittent — how long does it last? — is it brought on by hot, cold or sweet stimuli, or when eating? does pain keep child awake at night? is pain relieved by analgesics? | The symptoms of toothache give an indication of the probable pathology of pulp, e.g. intermittent pain of short duration brought on by hot, cold or sweet — pulp hyperaemia; spontaneous pain, severe, keeps child awake — acute pulpitis, abscess. | Unfortunately, the symptoms described by a child or by a parent may be vague and of little diagnostic value. |

| Information | Rationale | Notes |
|---|---|---|
| *PDH — Past dental history*:<br>Has dental care been regular or irregular in the past?<br>Has previous dental treatment been given elsewhere? If so, why has the parent changed dentist?<br>Has the child had any experience of dental treatment? If so, what treatment:<br>e.g. 'fillings'?<br>    extractions?<br>    local analgesia<br>    general anaesthesia? | The regularity of past dental care gives an indication of the parent's attitudes.<br>If a child is brought to a new dentist because he did not cooperate with a previous one, the reasons need to be pursued in such a way as to show the child that the dentist is interested and sympathetic, and that he will try to find a way of overcoming the problem. | When asking a child about previous experience of local analgesia, it is better to ask 'was your tooth made to go to sleep?' than 'did you have an injection?' or 'did you have a needle?', which would be considered threatening by many children. Similarly, when asking about general anaesthesia, 'did you go to sleep?' is better than 'did you have gas?' |
| Attitudes of the child to any of the above treatment (with a young child, the parent's opinion is relevant). | Any unfavourable attitudes to specific items of treatment must be taken into account in treatment planning. To pursue any form of treatment ignorant of the child's attitudes to that treatment reflects a lack of consideration for the child's feelings which is incompatible with the principles of good patient management. | The child's attitudes to previous treatment may be assessed by his response to a simple question like 'did you find it easy?' |
| Attitudes of the parent to dental treatment. | Parent's attitudes and expectations regarding dental treatment differ greatly; a treatment plan beyond their expectations should not be started without first explaining and justifying its value. | It may be anticipated that some parents would not appreciate the value of, for example, conservative treatment of primary teeth, or of preventive treatment. |
| *Medical history*<br>Congenital heart disease.<br>Rheumatic fever, chorea.<br>Blood disorder.<br>Respiratory tract disease.<br>Asthma.<br>Hepatitis, jaundice.<br>Gastro-intestinal disease.<br>Kidney or urinary tract disease.<br>Bone or joint disease.<br>Diabetes or other endocrine disease.<br>Skin disease.<br>Congenital abnormality.<br>Allergies, e.g. penicillin.<br>Recent or current medication.<br>Previous operations or serious illnesses.<br>Mental subnormality.<br>Epilepsy.<br>Family history of serious illness. | | |

found of examining the child, but if the reason for attendance was a routine 'check-up', postponement of the oral examination until the child's cooperation has been gained often is the most reasonable decision and the most successful in the long term.

## Radiographic examination

Sometimes the clinical examination provides all the necessary information about the patient, in which case radiographs are not required. More commonly, however, radiographs are required for one of the following reasons:

1. To diagnose dental caries in tooth surfaces not accessible to clinical examination.
2. To detect abnormalities in the developing dentition.
3. To investigate specific problems, for example the condition of periapical tissues associated with non-vital or traumatised teeth.

### Dental caries

Bite-wing radiographs are essential for the diagnosis of approximal surface caries. In a study of 5- to 7-year-old children, it was found that about two-thirds of the approximal surface lesions would not have been detected if radiographs had not been used (Murray and Majid, 1978). Approximal lesions may progress to form large cavities, which may even involve the pulp, before they are detectable clinically.

With the increasing use of fissure sealants in recent years, bite-wing radiographs have become important for the diagnosis of occlusal caries that might occur if sealants are defective (although early occlusal caries is not easily diagnosed on radiographs).

### Abnormalities in the developing dentition

An important aim in dentistry for children is to supervise the developing dentition and, if possible, to prevent or alleviate undesirable effects that might be caused by an abnormality in the dentition. Early detection of abnormalities requires a full radiographic survey.

Although it may be of interest to know of the existence of an abnormality during the primary dentition stage, it is of little practical importance at such a young age; therefore, it is normally preferable to wait until the early mixed dentition stage before obtaining the necessary radiographs.

A full radiographic examination of child patients at about the age of 7 to 8 years should be routine practice, and this may be achieved by one of the following combinations of radiographs:

1 a) Right and left rotated lateral oblique radiographs (bimolars) — to show maxillary and mandibular teeth distal to the canines.
  b) Nasal (standard) occlusal — to show the maxillary anterior region.
  c) Mandibular anterior occlusal — to show the mandibular anterior region. Abnormalities in this region are rare, and this view may be excluded unless there is a definite reason to include it.
2 a) Periapical radiographs — to show posterior teeth.
  b) Nasal occlusal and, possibly, mandibular anterior occlusal.

Usually, four periapical films are required (one for each posterior segment), but eight films may be required for older children. Because of this, and because intra-oral techniques require greater cooperation from the child than do extra-oral techniques, this approach is less convenient than bimolar radiography. Some dentists, however, routinely take molar periapicals and prefer canine and incisor periapicals to occlusal views (Kennedy, 1979).

3 a) Panoramic radiograph — to show the complete dentition.
  b) Nasal occlusal — to show the maxillary anterior region more clearly.

Panoramic radiography is a convenient method of obtaining a picture of the whole dentition on one film, but the equipment is expensive and therefore is available only in a minority of dental practices.

The anterior region of both jaws is the least well defined on panoramic radiographs, and teeth lying out of the line of the arch may not be detected. In the early mixed dentition, it is important to detect the presence of supernumerary teeth in the maxillary anterior regions, and therefore it is sensible to take a naso-occlusal radiograph (or a periapical) in addition to the panoramic radiograph.

### Specific problems

If the general radiographic survey is done by extra-oral radiography, selected periapical views may be required to show the periapical conditions of, for example, teeth with suspected pulp exposures, or of teeth that have been traumatised or received root canal treatment.

If an unerupted tooth or odontome is found in the radiographic survey, it may be necessary to determine whether it is placed labial or palatal to the roots of erupted teeth; this information is commonly required of an unerupted supernumerary tooth. The labio-palatal position may be determined by applying the principle of parallax to two periapical radiographs taken of the same area but at different angles; alternatively, a nasal occlusal and an off-centre periapical radiograph may be used.

A standard occlusal radiograph of the mandible may be useful in locating the bucco-lingual position of an unerupted mandibular tooth.

### Techniques

Brief details of recommended techniques are outlined in Table 1.2.

It is important to note that the rotated lateral oblique (Fig. 1.2) should show teeth distal to the canine in both the maxilla and the mandible. To obtain this view, it is essential to rotate the head by placing the tip of the patient's nose as well as the cheek in contact with the cassette; this rotation lifts the mandible on the side of the X-ray tube upwards, so that it does not become superimposed over the opposite canine and premolar region. It is convenient and economical to use one 18 × 13 cm film for views of both sides of the mouth; this can be done by using a lead rubber sheet to cover each half of the cassette in turn. This is called a bimolar radiograph (Bowdler Henry, 1955).

An alternative method of taking bimolar radiographs is to place the cassette on a flat surface and to sit the child so that he can place his head over it. A simple apparatus is available (Qualident Head Positioner, Orthomax Ltd.) which makes this method particularly easy to use (Fig. 1.3); it incorporates a board on which to place the cassette, a device for positioning the child's head correctly, and a lead rubber sheet that can be moved to cover each half of the cassette in turn.

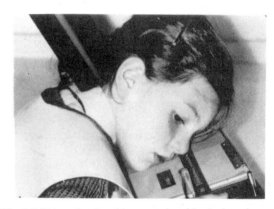

**Fig. 1.3** Using a head positioner to take a bimolar lateral oblique radiograph.

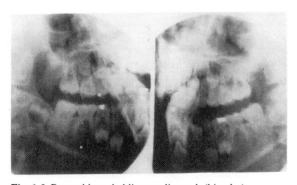

**Fig. 1.2** Rotated lateral oblique radiograph (bimolar).

## DIAGNOSIS

The information gathered from the clinical and radiographic examinations usually allows a diagnosis to be made. Sometimes, further diagnostic aids are required, for example pulp vitality tests for a traumatised tooth, or study models for orthodontic assessment. The diagnosis is a statement of any disease affecting the patient's oral health, or of any abnormality affecting dental development.

**Table 1.2** Radiographic techniques.

| | Bite-wing | Nasal-occlusal | Bimolar lateral oblique | Periapical |
|---|---|---|---|---|
| Head position | The imaginary line joining alar of nose to tragus of ear should be horizontal. | Alar-tragus line horizontal. | Sit the child sideways on the chair (armrest lowered). | Alar-tragus line horizontal. |
| Film size | For young child (e.g. under 5 yrs.)—2.2 × 3.5 cm. For older child—3.1 × 4.1 cm. Place the film in a bite-wing film holder—several types are available | 'occlusal' film 5.7 × 7.6 cm. | 13 × 18 cm film in cassette with intensifying screens | For young child—2.2 × 3.5 cm. For older child—3.1 × 4.1 cm. |
| Film position | Close to the lingual surfaces of maxillary and mandibular teeth, anterior border in line with the canines. Nearly vertical. If the corners of the film cause some discomfort they may be bent inwards. | Held between maxillary and mandibular anterior teeth. Longer dimension across the mouth, anterior border projecting a few mm beyond the incisal edges. | Rest the cassette on the chair's head-rest at an angle of about 45°. Position the child's head so that the nose and cheek touch the surface of the cassette and the lower border of the mandible lies parallel to its bottom edge. Ask the child to support the cassette with a hand. (For alternative method see text). | For incisors and canines, insert the film with its length running from the incisal edges of the teeth to the palate (or floor of the mouth), with its anterior border projecting a few mm beyond the incisal edges. For molars, place the film with its length running antero—posteriorly. Ask the child to support the film with a thumb or finger. |
| Direction of tube | Perpendicular to the film. | Between the tip and bridge of nose, at an angle of about +65°. | Just behind the angle of the mandible and just below the ear, aiming at the opposite premolar region at an angle of about +10°. | Perpendicular to a plane bisecting the angle formed by the long axis of the tooth and the plane of the film. |

| | maxillary teeth | mandibular teeth |
|---|---|---|
| prim. incisor | +45° | −10° |
| perm. incisor | +55° | −20° |
| prim. canine | +40° | −10° |
| perm. canine | +50° | −20° |
| molars | +20° | − 5° |

The exposure times are dependent on the type of X-ray machine and film used.
A protective lead-plastic apron should always be used.

The diagnosis defines the problem for which treatment must be planned.

## INTRODUCTORY TREATMENT

After having examined the child, a simple operative procedure should be introduce. Ideally, when the child has not presented with pain or any other complaint, the treatment should be a simple 'polish' using a brush or rubber cup in a slow-speed handpiece. The objectives are to introduce the child to the sensation of the dentist working in his mouth and to show him that this is a pleasant experience; this is especially important with the child who is attending for the first time. The Tell-Show-Do method (Ch. 2) is very effective. With the young child, brushing may be limited to a few incisors and take only a minute or two, the prime objective being to introduce the child happily to dentistry; whether plaque is removed or not is unimportant, and indeed prophylaxis paste usually is not used. With the older child, a full-mouth prophylaxis may be completed, and this treatment may conveniently be extended to the application of topical fluoride. Ideally, operative treatment involving injections or cavity preparation is not started at the first appointment; even the child with previous experience of dentistry elsewhere has, by this stage, been introduced to a sufficient number of new situations.

Unfortunately, children are often first taken to a dentist in pain and this form of introduction may not be possible. However, the important aim of influencing the child's long-term attitudes to dentistry should not be abandoned in the concern to treat pain. Certainly, immediate intervention is essential on some occasions but if intermittent pain has been tolerated for some time it is often preferable to prescribe analgesics to control any further episodes of pain, thus delaying operative treatment until the child's confidence has been obtained.

## CONCLUDING THE APPOINTMENT

Before dismissing the child, the dentist should give the parent a brief explanation of the treatment that is required. If restorations are required, this should be pointed out, but also it should be emphasised that attention to reparative treatment only is of little long-term benefit, and that prevention of further dental disease must also be an important aim. Perhaps it is enough at this first visit to make this one fundamental point about preventive treatment rather than to discuss in detail the methods that will be used. However, since oral hygiene instruction forms a part of the preventive plan, it is convenient to request that the child's brush be brought at the next visit.

Finally, some indication should be given to the parent of the probable length of the course of treatment; parents may become disillusioned if they expect to bring their child for two or three visits and later find that many more appointments are needed. Especially if the child is uncooperative and several introductory visits are envisaged during which little or no operative treatment will be

performed, the plan of action should be clearly explained to the parent (Hill and O'Mullane, 1979).

## SUMMARY OF THE FIRST APPOINTMENT

The recommended procedure for the first appointment may be summarised as follows:

1. Take the history
   a. social
   b. dental
   c. medical
2. Examine the child
   a. extra-oral
   b. intra-oral
3. Take radiographs if required
   a. to show dental caries — bite-wings
   b. to show the developing dentition (in patients over age 7 years)
      — rotated lateral obliques (bimolar)
        + nasal occlusal
        (+ mandibular anterior occlusal?)
        or panoramic + naso-occlusal
        or periapicals of posterior teeth
        + nasal occlusal
        (+ mandibular anterior occlusal?)
   c. to investigate specific problems
      — periapicals
4. Perform a simple operative procedure
   a. prophylaxis: incisors only (in young child) or full mouth, including removal of calculus if required.
   b. possibly topical fluoride treatment or other non-traumatic procedure.
   c. treat specific complaint if necessary.
5. Explain aims of treatment to parent
   a. emphasise the need for preventive as well as operative treatment.
   b. request that the child's toothbrush be brought at the next visit.
   c. give an estimate of the number of appointments required to complete treatment.

## TREATMENT PLANNING

Good treatment planning is at the very heart of good dentistry for children. Essential to good planning is a firm commitment to benefit the whole child, not merely his dentition, and to influence the child's attitudes to dentistry in addition to performing any necessary treatment. A course of treatment that is successful in completing operative treatment but that fails to establish or strengthen positive attitudes may be only of short-term benefit to the child; if negative attitudes are introduced more harm than good may be done. The essence of good dentistry for children is to plan and pursue treatment in such a way that the child benefits in the broadest sense, in the long term as well as in the short term.

To achieve these aims it is necessary to know more about the child than just the state of his dentition. Much of the necessary information is provided by the patient's social, dental and medical histories, and their influence on treatment planning has been noted on pages 6 and 7. Every child is different, and the most appropriate treatment plan for each individual patient can only be made on the basis of relevant background information. With this information, possible problems can be anticipated and treatment planned in such a way as to overcome or avoid them; without it, treatment can only proceed blindly, with the possibility of encountering unexpected problems. Thus, an adequate history is an essential requirement for good treatment planning.

An outline for treatment planning is presented below. The final plan should be recorded in note form, but should not be considered inflexible; it should be open to modification if necessary as treatment progresses.

| | Points to consider | Relevance in treatment planning |
|---|---|---|
| Behaviour management | The attitudes of the child and the parent to dental health, assessed by the regularity of past dental care, oral hygiene, etc. | The approach necessary to interest a family in dental health and to motivate them to practise preventive measures will inevitably be greatly influenced by their initial attitudes. |
| | Parent's attitudes to dental treatment. | Some parents do not value preventive or restorative dentistry, particularly for primary teeth. It would be necessary to change these attitudes before an ideal treatment plan could be made for their child. |
| | Child's attitudes to previous dental treatment; in particular, fears of specific items of treatment. | The selection of the most appropriate method of behaviour management must be based on a knowledge of the individual child's attitude to treatment. |
| Preventive treatment General | Caries experience. Medical history, especially congenital heart disease or history of rheumatic fever, bleeding disorders, debilitating disease with poor resistance to infection, mental or physical handicap. | All types of preventive treatment are especially important for patients with high caries experience and for those particularly at risk from dental diseases. |
| Oral hygiene instruction | Standard of oral hygiene, and state of gingival tissues. | If oral hygiene is poor and gingival inflammation is present, intensive oral hygiene instruction is required; if oral hygiene and gingival condition are good, re-emphasis and encouragement only may be required. |
| | Child's age. | When the child is less than about 6 years of age, or mentally or physically handicapped, the parent should be instructed in brushing the child's teeth. |
| Diet counselling | Caries rate. | Diet counselling is always important but is especially so if the child's caries rate is high. |
| Fluoride —tablets (or drops) | Parental interest. | Since parents must administer or supervise the use of the tablets, their interest is essential. |

| | Points to consider | Relevance in treatment planning |
|---|---|---|
| | Child's age. | Fluoride tablets are most strongly indicated for infants and young children; once started they may be continued to age 12–13 years (or be substituted by mouthrinsing at about 6–7 years of age). |
| —mouth-rinsing | Parental interest. | As above. |
| | Child's age. | Mouthrinsing is only feasible for children from about the age of 6–7 years, because younger children cannot manage the recommended procedure, which involves retaining solution in the mouth for 1–2 minutes. |
| —topical application | Is the child receiving systemic fluoride or using a mouthrinse regularly at home? | Application of topical fluoride or gel may not be justified for children receiving systemic fluoride or using a mouthrinse regularly, except for children with high caries rates or for those who are medically-at-risk, or mentally or physically handicapped. |
| Fissure sealing | Child's age. Caries rate. Morphology of pits and fissures. | Sealing of caries-free pits and fissures is particularly justified for newly erupted first permanent molars, especially for children with high caries rates (as assessed from the condition of the primary dentition) and for teeth with deep pits and fissures. |
| *Operative treatment* General | Medical history. | Precautions are sometimes necessary in the dental treatment of children with certain types of medical conditions (e.g. congenital heart disease, blood disorders). |
| Restorations | Depth of caries. | If caries is minimal or moderate, amalgam restorations usually are planned. If it is predicted that one or more teeth have pulp exposures, a decision must be made either to conserve by pulp treatment or to extract. |
| | Extent of caries. | Extensive lesions may be better restored with stainless steel crowns than with amalgam. |
| | Use of local analgesia. | Ideally, restorative dentistry is performed under local analgesia. However, if the child's attitudes are unfavourable, a decision must be made either:<br>(a) to reason with the child to change his attitude,<br>(b) to introduce some form of sedation,<br>(c) to pursue treatment without local analgesia (usually only possible if caries is minimal). |
| | Order of restoring teeth | If local analgesia is to be used, a maxillary premolar or primary molar should be chosen for the first restoration, as it is easiest to give a painless injection in this region. |
| Extractions | Are one or more teeth unsaveable, or have teeth already been extracted? | Extraction of primary molars usually should be accompanied either by 'balancing' extractions or by space maintenance. If a first permanent molar must be extracted, extraction of one or more of the other first permanent molars must be considered. |
| | Use of local analgesia or general anaesthesia. | A decision must be made to extract teeth under local analgesia (with or without sedation), or under general anaesthesia. The child's attitudes should be considered. |
| Orthodontic treatment | Crowding or spacing of:<br>(a) erupted teeth,<br>(b) unerupted teeth, i.e. availability of space in the arch for their eruption.<br>Developmental abnormalities.<br>Established malocclusion. | If there is crowding, extractions may be required immediately or be planned for the future. In cases of doubt, an orthodontist's opinion should be sought.<br><br>Some abnormalities should be treated early. Orthodontic treatment may be indicated. |

## REFERENCES

Beal J 1983 Social factors and preventive dentistry. In: Murray J J (ed) The prevention of dental disease. Oxford University Press, Oxford, ch 11

Bowdler Henry C 1955 A maxillostat. British Dental Journal 19:80–83

Hill F J, O'Mullane D M 1976 Preventive programme for the dental management of frightened children. Journal of Dentistry for Children 43:30–36

Kennedy D B 1979 Paediatric operative dentistry, 2nd edn. Wright, Bristol, ch 2

Murray J J, Majid Z A 1978 The prevalence and progression of approximal caries in the deciduous dentition in British children. British Dental Journal 145:161–164

Swallow J N, Jones J M, Morgan M F 1975 The effect of environment on a child's reaction to dentistry. Journal of Dentistry for Children 42:290–292

## RECOMMENDED READING

Holloway P J, Swallow J N 1975 Child dental health, 2nd edn. Wright, Bristol, ch 3

Wright G Z 1975 Behavior management in dentistry for children. Saunders, Philadelphia, ch 3 & 4

# 2

# Techniques of behaviour management

Behaviour shaping
Tell-show-do
Reinforcement
Desensitisation
Modelling
Hand-over-mouth

Sedation
  Oral route
  Intramuscular route
  Intravenous route
  Inhalational route
  Hypnosis

To obtain the cooperation of a child patient the dentist must not only establish good rapport with the child but also use effective techniques of behaviour management. Clearly, some knowledge of normal child development is essential, but this subject is outside the scope of this book and the reader is referred to the texts listed at the end of this Chapter.

Managing a child patient may be considered simply a matter of applying common sense, based on previous experiences with children but not on any formal knowledge of child psychology. Unfortunately, the application of common sense is not necessarily common practice. Therefore it is instructive to consider techniques that have proved successful in psychology and which can be applied in dentistry. Many dentists use these techniques intuitively, but when they are defined and described their basic principles can be applied consciously and, therefore, more effectively.

## BEHAVIOUR SHAPING

Psychologists use the term 'behaviour shaping' to refer to the process of influencing a patient's behaviour towards a desired ideal. An essential part of behaviour shaping is to define a series of steps on the path to the desired behaviour, and then to progress step by step to the goal. In relation to dentistry, it may be stated that ideal behaviour is shown by a patient who maintains excellent oral hygiene, exercises sensible diet control, and is relaxed and cooperative during operative treatment. It would be unrealistic to expect every patient to show this type of behaviour at the first appointment; but it would be wrong to accept as

unchangeable the behaviour of those who do not show it, or simply to hope that it will improve in time. The proper course of action is to plan treatment in such a way that the child's behaviour is gradually improved to the desired level. Only by so doing can the fundamental aims in dentistry for children be fulfilled: to influence positive attitudes and behaviour in addition to carrying out any necessary treatment.

For operative dentistry, behaviour shaping is based on a planned introduction of treatment procedures, so that the child is gradually trained to accept treatment in a relaxed and cooperative manner. Steps that may be defined for the introduction of treatment to an average school-aged child are:

1. Examination and prophylaxis.
2. Fissure sealant or topical fluoride application.
3. Small occlusal restoration in a primary tooth without local analgesia.
4. Infiltration analgesia and restoration.
5. Inferior dental nerve block and restoration.

The time spent on each step will depend on the child's behaviour. Thus, some children might require several short appointments at the early steps before being taken further, while others could be taken to step 5 within one or two appointments. Indeed, some children could be taken to step 5 at the first appointment, but this would not be considered good practice; even if the child accepts the treatment, such an approach rejects the principles of behaviour shaping and is less likely to succeed.

For very frightened young children, the following steps may be planned (Hill and O'Mullane, 1976):

15

1. Child to brush his teeth with his own tooth-brush at washbasin.
2. Mother, and then dentist, to brush child's teeth with his own brush at washbasin.
3. Child to sit on dental chair; examination and use of prophylaxis brush in slow-speed hand-piece.
4. Proceed as with normal child.

The gradual approach implicit in behaviour shaping may initially delay the progress of treatment, but when the child's full cooperation is obtained this delay is more than compensated, so that time spent initially can be regarded as a sound investment.

## TELL — SHOW — DO (TSD)

The essentials of TSD are to *tell* the child about the treatment to be carried out, to *show* him at least some part of how it will be done, and then to *do* it. The technique is used routinely in introducing a child to prophylaxis, which is always chosen as the first operative procedure. Thus, the child is told that his teeth are to be brushed, shown the 'special' brush and how it revolves in the handpiece, and then his teeth are brushed. To the TSD sequence should be added 'Praise', because good behaviour during this initial treatment, and indeed during any subsequent treatment, should immediately be reinforced (see below).

The transition from a brush to a bur is easily made; the bur may be introduced as a 'special cleaner' that cleans 'the little corners that the brush cannot reach'.

Some compromise is necessary in applying this method to the administration of local analgesia. Most dentists consider that the needle should not be shown, because most children (and adults too) are apprehensive about needles. Therefore the child is told that his tooth will be 'made to go to sleep', shown the surface analgesic on cotton wool, and the injection follows without further demonstration (Ch. 7).

For whatever treatment it is being employed, it is important to ensure a smooth continuity through the T-S-D stages. The explanations should not be lengthy and protracted, as this would tend to confuse the child and perhaps arouse anxiety; it should be done simply and casually. Similarly, the demonstration should be given briefly and in a matter-of-fact manner, so that the actual treatment follows without undue delay.

## REINFORCEMENT

Reinforcement may be defined as the strengthening of a pattern of behaviour, which increases the probability of that behaviour being displayed in the future. Psychologists who adhere to the social-learning theories of child development believe that a child's behaviour is a reflection of his responses to the rewards and punishments of his environment, and that a very important form of reward (and therefore a strong motivating factor for behaviour change) is the love and approval obtained first from his parents and later from his peers. Therefore, good behaviour by children in the dental situation, whether it be in brushing their teeth efficiently or in cooperating well in operative procedures, should be rewarded by a show of approval from the dentist. This approval is expected to reinforce the good behaviour, thus increasing the probability of it being repeated in subsequent treatment, because it becomes a normal pattern of behaviour for the child in that situation.

The dentist's approval should be shown frequently during treatment, whenever the child responds positively to directions (Rosenberg, 1974). Usually this approval is given verbally, but smiles and nods are also appropriate. The wording is not important and each dentist has his own favourite phrases ranging, for example, from a simple 'that's good', through 'well done, that's terrific' to 'you are one of my best patients'. The important point is that the child's good behaviour should be reinforced frequently.

The reward should be closely linked to the action. For example, if a child is asked to open his mouth wide and he responds well, he should receive an immediate sign of approval. Approval given only at the end of an appointment, for example 'we've finished now, you've been a very good boy' is not effective. Much worse, however, is to ignore the child's good cooperation during treatment; not only does this waste an excellent opportunity of strengthening that behaviour but may, by acting as a form of punishment, reduce the probability of that behaviour being repeated.

Another form of reward is a present, and this is justifiable at the end of a session provided it is given as a sign of approval of good behaviour. Presents should not be used to bribe children. Many types of suitable presents are available, for example, booklets and badges.

It is important to avoid reinforcement of poor behaviour. If a child is obstructive and the planned treatment cannot be completed, abrupt termination of treatment and return to the parent for consolation is very likely to reinforce that poor behaviour. It would be preferable to appear undisturbed and to pretend that treatment is completed (for example by placing a temporary dressing). The types of punishment that a dentist can use for poor behaviour are limited, other than the withdrawal of approval or other rewards. The dentist should not ridicule the child for his poor behaviour, or show his anger; he can only show the child that he is disappointed with him.

## DESENSITISATION

Desensitisation is one of the techniques used most frequently by psychologists in the treatment of fears. Classically, the technique involves three stages: first, training the patient to relax; second, constructing a hierarchy of fear-producing stimuli related to the patient's principal fear; and third, introducing each stimulus in the hierarchy in turn to the relaxed patient, starting with the stimulus that causes least fear and progressing to the next only when the patient no longer fears that stimulus (Wolpe and Lazarus, 1966). It is important to note that the patient must be helped to relax before his fear is overcome; simply repeating the stimulus many times increases rather than decreases fear. The technique has been used to overcome many types of fears, for example, fear of heights, of crowded places, of isolation, as well as fear of dentistry (Gale and Ayer, 1969).

To apply the technique in its classical form, a series of preliminary appointments is required to teach the patient how to relax. Although some dentists (especially those familiar with hypnosis) may be prepared to do this, and others may refer the patient to a psychologist, the basic concepts of the technique may be applied in dentistry without the preliminary appointments. It is important to know the basis of the child's fear, which may be a general fear of dentists, doctors, hospitals or clinics, or a more specific fear of 'the needle', 'the drill' or other aspect of dental treatment. When this information is known, a hierarchy of fear-producing stimuli can be constructed and worked through. If, for example, the child is frightened of the dental environment in general, desensitisation might include successive introduction of the child to the following stimuli:

1. Reception and waiting rooms.
2. Dentist and nurse.
3. Dental surgery.
4. Dental chair.
5. Oral examination.
6. Prophylaxis.

If, on the other hand, the child fears 'the drill', the selected stimuli might be:

1. Brushing the child's teeth with a prophylaxis brush held by hand.
2. Brushing with a prophylaxis brush in a slow-speed handpiece.
3. Using a finishing bur or stone in a slow-speed handpiece, revolving in the mouth but not in contact with teeth.
4. Applying the finishing bur or stone gently to a restoration or tooth surface.
5. Introducing a high-speed handpiece as in 3 and 4 above.

Desensitisation from fear of 'the needle' is more difficult; if this fear persists despite careful behaviour shaping during introductory appointments, some form of sedation may be considered (p. 18).

At each stage of a hierarchy, the child's fears are allayed by the kind, friendly and reassuring manner of the dentist and his staff, and positive behaviour shown by the child is strongly reinforced. When the child appears relaxed and contented, progress is made to the next stage. Some children's fears are quickly overcome in this way, allowing rapid progress through the hierarchy. On the other hand, others are more resistant, and this no doubt discourages many dentists from using the method.

## MODELLING

Modelling is another technique used by psychologists in the treatment of fears; for example, children frightened of dogs have been helped to overcome their fears by watching other children playing happily with dogs, the happy children being the models which the frightened children later imitated.

This simple technique may be applied to a variety of dental treatment situations but perhaps its most frequent application is in the introduction of an anxious child to oral examination in the dental chair. A parent or, preferably, another child is asked to act as the model, submitting to an examination and prophylaxis; the relaxed, co-operative behaviour of the model will, it is hoped, later be imitated by the anxious child. Tell-show-do and reinforcement should be used to supplement the modelling procedure; together with desensitisation, this is an effective approach to the problem of introducing simple treatment to the frightened child (Adelson and Goldfried, 1970).

## HAND-OVER-MOUTH

The 'hand-over-mouth' technique is generally regarded as being rather an extreme measure in dealing with an uncooperative child. It is rarely used in the U.K. but has its adherents in the U.S.A. (Levitas, 1974).

The technique involves restraining the protesting child gently but firmly in the dental chair, placing a hand (or towel) over his mouth to subdue his protests and, speaking quietly but clearly into his ear, telling him that the hand will be removed as soon as he stops crying (Craig, 1971). When the child responds favourably, the hand is removed immediately and he is praised. If protests start again, the procedure is repeated.

Such a technique cannot be popular with any dentist who cares for children and whose aim is to influence positive attitudes in addition to carrying out treatment. Its only possible justification might be in dealing with a spoilt child who has learned to manipulate his over-indulgent parents with temper tantrums, or with a defiant child who has found that silent but firm defiance always succeeds. Such children are not frightened; they simply do not wish to cooperate and know how to avoid doing so. Their behaviour usually soon becomes evident at the first appointment and is confirmed by the manner of their refusal to be examined. If such a child is picked up and placed on the chair or on a parent's lap, strong protests may be expected. The dentist should ignore these protests while examining the child; sometimes this simple show of authority by the dentist succeeds in establishing some basis for cooperation in the future. However, if the child behaves in a similar manner at the next visit, a decision has to be made about further action. It is in these cases that the hand-over-mouth technique may be justified. Until the child learns that the dentist is not impressed or deterred by tantrums or defiance, no treatment is possible. Furthermore, if the child's behaviour results in a rapid return to a consoling parent, that behaviour will be further reinforced.

The technique should never be used with frightened children, for whom desensitisation and other methods are appropriate. Correct assessment of the reasons for a child's uncooperative behaviour is therefore essential before using the hand-over-mouth technique.

## SEDATION

The great majority of children introduced to dentistry by the methods described above become relaxed and cooperative patients who readily accept most operative procedures. Unfortunately a minority remain, or become, uncooperative. The most common reason for lack of cooperation is fear, often of a specific procedure such as the injection or 'the drill'. If fear persists despite carefully conducted introductory appointments, some form of sedation may be helpful. In general, it may be said that sedation will be most effective with children who are genuinely frightened but who understand the need for treatment and who wish to be helped; children whose lack of cooperation has no rational basis and who simply do not wish to cooperate are less likely to respond favourably to any form of education.

It should be emphasised that by sedation is meant the allaying of anxiety. Although reducing anxiety tends to raise the patient's pain threshold, sedation does not produce analgesia. Therefore, the use of local analgesia is normally required, but this usually presents no problems when the patient is sedated. However sedation with nitrous oxide (p. 20) produces some analgesia in addition to sedation, and local analgesia is not always required.

It must also be emphasised that the sedated patient is conscious and in command of all normal protective reflexes, including the cough reflex. Therefore, sedation may be administered by the dentist who performs the dental treatment, in sharp contrast to anaesthesia which must not be administered by the person responsible for the dental treatment.

Sedation may be administered by the following routes:

1. Oral.
2. Intravenous.
3. Intramuscular.
4. Inhalational.

### Oral route

Many drugs and combinations of drugs have been used to sedate anxious children, including various barbiturates, chloral hydrate, hydroxyzine, meprobamate, promethazine and diazepam (Wright, 1975; Bennett, 1978). Unfortunately, few studies have been carried out to demonstrate their effectiveness with children; these studies have been reviewed by Barenie (1979).

Although it is simple and convenient to administer a drug orally, the effects are less predictable than when it is given by other routes, because of many factors that influence its absorption. When it is decided to administer a sedative orally, its use should not necessarily be abandoned if the desired effects are not obtained at the first attempt;

the dose may be increased until the appropriate dose for the individual patient is reached.

Diazepam is the drug that probably has been used most commonly in the U.K., either in a single dose 1 to 2 hours before treatment or, more commonly, in three doses as outlined in Table 2.1. It has been shown to be effective in helping apprehensive adults to accept dental treatment (Baird and Curson, 1970), but a recent study with children aged 4–13 years showed it to be ineffective (Lindsay and Yates, 1985). It might be expected to be more effective with teenaged children who wish to cooperate but who cannot control their fears.

Before prescribing a sedative, the dentist should gain the trust and confidence of the child. The sedative must be explained as something that will help him feel more relaxed so that the treatment may be done without worrying him. It is important that the child does not feel threatened by imagining that the sedative will force him into submission; rather he should feel that it is being used to help him. Unfortunately this approach based on trust and understanding cannot be used with very young, uncooperative children.

The cooperation of parents or guardians is also essential, since it is most convenient if they administer the sedative. Since the drug may cause drowsiness, it is preferable for the child not to attend school before the dental appointment.

### Intramuscular route

The advantage of administering a drug intramuscularly rather than orally is that its action is more rapid and its effect more predictable. A disadvantage, however, is that a nervous, uncooperative child inevitably finds the intramuscular injection an unpleasant procedure.

Various types of drugs have been used (Mussel-

**Table 2.1** Recommended dosages of diazepam for children.

|  | *Preparations* | *Dose* | |
|---|---|---|---|
| *Diazepam* (trade name 'Valium') | Diazepam tablets B.P. — 2 mg, 5 mg, 10 mg | On retiring to bed After breakfast | 5 mg 5 mg |
|  | Diazepam elixir — 2 mg/5 ml (teaspoon) | 1–2 hours before dental appointment | 5 mg |

man and McClure, 1975). An effective combination is promethazine hydrochloride (Phenergan) and pethidine. Promethazine is an antihistamine that has sedative and anti-emetic properties. Pethidine is a potent analgesic but has little sedative effect. In combination they provide sedation and analgesia, and the anti-emetic action of promethazine counteracts the nausea that may be produced by pethidine. The doses for intramuscular injection are pethidine 1.5 mg/kg body weight, and promethazine 0.75 mg/kg. The injection may be given in the upper, lateral quadrant of the buttock, the anterior aspect of the upper thigh, or the lateral aspect of the upper arm (Musselman and McClure, 1975; Bennett, 1978). The method is widely used in the U.S.A., particularly to produce deep sedation in very uncooperative young patients who generally cannot be adequately sedated by oral, intravenous or inhalational methods. In the U.K. such patients are usually treated under general anaesthesia.

### Intravenous route

The principal advantages of the intravenous route over the oral and intramuscular routes are that the injected drug has a very rapid effect and that the dose can be given in increments until the desired level of sedation is achieved.

Intravenously administered sedation for dental patients was introduced by Jorgensen and Leffingwell (1961), who used a mixture of pentobarbitone, pethidine and hyoscine. Later, diazepam became the drug of choice for intravenous sedation. Diazepam produces effective sedation, muscle relaxation and amnesia but it has the disadvantages that is only slowly eliminated from the body, and its injection into a vein is often painful. The more recently introduced midazolam has similar sedative, relaxant and amnesic properties to those of diazepam but it is more quickly eliminated from the body and does not cause pain on injection (McGimpsey et al, 1983).

Patients selected for intravenous sedation must be cooperative despite their anxieties, because they must be prepared to accept an intravenous injection. Their cooperation generally is based on trust and confidence in the dentist, and on their desire to receive treatment. For these and, perhaps, other reasons, the technique of intravenous sedation has been found to be more successful with adults than with children. However, some children can be successfully treated in this way (Healy and Hamilton, 1971).

To administer a drug intravenously requires a mastery of the technique of venipuncture, which is considered beyond the scope of this book. Midazolam is injected into a vein in the dorsum of the hand. The dose required to produce satisfactory sedation is about 0.1 mg/kg body weight; this is injected slowly, over a period of 1 to 2 minutes, during which time the child is spoken to in a relaxing and reassuring manner. Sedation is deepest immediately following the injection and for the next 10 minutes; during this period injections of local analgesia are given and treatment is commenced. There is complete or partial amnesia from the time of the intravenous injection; thus, the patient may remember the intravenous but not the intraoral injection, although he may have found the latter unpleasant. The depth of sedation becomes progressively lighter and the patient usually appears normal after about 1 hour. However, the drug may continue to have an effect for several hours; the patient should be required to rest for about 1 hour before leaving the surgery, and his parents should be instructed to keep him at home under supervision for the rest of the day. The need for a period of post-operative recovery, and the subsequent restriction of activities, are the main disadvantages of this technique.

Before inducing sedation by the intravenous or inhalational routes, it is important to ensure that 'a second appropriate person is present throughout' (General Dental Council, 1983). This person might be a suitably trained dental surgery assistant who is capable of monitoring the condition of the patient and of assisting the dentist in case of emergency. It is also essential to have, readily available, appropriate facilities for resuscitating a patient.

### Inhalational route

Sedation by inhalation of nitrous oxide and oxygen has become increasingly popular in recent years, pioneered principally by Langa (1968) who named the technique Relative Analgesia. This term was introduced by Guedel (1937) who, having described the stages of inhalation anaesthesia, divided the first stage (analgesia) into 'relative analgesia' and 'total analgesia'. Although nitrous oxide has analgesic properties, the principal aim of the technique is to sedate the patient, and for this reason the term 'conscious sedation' is sometimes preferred (Bennett, 1978). The sedated patient communicates freely with the dentist and is relaxed, fear having been reduced or eliminated. The pain threshold is raised, often to a point which allows simple conservative dentistry to be performed without added local analgesia. When local analgesia is required, an injection is usually accepted by patients who previously were afraid and would not accept it.

The levels of nitrous oxide analgesia have been described by Roberts (1983) as follows:

Plane 1: Moderate sedation
    and analgesia          5–25% $N_2O$
Plane 2: Dissociation sedation
    and analgesia          20–55% $N_2O$
Plane 3: Total analgesia   50–55% $N_2O$

Moderate analgesia is characterised by relaxation and mild analgesia; the patient may feel 'tingling' sensations in the toes, fingers or other parts of the body. At the lower levels of dissociation analgesia (about 30 per cent nitrous oxide), analgesia is more marked; the patient still reacts to pain but feels detached from and little concerned by it. The patient may report mild sensations of drowsiness, of detachment from his immediate environment, or of euphoria similar to that associated with alcoholic intoxication; these sensations are generally, but not always, regarded as pleasant. At higher levels of dissociation analgesia, these sensations become more marked and unpleasant, making such levels incompatible with relaxation. Thus, the desired level of sedation is within the zone of moderate analgesia or in the lower levels of dissociation analgesia, generally achieved by inhalation of between 15 and 35 per cent nitrous oxide. The concentration cannot be specified more precisely because patients vary considerably in their responses; the concentration administered is based on close observation of the patient's responses. However, in a related technique (Edmunds and Rosen, 1977), effective sedation has been reported with a fixed concentration of 25 per cent nitrous oxide, by using 'Entonox' (50 per cent nitrous oxide + 50 per cent oxygen) diluted with an equal volume of air.

*Technique*

Before using relative analgesia for the first time it is important to understand the principles of the technique, which have been fully discussed by Langa (1968), Bennett (1978) and Roberts (1983).

Specially designed continuous-flow machines are recommended for administering nitrous oxide and oxygen; they have several safety features, and are more convenient and economical to use than anaesthesia machines. The machines used most commonly in the U.K. are the Quantiflex 'RA' and 'MDM' machines. The 'RA' has separate controls to regulate the flow rates of nitrous oxide and oxygen; the 'MDM' has one control to regulate the gas mixture (that is, the proportions of nitrous oxide and oxygen) and another to regulate the total flow rate.

It is important to use a lightweight nosepiece. Three sizes are available, the smaller two being suitable for most children. The nosepiece has an exhaling valve and an air inlet. In the techniques recommended below for using both the 'RA' and 'MDM' machines, the air inlet is closed when nitrous oxide is introduced. Langa (1968) kept the air inlet one-quarter open. Provided that the dentist understands what he is doing it is not important which technique is used. However, if the gas mixture is diluted with air, a larger volume of nitrous oxide is required, which is an unnecessary waste of gas.

In the older nosepieces, the expiratory valve can be adjusted from an open to a closed position; in the newer nosepieces this valve is open and cannot be adjusted.

When using these standard types of nosepiece, expired gases pass through the expiratory valve into the surgery atmosphere, and it is therefore important to have adequate ventilation in the room. An 'anti-pollution' nosepiece is also available, which channels expired gases through the expiratory valve into a length of flexible tubing, the end of which is placed out of a window or through a hole in an outside wall.

Full cylinders of nitrous oxide and oxygen must

be connected to the machine in addition to the cylinders in use. Before using the machine, the pressures in the cylinders in use must be checked to confirm that they are not empty.

Before administering relative analgesia, it is important to ensure that a second appropriate person is present and that resuscitation equipment is readily available.

Success with nitrous oxide sedation is dependent on establishing close communication with, and gaining the cooperation of, the patient. Therefore, the method is most suitable for the same category of patient as might benefit from orally or intravenously administered sedation: the patient who is frightened of dentistry but who wishes to receive treatment. Very young, or mentally handicapped, children present special problems, but sedation sometimes can be successful if their attention and interest can be gained. For these, or for particularly nervous patients, an orally administered sedative may be helpful in overcoming the initial fear of the inhalation method itself.

An important advantage of inhalational sedation over intravenous diazepam is that the patient recovers rapidly and can be dismissed within 5 minutes of the termination of treatment, with no

## Technique: relative analgesia

| Procedure | Method | Rationale | Notes |
|---|---|---|---|
| *Introductory appt.* | | | |
| 1. Prepare the patient. | Explain the technique in terms that the child can understand: e.g. 'happy air', 'magic wind', 'helps you to feel good, relaxed, happy'. | Good psychological preparation is essential. The child's attention, interest and cooperation must be obtained before the technique can be introduced. | It cannot be emphasised too strongly that the success of the technique is greatly dependent on the dentist's participation in relaxing the patient. It is strongly recommended that the dentist should experience relative analgesia, so that he can describe the sensations accurately to his patients. |
| | Emphasise that he will not go to sleep. Mention that many children have tried it, as well as the dentist and nurse; all think 'it's great'. | | |
| | Reassure the child that no dental treatment will be done at this appointment. | Removing the threat of treatment increases the chances of the child accepting the procedure. | Sometimes treatment is essential and ideal introduction is not possible. |
| 2. Fill the reservoir bag with $O_2$. Open the air inlet on the nosepiece. | Allow the bag to fill slowly, or fill quickly by using the '$O_2$ flush' control. | | If using an old type of nosepiece, the expiratory valve should be fully open. |
| | | An open air inlet ensures an adequate supply of air to breathe. | |
| 3. Introduce the nosepiece | Position the nosepiece gently on the child's nose and ask him to 'make it comfortable'. Adjust the position and the tension of the tubes behind the chair in such a way that the nosepiece is held securely but not tightly on the patient's nose. | Allowing the child to position the nosepiece helps him to feel that he has control over the situation and is not being restrained. | |
| | Give praise and suggestions of pleasant, relaxing sensations, while the child breathes $O_2$ and air. | It is important to have the child comfortably relaxed even before the $N_2O$ is introduced. | |
| 4. Set $O_2$ flow rate to about 4 litres/min. Close the air inlet. | Observe the reservoir bag to check that flow rate is adequate; increase if necessary. Give the child encouragement, reassurance and praise as appropriate. | A volume of 4 litres/min. of gas is usually adequate for comfortable breathing by children (adults require 6–8 litres/min.). The flow rate should be sufficient to prevent the reservoir bag from emptying. | |

| *Procedure* | *Method* | *Rationale* | *Notes* |
|---|---|---|---|
| 5. Introduce $N_2O$ | Introduce $N_2O$ only if the child is cooperating.<br>'RA' machine — Keep $O_2$ flow at 4 litres/min. Introduce $N_2O$ at 0.5 litres/min.<br>'MDM' machine — Set gas mixture control to about 90% $O_2$ (i.e. 10% $N_2O$); the total flow rate remains constant. | If the child is not cooperating, further psychological preparation is advisable before proceeding. | 4 litres/min $O_2$ + 0.5 litres/min $N_2O$ = 11% $N_2O$. This does not take into account leakage around the nosepiece, or mouthbreathing. |
| 6. Inform and make suggestions about sensations to be expected. | Sit near the child and speak quietly and calmly into his ear with a soothing voice.<br>*Inform* the child that he *may* smell the 'happy air'; *suggest* that it is a 'nice' smell.<br>*Inform* him that he *may* feel slight tingling in the toes, fingers or other parts; *suggest* that it is a 'funny feeling'.<br>*Inform* that the whole body *may* feel very light, or very heavy; *suggest* that it is a 'lovely feeling', like 'floating in the clouds' or 'lying comfortably in bed'.<br>From time to time, ask the patient *what* he feels. Reinforce all the pleasant sensations described. | Since patients' responses differ, it is wise to use the word 'may' rather than 'will', and to suggest alternative sensations.<br>Asking the child *what* he feels is better than to ask *how* he feels; the latter suggests that he may not feel well. | Verbal communication is essential, but it is also helpful to maintain physical communication with the child by placing a hand on his shoulder from time to time. |
| 7. Increase the proportion of $N_2O$ if desired. | If the expected sensations are not reported within about 2 minutes, or to deepen the level of sedation, increase the concentration of $N_2O$.<br>'RA' machine — increase $N_2O$ by 0.5, litres/min. and, if desired after 1–2 mins., by another 0.5 litres/min. to total 1.5 litres/min.<br>'MDM' machine — set gas mixture to 80% $O_2$ and, if desired after 1–2 mins., to 70% $O_2$. | It is important:-<br>i) to increase the concentration of $N_2O$ gradually,<br>ii) to allow at least 1 minute for the new concentration to have its effect,<br>iii) to check on the effect by observing and by questioning the patient. | 1.5 litres min. $N_2O$ + 4 litres/min. $O_2$, with *no* air dilution produces $N_2O$ concentration of 30%. |
| 8. Terminate the session | When the patient has enjoyed the experience for 1–2 minutes, the session may be terminated. Before doing so, suggest to the child that at subsequent visits he will again feel happy and relaxed, and that he will not be worried by any dental treatment.<br>Reduce $N_2O$ to zero and give 100% $O_2$ for at least 2 minutes. | As $N_2O$ is rapidly eliminated through the lungs, the relative concentration of $O_2$ in the lung alveoli might fall to a hypoxic level if $O_2$ is not administered. | The patient may be shown that mouthbreathing lightens the level of sedation. Knowledge that they have this control gives some patients added confidence. |

4ℓ $O_2$ : 0·5ℓ $N_2O$ = 11%
1ℓ $N_2O$
4ℓ $O_2$ : 1·5ℓ $N_2O$ = 30%

(*Continued overleaf*)

| Procedure | Method | Rationale | Notes |
|---|---|---|---|
| *Subsequent appointments* | | | |
| 1. Prepare the patient. | Remind the child of the pleasant sensations experienced at the last visit. | | |
| 2, 3, 4 | As at introductory appointment. | | |
| 5. Introduce N₂O | Set the flow rate and $N_2O$ concentration at the level found satisfactory at the introductory appointment. | $N_2O$ need not be increased gradually as at the introductory appointment. | |
| 6. Inform and make suggestions about sensations. | Inform the child that the sensations will begin to be noted in about 1 minute. Repeat the suggestions made at the last visit. | Continued close communication with the child is essential. | |
| 7. Proceed with dental treatment. | When the patient is comfortably sedated, start dental treatment. Suggest that the treatment will not worry him, because he is so 'comfortable', 'happy' or other appropriate suggestion. Local analgesia may not be required for conservative dentistry. If local analgesia is required:- Introduce with care if this is known to have caused anxiety previously. Inform the child, in a casual manner, that it will be given, and suggest that it will not worry him. Regularly reinforce good behaviour with praise. When treatment is completed, reduce $N_2O$ to zero and give 100% $O_2$ for at least 2 minutes. | The pain threshold may be sufficiently elevated in the sedated patient to obviate the need for local analgesia. The dentist should not use sedation to break faith with the child by carrying out treatment without his consent. | If the degree of sedation is not adequate, further increments of about 5% $N_2O$ may be added. Beyond about 40% $N_2O$, symptoms of dissociation may be unpleasant. |

limitations on the activities he may undertake during the rest of the day. In addition, most (but not all) children prefer the nosepiece to an intravenous injection.

No special instructions need be given to a parent bringing a child for nitrous oxide sedation, but to reduce even further the slight possibility of vomiting, the parent may be advised to give the child no more than a light meal 2 or 3 hours before the dental appointment. Contra-indications are few, but include upper respiratory infections (e.g. the common cold) and pulmonary disease. Clearly, nasal obstruction due to any cause, if it prevents easy breathing through the nose, makes the method difficult or impossible to use. If the patient is under psychiatric care, it is prudent to consult with the psychiatrist before proceeding with this or with any other form of sedation.

## HYPNOSIS

Hypnosis has been defined as 'a particular state of mind which is usually induced in one person by another...a state of mind in which suggestions are not only more readily accepted than in the waking state but are also acted upon more powerfully than would be possible under normal conditions' (Hartland, 1971).

Hypnosis has long been a controversial and misunderstood subject, shrouded by an aura of mysticism which has been encouraged by public entertainers. However, much progress has been made during the last 20 or 30 years in the scientific investigation of hypnosis, and it now holds an accepted place in medical and dental practice.

It is estimated that 90 per cent of individuals can be induced into a light hypnotic trance, which is characterised by relaxation and reduction of anxiety; 70 per cent of these individuals can be deepened to a medium trance, in which some analgesia may be produced; and a further 20 per cent of these can reach a deep trance in which considerable analgesia is possible. Hypnosis can only be induced in individuals who wish to co-operate. Although this might suggest that children are often unsuitable subjects, the reverse is the case. The apparent paradox is explained by the fact that children generally are more amenable to persuasion and suggestion than adults, and more accustomed to accepting instructions without question. It is, however, essential to gain their confidence and to hold their attention, and this may not be possible with very young, frightened or timid children.

Hypnosis is used most commonly in dentistry as a method of helping the anxious patient to relax. A light trance is usually sufficient to achieve this objective; the relaxed patient can then accept treatment procedures which previously were unacceptable. Some patients may be taken to deeper levels, at which sufficient analgesia of teeth or oral tissues may be produced to perform treatment without the need for injection of a local analgesic. Other indications for hypnosis include helping the patient who 'gags' when anything is placed in his mouth; encouraging children to wear orthodontic appliances; and introducing children to inhalational sedation or to general anaesthesia.

No doubt many dentists relax their patients by using a calm, kind, understanding approach, without the aid of hypnosis, and the depth of relaxation they achieve may be similar to that of a light hypnotic trance. However, techniques that have been established for the induction of hypnosis are more precise and more likely to be effective with most anxious patients. Various techniques have been described by Hartland (1971), Lampshire (1975) and Smith (1977).

Before proceeding to induce hypnosis, the dentist must prepare the patient by explaining what is to be done. Although adults require careful preparation to correct misconceptions and to remove suspicions and fears of hypnosis, children require only minimal preparation. The word 'hypnosis' need not be used with children. Young children may be told that they will have a special kind of sleep, when their eyes will be closed as if they were asleep but that it will be different because they will hear everything that the dentist says and will be able to talk without waking up. Older children need only be informed that the purpose is to help them to relax so that their worries about dental treatment may be overcome. Parents may be informed that this form of deep relaxation is called 'hypnosis', but it is not essential to offer this information. It is clear that both the child and the parent must have trust in the dentist.

As with inhalational sedation, the ideal approach is to devote the first session to introducing the child to hypnosis, having informed him that no dental treatment will be performed; removing the anxiety about impending treatment increases the chances of success. With the reassurance of a pleasant experience, together with the use of post-hypnotic suggestion, hypnosis is induced more easily and more rapidly at subsequent meetings.

REFERENCES

Adelson R, Goldfried M R 1970 Modelling and the fearful child patient. Journal of Dentistry for Children 37:476–489
Baird E S, Curson I 1970 Orally-administered diazepam in conservative dentistry. British Dental Journal 128:25–27
Barenie J T 1979 Premedication for behaviour control. In: Ripa LW, Barenie J T Management of dental behaviour in children. PSG Publishing Co., Littleton, Mass., ch 7–10
Bennett C R 1978 Conscious sedation in dental practice, 2nd edn. Mosby, St. Louis

Craig W 1971 Hand over mouth technique. Journal of Dentistry for Children 38:387–389
Edmunds D H, Rosen M 1977 Sedation for conservative dentistry: further studies on inhalation sedation with 25 per cent nitrous oxide. Journal of Dentistry 5:245–251
Gale E N, Ayer W A 1969 Treatment of dental phobias. Journal of the American Dental Association 78:1304–1307
General Dental Council 1983 Notice for the guidance of dentists: general anaesthesia and sedation

Guedel A E 1937 Inhalational anaesthesia. Macmillan, New York

Hartland J 1971 Medical and dental hypnosis and its clinical applications, 2nd edn. Baillière Tindall, London

Healy T E J, Hamilton M C 1971 Intravenous diazepam in the apprehensive child. British Dental Journal 130:25–27

Hill F J, O'Mullane D M 1976 Preventive programme for the dental management of frightened children. Journal of Dentistry for Children 43:30–36

Jorgensen N B, Leffingwell F 1961 Premedication in dentistry. Dental Clinics of North America (July) 299–308

Lampshire E L 1975 Hypnosis in dentistry for children. In: Wright G Z (ed) Behaviour management in dentistry for children. Saunders, Philadelphia, ch 6

Langa H 1968 Relative analgesia in dental practice. Saunders, Philadelphia

Levitas T C 1974 Home: hand over mouth exercise. Journal of Dentistry for Children 41:178–182

Lindsay S J E, Yates J A 1985 The effectiveness of oral diazepam in anxious child dental patients. British Dental Journal 159:149–153

McGimpsey J G, Kawar P, Gamble J A S, Browne E S, Dundee J W 1983 Midazolam in dentistry. British Dental Journal 155:47–50

Musselman R J, McClure D B 1975 Pharmacotherapeutic approaches to behaviour management. In: Wright G Z (ed) Behaviour management in dentistry for children. Saunders, Philadelphia, ch 8

Roberts G J 1983 Relative analgesia in clinical practice. In: Anaesthesia and sedation in dentistry. Coplans M P, Green R A (eds) Elsevier, Amsterdam, ch 10

Rosenberg H M 1974 Behaviour modification for the child dental patient. Journal of Dentistry for Children 41:111–114

Smith S R 1977 A primer of hypnosis. British Society of Medical and Dental Hypnosis, London

Wolpe J, Lazarus A A 1966 Behaviour therapy techniques: a guide to the treatment of neuroses. Pergamon, Oxford

## RECOMMENDED READING

(Behaviour Management)

Bennett A E 1976 Communication between doctors and patients. Oxford University Press, Oxford

Burns R B 1982 Children and dentists: some psychological issues. Part 1: applications of behaviour modification. Proceedings of the British Paedodontic Society 12:9–11

Christen A G 1977 Piagetan psychology: some principles helpful in treating the child dental patient. Journal of Dentistry for Children 44:48–52

Ingersoll B D 1982 Behavioral aspects in dentistry. Appleton-Century-Crofts, New York

Kent G 1984 The psychology of dental care. Wright, Bristol

Kreinces G H 1975 Ginott psychology applied to pedodontics. Journal of Dentistry for Children 42:119–122

Ripa L W, Barenie J T 1979 Management of dental behaviour in children. PSG, Littleton, Mass.

Wright G Z 1979 Behavior management in dentistry for children. Saunders, Philadelphia, ch 5

(Psychological Development)

Alpern G 1975 Child development: basic concepts and clinical considerations. In: Wright G Z (ed) Behavior management in dentistry for children. Saunders, Philadelphia, ch 2

Blain S M 1982 Behaviour. In: Barber T K, Luke L S Pediatric Dentistry. Wright, Bristol, ch 4

Kenna M D, Smith B A 1985 Psychologic growth and development. In: Braham R L, Morris M E (eds) Textbook of pediatric dentistry, 2nd edn. Williams and Wilkins, Baltimore, ch 3

Gesell A L 1954 The first five years of life. Methuen, London

Gesell A L, Ilg F J 1946 The child from five to ten. Hamilton, London

Holloway P J, Swallow J N 1975 Child dental health, 2nd edn. Wright, Bristol, ch 2

Lowrey G H 1973 Growth and development of children, 6th edn. Year Book Medical Publishers, Chicago

Sarles R M 1981 Psychologic growth and development. In: Forrester D J Pediatric dental medicine. Lea and Febiger, Philadelphia, ch 3

Sheridan M D 1975 From birth to five years, 3rd edn. NFER-Nelson, Windsor

# PART TWO

# Treatment of dental caries
# — preventive methods

# 3

# Dental health education

The Individual
    Toothbrushing instruction
    Flossing instruction
    Diet counselling

The Community
    Dental health campaigns
    Education in primary schools
    Education in secondary schools
    Education in ante- and post-natal clinics

It is generally accepted that dental caries is initiated by acids produced during the bacterial degradation of dietary carbohydrate in the dental plaque. It follows that two important methods of preventing dental caries must be to control dietary carbohydrate and to remove dental plaque from the teeth. It should be an important aim of every dentist to educate his patients about these methods, and, indeed, of the dental profession to educate the public at large. To be effective, methods used in dental health education should be planned and carried out skilfully. The aim must be not only to instruct, but also to persuade; success depends greatly on the sincerity and interest shown by members of the dental team.

## DENTAL HEALTH EDUCATION OF THE INDIVIDUAL

### Toothbrushing instruction

Although more than 50 per cent of children in the U.K. claim to brush their teeth at least twice a day, the majority have debris on their teeth (Todd and Dodd, 1985); this indicates that toothbrushing generally is done inefficiently. In teaching children how to brush their teeth, the aim must be to instruct and to encourage them to remove all debris and plaque from all accessible tooth surfaces.

A suggested method is outlined below.

It is not easy to master an efficient technique of

## Technique: toothbrushing instruction

| Procedure | Method | Rationale | Notes |
|---|---|---|---|
| 1. Assess oral cleanliness. | Examine in turn the following tooth surfaces:<br><br>buccal  buccal        buccal<br>6      1            6<br><br>6           1   6<br>lingual    buccal  lingual<br>Rest a probe against the tooth surface in the distal embrasure, with its tip at the gingival margin. Draw the probe mesially, keeping it in contact with the tooth surface. Observe the distribution of debris, and score as follows:<br>  0 — no debris.<br>  1 — debris within gingival 1/3 only.<br>  2 — debris beyond gingival 1/3 but within gingival 2/3.<br>  3 — debris beyond gingival 2/3 (i.e. covering most of surface). | An assessment of the patient's oral cleanliness provides a baseline against which the effects of instruction can be evaluated. An objective assessment is preferred to a simple statement of 'good', 'fair' or 'poor'. | The method outlined is based on the Oral Debris Index described by Greene and Vermillion (1964). |

| Procedure | Method | Rationale | Notes |
|---|---|---|---|
| | Record results, e.g. $\dfrac{1 \quad 1}{2 \quad \| 2} \; \dfrac{\| \; 2}{2}$ | Recording the results in this way indicates where the emphasis in instruction needs to be given:- e.g. $\dfrac{0 \quad 0}{2 \quad \|0} \; \dfrac{\| \; 0}{2}$ instruction required only in cleaning lingual of mandibular molars. $\dfrac{2 \quad 0}{2 \quad \|0} \; \dfrac{\| \; 0}{0}$ instruction required only in cleaning right side of mouth. $\dfrac{2 \quad 1}{2 \quad \|1} \; \dfrac{\| \; 2}{2}$ general instruction required. | If the specific tooth is not present in the mouth, use the tooth just mesial or distal to it — regions of the mouth are more important than specific teeth. Debris scores recorded in the patient's notes can be of value in motivating the patient, by showing how toothbrushing has improved at subsequent visits. |
| 2. Assess tooth-brushing technique. | Observe the child brushing his own teeth, ideally with his own toothbrush. Note: 1. whether all surfaces of teeth are brushed. 2. whether teeth are brushed in any particular order. 3. whether any specific technique is used. | Instruction should be tailored to the needs of the individual patient. Observing the patient's technique indicates whether full instruction is required or whether attention need be given only to specific aspects. | It has been recommended (Ch. 1) that, at the first visit, the child be asked to bring his toothbrush for the next appointment. Not only will the child brush more comfortably with his own brush but the adequacy of his brush can be assessed. Disposable brushes should be available for those who forget to bring their own. |
| 3. Explain the reasons for tooth-brushing. | According to the child's age and intelligence, give a brief explanation of the cause of decay. Indicate the role of 'germs', plaque and foods. Use models, posters or extracted teeth to illustrate the progress of caries. | A child can only be persuaded to brush his teeth if he sees it as something which will be of benefit to him. | |
| 4. Start instruction. | (Assuming that the child's toothbrushing efficiency is poor, as assessed by the state of oral cleanliness and the observed toothbrushing technique). On a model, demonstrate that 'back' teeth have 3 'sides' — cheek, tongue and biting surfaces — and that 'front' teeth have 2 'sides' (Fig. 3.1a). Explain that all these 'sides' need to be brushed. So as not to miss any, a system is needed — suggest a starting point and an order for brushing all his teeth (Fig. 3.1b). Ask the child to demonstrate the suggested system on the model and then in his own mouth. | It is important to give the child a mental picture of what he must brush, and to emphasise the need for a systematic approach. | Ideally, a parent should be present to listen and observe; a good parent will remind the child at home of the dentist's instructions. It is reasonable to exclude mention of approximal surfaces, since a toothbrush cannot be applied to these surfaces. |
| 5. Give advice to the child and/or parent: toothbrush | Recommend a multi-tufted brush, with a head approx. 2 cm long. | Fine filament brushes are more likely to penetrate interdentally and into the gingival crevices. | Parents often provide their child with too large a brush. |

| Procedure | Method | Rationale | Notes |
|---|---|---|---|
| toothpaste | Recommend a fluoride-containing toothpaste. | Fluoride-containing toothpastes are effective in reducing caries incidence. | Most toothpastes on the market in Britain now contain fluoride. |
| frequency | Recommend that teeth are brushed after breakfast, and last thing at night before going to bed. | 'Brush after breakfast and before going to bed' has been an accepted dental health message for many years. | It is more important to remove plaque thoroughly once a day than to brush inefficiently more often. |
| duration | Advise the child to take 2 to 3 minutes for brushing. | Thorough toothbrushing cannot be accomplished very hurriedly. | A systematic and efficient technique is more important than the duration of brushing. |
| 6. (At the next visit) Evaluate progress. | Assess the state of oral cleanliness, as described above. Note any improvements and praise the child. Encourage rather than criticise. | Efficient toothbrushing is not easy. Rapid improvement should not be expected — the child should be given time to improve gradually. | |
| 7. Introduce a self-assessment method. | With a cotton pledget, apply disclosing solution to all surfaces of the teeth (Fig. 3.1c). Alternatively ask the child to chew a disclosing tablet. Demonstrate the disclosed plaque to the child, then ask him to brush it off and to check his efficiency. | | |
| 8. Give more detailed instruction on technique | If the child uses a recognisable technique, develop that technique to a greater level of efficiency. If a haphazard technique is used, introduce either a *gentle* scrubbing action, or the Bass technique, or any other. | There is no evidence that any particular technique is more efficient than others. Especially with children, who may become discouraged by a difficult exercise, it is more important to emphasise the need to reach all tooth surfaces than to insist on a particular technique. | |
| | Recommend the occasional use of a disclosing tablet at home. | | Parental interest and cooperation are essential if disclosing tablets are to be of any value in home use. |
| 9. (At subsequent visit) | | | |
| Evaluate progress and reinforce previous instruction. | Assess oral cleanliness and toothbrushing technique as before. Instruct as necessary to maintain standards or to improve in specific aspects. Reinforce good performance by praising and giving an appropriate reward (e.g. a badge). | Good behaviour, if reinforced, is more likely to be continued. | |

*(illustrations overleaf)*

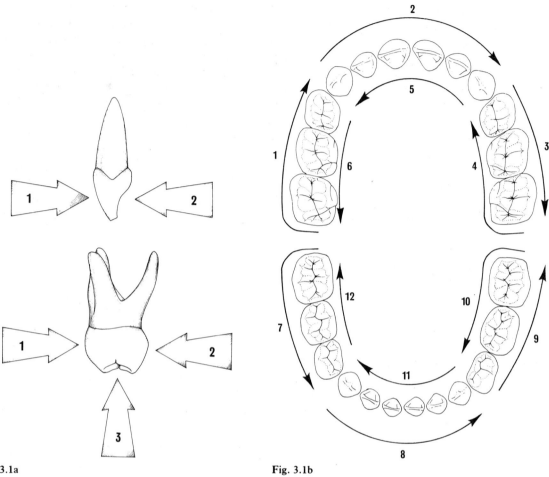

Fig. 3.1a

Fig. 3.1b

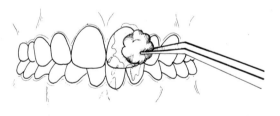

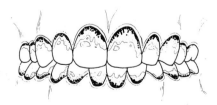

Fig. 3.1c

toothbrushing, and some children do not have the manual dexterity to succeed. This is especially the case with young children below the age or 5 to 6 years, and with the mentally or physically handicappcd. To help such patients, the dentist must involve a parent (or guardian), who must be encouraged to accept responsibility. Children should be encouraged to brush their own teeth, but also to allow parents to help. Instruction concerning technique should then be directed at the parent. Electric toothbrushes may also be useful for such patients.

Several toothbrushing techniques have been proposed; these are summarised in Table 3.1 and illustrated in Figure 3.2. There is no evidence that one technique is superior to others in removing dental plaque, although it might be expected that the Scrub method would not penetrate the gingival sulcus or interdental areas as readily as others. All except the Scrub method require some manual dexterity. To insist on a method that the child finds difficult risks discouraging the child from brushing at all. It is usually wiser to start with the Scrub technique and to introduce one of the other techniques only after some progress has been made in developing the child's interest and co-operation. The Bass technique is currently in favour in the U.K. and the U.S.A.. If the parent brushes the child's teeth, the Bass method may be recommended; the child may learn to imitate the technique.

If not instructed, a parent usually will face the child to brush his teeth. A much better approach is as illustrated in Figure 3.3; this provides good support for the child's head and gives the parent much greater control. The parent should be instructed to use the fingers of the left hand to retract the child's cheeks and lips as required, to improve access for the toothbrush; most parents will not do this unless instructed, using their left hands only to support the child's head. Parents should be advised to start brushing their child's teeth as soon as the first tooth erupts, so that toothbrushing becomes accepted as part of the normal bathroom routine.

The relationship between toothbrushing and

**Table 3.1** Summary of toothbrushing techniques

| Method | Starting position Tips of bristles | Direction of bristles | Movements* |
|---|---|---|---|
| Scrub | On gingival margin | Horizontal | Scrub in antero-posterior direction, keeping brush horizontal. |
| Roll | On gingival margin | Pointing apically, parallel to the long axis of the teeth. | Roll brush occlusally, maintaining contact with gingiva, then with tooth surface. |
| Bass | On gingival margin | Pointing apically, about 45° to the long axis of the teeth. | Vibrate the brush, not changing the position of the bristles. |
| Stillman | On gingival margin | Pointing apically, about 45° to the long axis of the teeth | Apply pressure to blanch the gingiva, then remove. Repeat several times. Slightly rotate the brush occlusally during the procedure. |
| Modified Stillman | On gingival margin | Pointing apically, about 45° to the long axis of the teeth | Apply pressure as in Stillman method, but at the same time vibrate the brush and gradually move it occlusally. |
| Fones | On gingival margin | Horizontal | With the teeth in occlusion, move the brush in a rotary motion against the maxillary and mandibular tooth surfaces and gingival margins. |
| Charters | Level with occlusal surfaces of teeth | Pointing occlusally, about 45° to the long axis of the teeth. | Vibrate the brush while moving it apically to the gingival margin. |

* For occlusal surfaces, a vigorous scrubbing action is recommended, except by Charters, who recommends small rotary movements to encourage the bristles to penetrate pits and fissures.

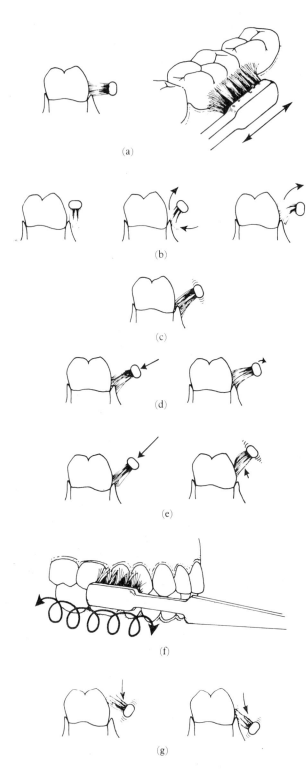

gingivitis is easy to demonstrate: every dentist has noted marginal gingivitis associated with plaque deposits in his patients, and the resolution of the gingivitis on the institution of efficient tooth-brushing. This relationship has been confirmed in clinical studies with adults and with children (Koch and Lindhe, 1965). However, the relationship between toothbrushing and dental caries is less obvious. With individual patients, the introduction of efficient toothbrushing may be seen to be followed by the arrest of, for example, early cervical lesions, but various types of studies with groups of children have shown only a weak relationship between oral hygiene and dental caries (Andlaw, 1978; Sutcliffe, 1983). It is probable that toothbrushing must be done very efficiently to have an effect in preventing dental caries; in addition, its effect is limited by the fact that tooth-brush bristles cannot penetrate deep pits or fissures, or interdental spaces.

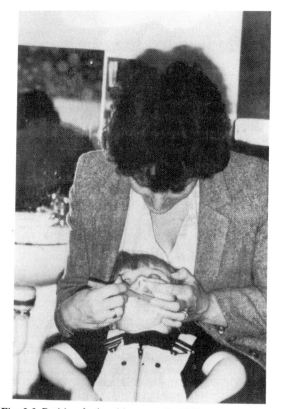

**Fig. 3.2** Toothbrushing techniques: (a) Scrub (b) Roll (c) Bass (d) Stillman (e) Modified Stillman (f) Fones (g) Charters.

**Fig. 3.3** Position for brushing a small child's teeth.

## Flossing instruction

The use of dental floss enables plaque to be removed from approximal tooth surfaces that are inaccessible to the toothbrush. Ideally, therefore, flossing should accompany toothbrushing as part of normal oral hygiene practice. However, flossing is a difficult technique, requiring considerable practice before it is mastered. Most children need constant encouragement to maintain an adequate standard of toothbrushing, and it would be unreasonable to expect all children to perform an additional procedure. Therefore, flossing should only be introduced to children who use a toothbrush easily, efficiently and with some enthusiasm. They may be shown how to use floss on anterior teeth first, later extending to posterior teeth. Alternatively, a motivated parent who uses floss may be encouraged to floss the child's teeth. It is important for the dentist or hygienist to supervise the procedure periodically, because a poor flossing technique can do more harm than good.

The following advice may be given to the child and parent (illustrations follow on p. 36):

1. Use unwaxed floss. Waxed floss may leave a layer of wax on the tooth surface that may inhibit the uptake of fluoride from toothpaste or from topical treatments.
2. Cut off a length of about 30 to 40 cm of floss and lightly wrap the ends around the middle fingers (Fig. 3.4a, b).
3. The tips of the fingers or thumbs controlling the floss should not be more than about 2 cm apart, to give maximum control (Fig. 3.4c, d).
4. Pass the floss gently through the contact points by moving the floss bucco-lingually until it slides through slowly. Avoid forcing it through roughly which would traumatise the interdental papilla.
5. Move the floss gently occluso-gingivally and bucco-lingually against each approximal surface; the floss should be allowed to spread just below the gingival margin (Fig. 3.4e, f).
6. After flossing all the teeth, rinse the mouth vigorously to remove the plaque and debris dislodged from the interdental spaces.

The effect of flossing on dental caries has been investigated in only one study, which has shown that caries incidence was reduced in approximal surfaces of primary molars that were flossed daily for 20 months by research assistants (Wright, Banting and Feasby, 1977).

## Diet counselling

A good, balanced, diet is essential for optimal general health; this is important for the mother and fetus during pregnancy and for the growing child. However, there is no evidence that nutritional deficiencies during the period of tooth development affect the teeth or oral soft tissues in such a way as to make them later more susceptible to dental disease. Other than the possible supplementation of the diet with fluoride (Ch. 4) there are no specific recommendations that need be given concerning the nutritional value of the diet and its relation to oral health.

The most important factor in the relationship of diet and dental health is the frequency of consumption of foods containing refined carbohydrate. After eating a carbohydrate-containing food, acid is produced in the dental plaque (Stephan, 1940). When acid depresses plaque pH below about pH 5.5, enamel demineralisation may occur, and this is generally accepted as being the first stage in the initiation of dental caries. The more frequently that acidic conditions below pH 5.5 are produced in the plaque the more rapidly will caries be initiated and progress; this relationship has been demonstrated in a variety of studies (Andlaw, 1977). Thus, the most important aim in diet counselling in relation to dental health is to encourage the patient to control the frequency of eating carbohydrate-containing foods.

Although oral bacteria can break down many carbohydrates to acid, sucrose is particularly implicated in dental caries (Rugg-Gunn and Edgar, 1984). Unfortunately, sucrose is a constituent of the majority of snack foods.

The problems of diet counselling are formidable. Many people have acquired at an early age the habit of frequent eating of sweets and snack foods, and consider this to be normal and acceptable behaviour. For an individual patient to change these habits requires him to undergo a fundamental change in attitude; for the dentist (or his ancillary) to achieve this presents a considerable

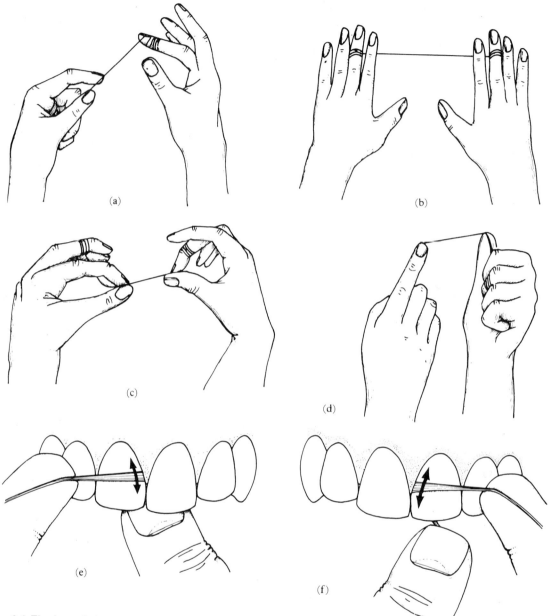

**Fig. 3.4** Flossing technique.

challenge. To have any chance of success, the methods used in diet counselling should be planned not only to give information but also to persuade the child and parent to act on this information. At least for the younger children, parental involvement is essential.

It is easy to explain the reasons for controlling the frequency of eating: the child and parent may be given a brief outline (perhaps with visual aids) of the production of acid on the tooth, including the interaction of 'germs' and food in the plaque. Although such an exercise at least fulfils the dentist's responsibility to inform his patient, it usually has limited impact and therefore may not motivate the patient to improve his diet habits. No known method is certain to have the desired effect, but the use of a diet sheet, on which the parent is asked to record the child's diet for a number of days, is recommended. The advantages of this method are that the parent (and child if old enough) becomes actively involved in recording the diet, and that the advice subsequently given is more personal, being based on the child's own diet.

Various diet record sheets have been designed (Nizel, 1980; Nikiforuk, 1985), varying considerably in their complexity. A simple diet sheet is illustrated on this page.

It is most important to be tactful in introducing the diet sheet to parents. It should be introduced as a means of helping them more effectively; this is printed on the sheet but should be emphasised verbally. If introduced in this way, most parents are pleased to cooperate, but a careless approach might antagonise them by giving the impression that their care of the child is to be criticised.

When the completed diet sheet is returned by the patient, there are two principal ways of proceeding. The simpler but perhaps the less effective way is for the dentist to peruse the information in the presence of the child and parent, and to comment and advise on the good or bad points that emerge from it. Another approach is to receive the sheet, expressing thanks for their interest and help in completing it, and to inform them that the diet will be analysed in time for their next visit. At the next visit, the results of the analysis are presented, accompanied by written recommendations (see over leaf). The advantages of this approach are that a more objective assessment of the diet is given, and that the care and interest of the dentist or hygienist are more clearly demonstrated to the parent; both of these are strong motivational factors.

Several methods of analysing diet records have been proposed. A very simple method is outlined overleaf. A more detailed method has been used by Holloway, Booth and Wragg (1969), and other methods have been described by Nizel (1980) and Nikiforuk (1985).

The simplest type of analysis is adequate if the aim is specifically to recommend control of the frequency of eating. If the aim were to give broader nutritional advice, a more detailed analysis would be required.

## DIET RECORD SHEET

Dental decay is caused by acids which are formed by bacteria (germs) acting on food particles on the tooth surface.

FOOD + BACTERIA → ACIDS → DECAY

The information requested below will enable us to estimate the severity of the attack on the teeth, and will help us to advise you on how this attack may be reduced.

Please record all foods and drinks taken each day for *THREE DAYS* including 'extras' eaten between meals.

Include one weekend day, if possible.

Estimate the approximate amounts of the foods eaten as follows:

vegetables, puddings,
   sugar, cereals ..................... teaspoons or tablespoons
bread, cheese ........................ slices
drinks ............................... tumblers or cups
meat, fish ........................... size of portions

fruits, sweets, biscuits,
   chocolates ....................... type and number

NAME:                           date of birth:
Ist Day – Date .....................

                           *Food or drink    Quantity*
Breakfast

Between breakfast
  and lunch

Lunch

Between lunch
  and tea

Tea

After tea

(Space for the 2nd and 3rd day diet records is provided on the reverse side of the sheet)

*Simple method of analysing the diet record*

'Exposures of teeth to acid attack' are scored as follows:

| Meals | Score | Between Meals | Score |
|---|---|---|---|
| Average meal | 2 | Non-cariogenic item (e.g. cheese, carrot, nuts) | 0 |
| Meal followed by toothbrushing | 1 | Item eaten within 5 mins (e.g. sweet or biscuit or bar of chocolate) | 1 |
| | | Item eaten over longer period (e.g. packet of sweets) | 2 |

The scoring system is arbitrary and unscientific, but is based on available information about the cariogenicity of foods. The scores are entered on the Diet Analysis and Recommendations sheet. The contribution of between-meal snacks is clearly highlighted, as is the reduction that can be achieved in the total number of exposures of the teeth to attack. It is hoped that the size of the reduction will impress the parent as something worth achieving.

In giving recommendations, the following guidelines are suggested:

1. First, praise good points in the diet. The aim must be to encourage rather than to criticise.
2. Emphasise the danger of between-meal snacks, and comment on between-meal items in the child's diet.
3. Recommend substitution of non-cariogenic between-meal foods for cariogenic items. Based on research evidence, only meats, cheese, carrots and nuts can be classified as non-cariogenic. In the past, apples would have been included in this list, but more recent evidence does not allow this (Rugg-Gunn, Edgar and Jenkins, 1978). However, apples and other fruits, and potato crisps, are still to be preferred to sweets, biscuits and cakes.
4. Emphasise the desirability of eating good, nutritious meals.
5. Encourage toothbrushing after meals whenever possible.
6. Point out that a diet which controls dental caries also controls overweight, which is a common problem with school children.
7. Sweets are a special problem. Advise that they should be consumed at the end of a meal rather than between meals. To advise complete elimination of sweets is not realistic in most cases.

Ideally, diet counselling should be given to mothers immediately after the birth of a child: it is easier to establish good habits than to change bad habits later. In particular, mothers should be warned against allowing infants to drink *ad lib* from a feeding bottle or reservoir-type pacifier, especially at night (unless the drink is water). Rampant caries of the infant's dentition results from prolonged exposure of the teeth to fruit juices or even milk. Particularly popular with infants are proprietary vitamin syrups, which have a high sugar content and are highly acidic.

## DENTAL HEALTH EDUCATION OF THE COMMUNITY

Dental health education has been pursued within communities in various ways which are briefly discussed below. Any efforts that are made in community dental health education depend largely on the manpower and financial resources of the community and on the priority given to such activities in relation to other commitments of the dental service.

To be understood, the dental health message must be kept simple. It is generally agreed that the following four points should be included:

1. Avoid eating sweet, sticky, between-meal snacks.

DIET ANALYSIS AND RECOMMENDATION

| Day | Exposures of teeth to acid attack | |
|---|---|---|
| | Recorded diet | Recommended diet |
| 1 Meals | | |
| Between meals | | |
| 2 Meals | | |
| Between meals | | |
| 3 Meals | | |
| Between meals | | |

Total number of acid attacks:

*Note*: If the recommendations are followed, the acid attack on (Child's name) teeth can be reduced by ........................
*Recommendations*:

2. Brush the teeth thoroughly at least once a day with a fluoride toothpaste.
3. Support the fluoridation of water supplies.
4. Visit the dentist for regular check-ups.

## Dental health campaigns

Dental health campaigns have been mounted from time to time with varying degrees of ingenuity but always with great enthusiasm (Davis and Land, 1962; Dowell, 1965). Some campaigns have been directed at specific groups (e.g. schoolchildren), others at a whole community. These campaigns always succeed in stimulating interest, but their effects on the dental health of the community are uncertain; any reported improvements have been of short duration (Finlayson and Wilson, 1962).

## Dental health education in schools

Dental health education is most commonly directed at school children; primary schoolchildren, in particular, have long been a favourite target group. Short-term improvements have been reported in dental health knowledge and in oral cleanliness (Addy and Edmunds, 1977; Furniss, 1978; Howat et al, 1984; Hodge et al, 1985), but

these improvements are generally not maintained (Rayner and Cohen, 1971). Regular reinforcement, no doubt, is important and greater benefits might be obtained if parents could be involved. Unfortunately this is usually not practicable.

In recent years there has been a change of approach to dental health education in schools. The emphasis has turned towards developing programmes that can be integrated into normal school work and be used by school teachers. Several programmes have been developed and tested in the U.K.: in primary schools (McIntyre, Wight and Blinkhorn, 1984; Towner, 1984), in secondary schools (Craft et al, 1981; Arnold and Doyle, 1984) and in pre-school groups (Croucher et al, 1985). In general, these studies have shown that programmes can be devised that are well received by teachers and children, that knowledge of dental health can be increased, and that some improvement in dental health behaviour (reflected by improved oral cleanliness and gingival health) can be obtained. Follow-up in some secondary schools several months after a programme ended showed that some of the improvements were maintained (Craft, Croucher and Dickinson, 1981) but the evidence regarding long-term benefits is inconclusive (Arnold and Doyle, 1984).

## REFERENCES

Arnold C, Doyle A J 1984 Evaluation of the dental health education programme 'Natural Nashers'. Community Dental Health 1:141–147

Craft M, Croucher R E, Dickinson J 1981 Preventive dental health in adolescents: short and long term pupil response to trials of an integrated curriculum package. Community Dentistry and Oral Epidemiology 9:199–206

Croucher R E, Rodgers A I, Franklin A J and Craft M H 1985 Results and issues arising from an evaluation of community dental health education: the case of the 'Good Teeth' programme. Community Dental Health 2: 89–97

Health Education Council 1985 The scientific basis of dental health education: a policy document

Hodge H, Buchanan M, Jones J, O'Donnell P 1985 The evaluation of the infant dental health education programme developed in Sefton Community Dental Health 2:175–185

Holloway P H, Booth E M, Wragg K A 1969 Dietary counselling in the control of dental caries. British Dental Journal 126:161–165

Howat A P, Craft M, Croucher R, Rock W P, Foster T D 1984 Dental health education: a school visits programme for dental students. Community Dental Health 2:23–32

Koch G, Lindhe J 1965 The effect of supervised oral hygiene on the gingiva of children: the effect of toothbrushing. Odontologisk Revy 16:327–335

Maddick I, Downton D 1970 Project work in teaching dental health. Journal of School Health 40:197–199

McIntyre J, Wight C, Blinkhorn A S 1984 A reassessment of Lothian Health Board's dental health education programme for primary schools. Community Dental Health 2:99–108

Nikiforuk G 1985 Understanding dental caries, 2: Prevention-basic and clinical aspects. Karger, Basel, ch 8

Nizel A E 1980 Nutrition in preventive dentistry, science and practice 2nd edn. Saunders, Philadelphia

Rayner J F, Cohen L K 1971 School dental health education. In: Richards N D, Cohen I K (eds) Social sciences and dentistry: a clinical bibliography. Sigthoff, The Hague, p 286

Rugg-Gunn A J, Edgar W M 1984 Sugar and dental health: a review of the evidence. Community Dental Health 1:85–92

Rugg-Gunn A J, Edgar W M, Jenkins G N 1978 The effect of eating some British snacks upon the pH of human dental plaque. British Dental Journal 145:95–100

Stephan R M 1940 Changes in the hydrogen ion concentration on tooth surfaces and in carious lesions. Journal of the American Dental Association 27:718–723

Sutcliffe P 1983 Oral cleanliness and dental caries. In: Murray J J (ed) The prevention of dental disease. Oxford University Press, Oxford ch 4

Todd J E, Dodd T 1985 Children's dental health in the United Kingdom 1983. Her Majesty's Stationery Office, London, p65 and p76

Towner E M L 1984 The 'Gleam Team' programme: development and evaluation of a dental health education package for infant schools. Community Dental Health 1:181–191

Wright G Z, Banting D W, Feasby G H 1977 The effect of interdental flossing on the incidence of proximal caries in children. Journal of Dental Research 56:574–578

## RECOMMENDED READING

Forrest R O 1976 Preventive dentistry. Wright, Bristol, ch 3

Murray J J (ed) 1983 The prevention of dental disease. Oxford University Press, Oxford

# 4

# Fluorides

## TOXICITY

Fluoride is a potentially toxic substance. Since it is utilised in various forms for caries prevention, it is important to know the amount of fluoride used and the safety margins involved with each form of treatment (Heifetz and Horowitz, 1984).

The information on toxic doses given in this chapter is based on the data presented in Table 4.1. The 'certainly lethal dose' of fluoride is generally accepted to be 32–64 mg fluoride per kilogram body weight (Hodge and Smith, 1965); the calculations in Table 4.1 are based on the lower limit of 32 mg/kg.

The dose that might cause gastro-intestinal symptoms (nausea, hypersalivation, abdominal pains, vomiting, diarrhoea) appears to be about 1 mg fluoride per kilogram body weight, although only very minor symptoms occur with doses below 5 mg/kg (Spoerke, Bennett and Gullekson, 1980).

The risk of overdosage is extremely small, but is important to take appropriate action if it is suspected. If the amount of fluoride product that has been ingested can be estimated (e.g. number of

**Table 4.2** The amount of fluoride contained in various fluoride products.

| Product | Amount of fluoride |
|---|---|
| Tablets | 0.25, 0.5 or 1.0 mg per tablet |
| Drops | |
|   Fluorigard (Colgate Hoyt) | 3.8 mg/ml |
|   Fluordrops (En-de-Kay) | 1.7 mg/ml |
| Rinses | |
|   Fluorigard (Colgate Hoyt) | 0.23 mg/ml |
|   Colgate Point Two | 0.9 mg/ml |
|   Fluorinse (En-de-Kay)* | 9.0 mg/ml |
| Gel (APF) | 12.3 mg/ml |

* This product is diluted before use

tablets, or volume of mouthrinse), the amount of fluoride ingested can be calculated from the information given in Table 4.2.

When overdosage is suspected the following action is recommended (Bayless and Tinanoff, 1985):

If less than 5 mg F/kg has been ingested: give the child milk to drink and keep the child under observation.

If more than 5 mg F/kg has been ingested: induce vomiting if possible, give milk and refer to hospital.

## METHODS FOR THE INDIVIDUAL PATIENT

### Methods administered by dental personnel

*Topical application of solution or gel*

The idea of applying fluoride solution to teeth closely followed the demonstration in the U.S.A. of the caries-preventive effect of fluoride when

**Table 4.1** The amount of fluoride required to cause gastro-intestinal symptoms or lethal poisoning.

| Age (years) | Weight (kg) | mg F to cause gast.-int. symptoms* | mg F to cause lethal poisoning[†] |
|---|---|---|---|
| 2 | 10 | 10 | 320 |
| 3 | 14 | 14 | 448 |
| 4 | 18 | 18 | 576 |
| 5 | 20 | 20 | 640 |
| 8 | 25 | 25 | 800 |
| 10 | 30 | 30 | 960 |
| 15 | 45 | 45 | 1440 |

* Dose: 1 mg F/kg (Spoerke, Bennett and Gullekson, 1980)
† Dose: 32 mg F/kg (Hodge and Smith, 1965)

present in public water supplies. The first topical fluoride technique that was shown to be effective involved the use of neutral 2 per cent sodium fluoride solution (Knutson, 1948). A disadvantage of this technique was that a series of four applications at about weekly intervals was required. The search for more effective agents led to the introduction of 8 per cent stannous fluoride solution (Gish, Muhler and Howell, 1962). However, stannous fluoride has certain disadvantages: it is unstable in solution (which makes it necessary to prepare a fresh solution for each treatment), and it produces a brown stain in hypomineralised or demineralised enamel (for example, in early carious lesions and at the margins of restorations); this stain is unsightly if it occurs in anterior teeth.

It has been claimed that the stain produced in early lesions is an advantage because it discloses the lesion and demonstrates its arrest (Forrest, 1976). However, acidulated phosphate-fluoride (APF) is now generally used for topical applications. The composition of APF is 2 per cent sodium fluoride and 0.3 per cent hydrofluoric acid in 0.1 M orthophosphoric acid; the pH is about 3.3.

The development of APF was reviewed by Brudevold and DePaola (1966), who pointed out that the presence of phosphate enhances fluoride uptake into enamel while preventing precipitation of calcium fluoride and dissolution of enamel,

both of which were considered to be undesirable reactions that would occur in the absence of phosphate. However, it is now known that calcium fluoride is formed within the enamel and, by dissolving slowly, releases fluoride ions; although some fluoride is lost from the enamel, some remains and promotes the formation of fluorapatite (Mellberg and Ripa, 1983).

APF is available in solution or gel form, and is stable when stored in plastic or polythene containers. Its taste is less disagreeable than that of stannous fluoride, and is improved by the addition of flavouring agents. It does not stain enamel.

Solution or gel may be applied to the teeth either directly with a cotton applicator (direct technique), or indirectly in a tray (indirect technique). In addition, a varnish is available containing 5 per cent sodium fluoride (p. 46), which is applied by the direct technique.

It was only with the advent of APF gels that the indirect method became popular, since gels are particularly easy to use in a tray. This method is quicker than the direct method and therefore is usually preferred. However, the direct method is often better with a young, nervous child who may not tolerate a tray; direct application of solution, gel or varnish is a simple procedure that is useful in introducing the child to dental treatment. In addition, when treating a mixed dentition in which primary molars are missing, it may be

## Technique: topical fluoride application

*A. Direct technique: solution, gel or varnish*

| Procedure | Method | Rationale | Notes |
|---|---|---|---|
| 1. Ask the child to brush his teeth | Supervise the child brushing his teeth (and flossing if normally done). | Food debris must be removed before fluoride application. Even if oral hygiene is satisfactory, observing the child brushing at this stage provides an opportunity to reinforce good technique. | Until recently, a full prophylaxis has been considered to be an integral part of the topical fluoride technique. However, sufficient evidence now exists to show that it is not necessary (Ripa, 1984). |
| 2. Isolate teeth | Use saliva ejector, cotton wool rolls and/or absorbent pads to isolate the teeth to be treated. Isolate either one quadrant of teeth or a ½ mouth (maxillary and mandibular teeth on one side) or a ⅓ mouth (maxillary and mandibular primary and/or permanent molars on one side, or maxillary and mandibular incisors and canines). | Isolation allows the teeth to be dried and prevents dilution of the applied fluoride by saliva. The number of teeth that can be comfortably isolated depends on the patient. In general, quadrant isolation is most appropriate for young children: ½ mouth for teenagers; ⅓ mouth for mixed dentition-age children. | |

| Procedure | Method | Rationale | Notes |
|---|---|---|---|
| 3. Dry the isolated teeth | Dry the isolated teeth with compressed air. | Saliva on the tooth surface would dilute the solution or gel. | |
| 4. Apply solution, gel or varnish | With a cotton bud, or pledget held in tweezers, apply solution, gel or varnish to all tooth surfaces, working it especially into the interstitial spaces from buccal and lingual sides. Keep cotton wool rolls away from the teeth. Keep the teeth covered with solution or gel for 4 minutes.<br>If using varnish, allow to dry for 1–2 minutes. | Solution or gel would be absorbed by cotton wool rolls. A 4-minute application has become accepted as standard practice. | It is not known whether a shorter application would be equally effective, or a longer application more effective. |
| 5. (After 4 minutes) Remove solution or gel from accessible tooth surfaces | With cotton wool roll or gauze, wipe solution or gel from accessible tooth surfaces but do not attempt to remove it from approximal surfaces. | The amount of solution or gel placed on the teeth is small, but it is undesirable for the child to ingest an unnecessary dose of fluoride. Moreover, the taste is often considered to be unpleasant. | Although there is no evidence to prove it, more prolonged exposure of approximal surfaces to fluoride may be beneficial. |
| | Instruct the child to expectorate thoroughly but not to rinse. | It is desirable to expectorate residual fluoride. | |

Isolate another quadrant or ⅓ mouth, or the other ½ mouth, and repeat the treatment.
At the end of treatment, advise the patient not to eat or drink for ½ hour, to prolong contact of fluoride with approximal surfaces of the teeth.

## B. Indirect (tray) technique: gel

| Procedure | Method | Rationale | Notes |
|---|---|---|---|
| 1. Ask the child to brush his teeth | See procedure 1, direct technique. | | |
| 2. Select and prepare a tray | Select a tray and check that it is the correct size by trying it in the mouth.<br>Place the correct-sized absorbent insert into the tray and place only enough gel to cover the base of the tray (2–3 ml) | Enough gel should be used to cover the teeth, but over-filling would result in it being squeezed out of the tray, which is not only unpleasant for the patient but may also be toxic (p. 41). | Various types of tray are available. A close-fitting tray with a disposable absorbent insert is recommended (e.g. the air-cushion tray). |
| 3. Dry the teeth | Isolate the maxillary or mandibular arch by retracting the cheeks, ideally with the plastic cheek retractor that is included in some kits (Fig. 4.1a, b) and dry with compressed air.<br>Do not place a saliva ejector at this stage, or cotton wool rolls. | A saliva ejector or cotton wool rolls would obstruct the placement of the tray. | It has to be accepted that drying of lingual surfaces of of mandibular teeth may be incomplete. |

| Procedure | Method | Rationale | Notes |
|---|---|---|---|
| 4. Insert the tray | Sit the patient nearly upright. | If the patient is reclined, any excess solution or gel extruding from the tray would flow into the throat. | |
| | Keeping the cheeks away from the dry teeth, insert the tray. If using a plastic cheek retractor, remove it after inserting the tray. Apply finger pressure on the tray or, if using the 'air-cushion' tray, ask the child to apply pressure by closing his mouth gently on the tray. | Pressure squeezes gel into the interstitial spaces. | It is feasible (but not when using the rather bulky 'air-cushion' trays), to treat both arches at the same time, in which case, after inserting the first tray, teeth in the other arch are isolated and dried and a second tray inserted. Alternatively, it is possible to use upper and lower trays that are hinged together and therefore inserted at the same time. |
| | Insert a saliva ejector. If using the 'air-cushion' tray, attach a suction tube to the tray, instead of, or in addition to, the saliva ejector. | Suction is desirable to remove any excess gel extruding from the tray, and to avoid possible dilution of of the gel by saliva. | The 'air-cushion' tray incorporates an attachment for connection to suction apparatus. |
| 5. (After 4 minutes) Remove the tray and remove excess gel. | Remove the tray from the mouth. Before allowing the patient to close his mouth, remove the paper insert that will have remained on the teeth, and wipe excess gel from accessible surfaces with a cotton wool roll or gauze. Do not attempt to remove remaining gel from interstitial spaces. Instruct the patient to expectorate thoroughly but not to rinse. | Many children find the taste of solution or gel unpleasant; a considerable excess of gel usually remains after removal of the tray. Longer exposure of approximal tooth surfaces to fluoride may be beneficial. | The amount of solution wetting the teeth is not excessive; its removal is therefore unnecessary. |

Isolate the other arch and repeat the treatment.
At the end of treatment, advise the patient not to eat or drink for ½ hour, to prolong exposure of the teeth to fluoride.

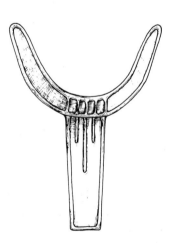

Fig. 4.1a

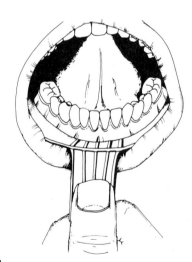

Fig. 4.1b

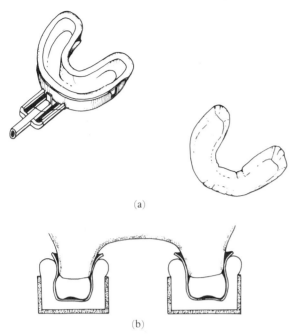

(a)

(b)

**Fig. 4.2** (a) 'Air cushion' tray and insert. (b) Close adaptation to the teeth

**Table 4.3** Volumes of APF or gel (12.3 mg F/ml) required to cause gastro-intestinal or lethal fluoride poisoning (based on data given in Table 4.1)

| Age (yrs) | Gast.-int. symptoms volume (ml) | Lethal poisoning volume (ml) |
|---|---|---|
| 5 | 1.6 | 52 |
| 10 | 2.4 | 78 |
| 15 | 3.7 | 117 |

preferable to apply fluoride directly to permanent incisors and first molars only.

Various types of tray are available. Some trays are supplied with disposable absorbent paper or sponge inserts to help retain solution or gel. One type of tray incorporates an air-filled rubber membrane on which a paper insert is placed (Fig. 4.2a); this 'air cushion' tray is highly recommended because, when pressure is exerted on it, it becomes closely adapted to the teeth and squeezes solution or gel into the interstitial spaces (Fig. 4.2b). It has been shown that this type of tray distributes gel over tooth surfaces more efficiently than other types of tray that are currently available (McCall et al, 1984).*

It should be remembered that APF contains a high concentration of fluoride (12.3 mg/ml); even a small bottle (200 ml) contains a potentially lethal dose (Table 4.1). The required quantity of gel should be dispensed directly into the tray and this should be kept out of the child's reach, because ingestion of relatively small quantities (e.g. 1.6 ml by a 5-year-old child) may cause gastro-intestinal

symptoms. Care should be taken to avoid using unnecessarily large amounts (2–3 ml is sufficient), suction apparatus should be used during the 4-minute application period, and excess gel should be wiped from accessible tooth surfaces before asking the child to expectorate thoroughly. If these precautions are taken (as described in the technique section above), it is difficult to envisage how patients can possibly ingest the large amounts of gel ingested by some of the subjects in the study of Ekstrand et al (1981). This conclusion is supported by the results of studies which investigated the retention of fluoride following topical fluoride treatment (McCall et al, 1983; LeCompte and Doyle, 1985; Tyler and Andlaw, 1987).

The effectiveness of topical fluoride treatment has been reviewed by Brudevold and Naujoks (1978). APF solution and gel appear to be equally effective. Of eight clinical trials in which APF solution was applied once or twice a year by the direct method to permanent teeth of children, two showed no effect but the others showed 28 to 55 per cent fewer carious surfaces after periods of 2 or 3 years. Similarly, studies with APF gel applied in trays showed reductions of 20 to 40 per cent; there do not appear to have been any studies done of the direct application of gel. These percentage reductions reflected average differences of about one tooth surface per child per year; in no study was the difference as great as two surfaces per child. Another useful review is by Ripa (1981).

Relatively few studies have tested the effectiveness of applying fluorides to the primary dentition. Neutral 2 per cent sodium fluoride and 4 per cent stannous fluoride solutions have been used, but not APF. In general, the results indicated modest reductions in caries (McDonald and Muhler, 1957).

Most topical fluoride studies have been conducted in areas served by water supplies contain-

---

* Unfortunately this tray is no longer available in the U.K.

ing low concentrations of fluoride. The few studies conducted in fluoridated areas have given conflicting results, and it may be concluded that topical fluoride treatment is not justified for lifelong residents of fluoridated areas, unless they show signs of caries activity and can be classified as 'high-risk' patients for this or other reasons (p. 49). When fluoride is introduced into a public water supply, topical fluoride treatment may be continued for children whose teeth were erupted when fluoridation began.

In recent years the use of fluoride-containing toothpastes has increased greatly, but little is known of the value of topical fluoride treatment to children who use fluoride toothpastes. A recent 3-year study showed that twice-yearly applications of APF gel was of little benefit to 11 to 12-year-old children who used fluoride toothpaste (Mainwaring and Naylor, 1978). However, the gel was not professionally applied; it was applied by the children themselves in plastic trays. Further evidence is required on this matter, but it is probable that only children with high caries rates benefit significantly from topical application if they already use a fluoride toothpaste regularly.

Newly erupted teeth derive more benefit from topical fluoride than more mature teeth; this indicates the importance of treating teeth soon after their eruption. Thus, topical fluoride treatment could be started at about the age of 3 years, soon after the primary molars erupt. However, because of the practical difficulties of performing the technique efficiently for such young children, and because systemic fluoride is of more value at this age (p. 47), topical fluoride treatment, if indicated, is often delayed until the permanent teeth erupt at the age of 6 or 7 years; thereafter, twice-yearly application may be continued up to late adolescence. Continuation into adult life generally is not justified; the few studies of fluoride application to adults' teeth give no clear evidence of its value. However, it can be justified for adults who show evidence of continued high caries activity.

## Fluoride varnishes

Fluoride varnish remains in contact with enamel for longer periods of time than do solution or gel. Varnishes that are currently available in the U.K. contain 5 per cent sodium fluoride (Duraphat), and 0.7 per cent fluorsilane (Fluor Protector).

Since varnish dries quickly after application to the teeth, it is particularly useful when treating young children. It is also convenient to use when treating specific sites of caries activity, for example early enamel demineralisation at the cervical margins of teeth in older children and adults.

Clinical trials of fluoride varnishes have indicated that they are effective in preventing dental caries (Clark, 1982; Modeer, Twetman and Bergstrand, 1984). Although the results have been variable and varnish has not been directly compared with solution or gel, the evidence suggests that varnish is at least as effective.

## Prophylaxis paste

Various fluorides have been incorporated into prophylaxis pastes: sodium fluoride, stannous fluoride, APF, sodium monofluorophosphate, and stannous hexafluorozirconate. Clinical trials to test the efficacy of these pastes in preventing dental caries have given variable results (Horowitz, 1970; Murray and Rugg-Gunn, 1982) and therefore it is concluded that prophylaxis with such pastes should not be considered as an alternative treatment to the application of solution, gel or varnish. However, there are no contra-indications to using a fluoride-containing paste to clean teeth before application of solution, gel or varnish.

## Methods administered by the patient (or parent)

### Fluoride toothpaste

Since 97 per cent of the toothpastes currently marketed in the U.K. contain fluoride, most people who use toothpaste give themselves a topical fluoride treatment when they brush their teeth.

A large number of clinical trials have been conducted with children of toothpastes containing either sodium fluoride, stannous fluoride, amine fluoride, APF and sodium monofluorophosphate. The results are fairly consistent in showing reductions of about 15 to 30 per cent in the number of tooth surfaces becoming carious over periods of 2 to 3 years; in most studies these reductions reflected the prevention of caries in about 1 surface per child per year (Murray and Rugg-Gunn, 1982; Fehr and Moller, 1978). There is no firm evidence that one type of fluoride toothpaste is more effective than others.

Most toothpastes contain 0.1 per cent fluoride; therefore 1 g of toothpaste contains 1 mg fluoride. The average amount of toothpaste used by children below 7 years of age ranges from about 0.4 to 1.4 g, and the average proportion ingested ranges from 14 to 35 per cent (Barnhart et al, 1974). Thus, fluoride ingestion can be estimated to range from 0.06 to 0.5 mg.

Concern has been expressed about toothpaste ingestion by young children who do not rinse or expectorate efficiently after brushing. The great majority of children ingest less than 0.25 g of toothpaste (Barnhart et al, 1974; Baxter, 1980), but the occasional child ingests as much as 1 g of paste, containing 1 mg of fluoride (Hargreaves, Ingram and Wagg, 1972). Excessive ingestion of toothpaste clearly is undesirable for children already receiving systemic fluoride. Parents should be advised to supervise toothbrushing by young children, and to limit the amount placed on the brush to about the size of a small pea.

The concern about excessive toothpaste ingestion centres on the possibility of causing mottling of developing enamel. However, there is no evidence that ingestion of fluoride toothpaste *per se* causes mottling; indeed, in a study investigating this possibility, fewer developmental defects of enamel were found in children who used a toothpaste containing more than twice the normal concentration of fluoride (0.24%) than in children who used a fluoride-free toothpaste (Houwink and Wagg, 1979).

### Fluoride tablets and drops

In areas served by low-fluoride water supplies, tablets and drops provide a method for systemic administration of fluoride. In theory, this form of administration has the advantage over water fluoridation that it allows specific doses of fluoride to be given. In practice, it is difficult to sustain the interest of even the most highly motivated families for the long-term comsumption that is necessary.

Table 4.4 Recommended dosage of fluoride tablets and drops (mg F/day), related to the concentration of fluoride in the drinking water (Dowell and Joyston-Bechal, 1981).

| age (years) | water F (ppm) | | |
|---|---|---|---|
| | <0.3 | 0.3–0.7 | >0.7 |
| <2 | 0.25 | 0 | 0 |
| 2–4 | 0.50 | 0.25 | 0 |
| >4 | 1.0 | 0.5 | 0 |

The following preparations are currently available in the U.K.:

*Fluoride drops.* These contain sodium fluoride, but the amount delivered in each drop varies; for example, one preparation delivers 0.125 mg fluoride per drop, and another 0.033 mg per drop.

*Fluoride tablets.* These contain either 0.5 mg fluoride (1.1 mg sodium fluoride) or 1 mg fluoride (2.2 mg sodium fluoride). Tablets are prepared with various flavours.

For delivering doses of 0.25 mg the drops are most convenient; the appropriate number of drops are added to the baby's food or drink each day. When doses of 0.5 mg are required, drops may be continued, but when the child is old enough to suck or chew tablets he should be encouraged to do so because there is strong evidence that fluoride in tablets can exert a topical as well as a systemic effect.

The dosage recommended for use in the U.K. was proposed by the Dental Health Committee of the British Dental Association (Dowell and Joyston-Bechal, 1981). Their recommendations, given in Table 4.4, are identical to those of the American Dental Association (1982) and of the American Academy of Pediatrics (1979) except that the maximum dose of 1 mg is recommended from the age of 4 years instead of from the age of 3 years.

*Period of fluoride supplementation*: There has been controversy about the desirability of starting fluoride supplementation during pregnancy. Although fluoride passes through the placenta, the concentration that reaches the foetus is much lower than that of the maternal blood. The general consensus of opinion is that there is no indication for starting fluoride administration before birth.

An important period for fluoride supplementation is from birth to the age of 5 or 6 years, during which time enamel of all primary and permanent teeth (other than third molars) is formed. Studies in which fluoride was administered during this period have shown considerable reductions of dental caries in primary and permanent teeth (Binder, Driscoll and Schutzmann-sky, 1978).

Another important period for fluoride supplementation is from the age of 5 to 6 years to the age of 12 to 14 years; this is the pre-eruptive maturation phase of premolars and second molars, during which time fluoride is taken up from the tissue fluids. Studies of fluoride administration starting at age 6 or 7 years and continuing for up to 8 years have shown significant caries reductions (Marthaler, 1969). However, some parents are reluctant to continue giving tablets throughout the child's school years because they do not want their child to develop a habit of self-medication that might persist into adolescence and even into adult life. If the patient is classified as 'high risk' (p. 49) encouragement to continue taking tablets is justified but, if not, it is not unreasonable to discontinue tablet administration and to transfer to a mouthrinsing regime a few years later when permanent teeth start to erupt (p. 48).

*Problems in administering tablets and drops*: A serious drawback limiting the use of fluoride tablets and drops in dental practice is the need to have the intelligent cooperation of the child's parents. They must by highly motivated to administer fluoride daily for several years, and they must be careful and responsible in storing the tablets in a safe place, out of children's reach. Fluoride drops are dispensed in bottles containing 30 ml of 0.38 per cent fluoride, or 60 ml of 0.17 per cent fluoride. Reference to Table 4.5 shows that gastrointestinal symptoms might be caused if a 5-year-old child consumes about one-sixth of the contents of a 30 ml bottle, or if a 10-year-old child con-

sumes about a quarter; but there is a considerable safety margin before reaching the lethal dose.

Fluoride tablets are usually dispensed in quantities of 120 tablets, in bottles with child-proof lids. Again, reference to Table 4.5 shows that unpleasant symptoms could occur if an overdose were taken, but that it would be necessary to consume the contents of several bottles to reach a lethal dose.

### Fluoride mouthrinses

Mouthrinsing with a fluoride solution has emerged during the last 10 to 15 years as a simple and convenient method of topical fluoride application.

The solutions most commonly available are flavoured neutral sodium fluoride solutions; a 0.05 per cent solution (0.023 per cent fluoride) is recommended for daily use, and a 0.2 per cent solution (0.09 per cent fluoride) for weekly or fortnightly use.

*Method.* The child and parent should be given the following instructions:

1. Clean teeth thoroughly in the usual way.
2. Take about 10 ml of solution into the mouth and gently 'swish' the solution between the teeth for at least 1 minute.
3. Spit the solution into a basin after the 1-minute period, do not swallow it.
4. Do not eat or drink for at least half an hour.

Whether the 0.05 per cent sodium fluoride solution is used daily or the 0.2 per cent weekly is for the child and parent to decide; there is no evidence that one or the other regime is more effective. The parent should be advised to select a specific time every day or week, so that it is not forgotten.

Clinical trials of mouthrinsing have been conducted in schools, where it could be supervised. Various solutions have been tested, including neutral sodium fluoride, APF, stannous fluoride and amine fluoride solutions. Studies in several countries have shown that daily or weekly mouthrinsing reduces the incidence of dental caries by about 40 per cent over periods of 2 to 3 years in non-fluoridated areas; these reductions reflect the prevention of caries in about one tooth surface per child per year (Birkeland and Torell, 1978). More

**Table 4.5** Volume of fluoride drops (3.8 mg F/ml) and number of tablets (1 mg F/tab) required to cause gastrointestinal symptoms or lethal fluoride poisoning (based on data given in Table 4.1)

| Age (yrs) | Gast.-int. symptoms | | Lethal poisoning | |
|---|---|---|---|---|
| | drops (ml) | tablets | drops (ml) | tablets |
| 2 | 3 | 10 | 84 | 320 |
| 5 | 5 | 20 | 168 | 640 |
| 10 | 8 | 30 | 252 | 960 |

recently it has been shown that fluoride rinsing can also benefit children living in a fluoridated area (Driscoll et al, 1982).

Many of the early trials of fluoride mouth-rinsing were conducted before fluoride toothpastes were widely available, but more recent studies have shown that rinsing with a fluoride solution reduces caries incidence in children who, it can be assumed, used fluoride toothpaste at home (Ripa et al, 1983). However, in studies involving brushing with a mouthrinsing solution, little additional benefit was gained by children who rinsed after brushing compared to those who only brushed or rinsed (Ashley et al, 1977; Blinkhorn et al, 1983); but it should be noted that children in the latter study rinsed for only 30 seconds. It is possible that only children with high caries rates benefit significantly from using a fluoride mouthrinse in addition to brushing their teeth with a fluoride toothpaste.

Mouthrinsing may be introduced when a child is 6–7 years of age and able to rinse correctly; primary molars and, especially, newly-erupting permanent incisors and first molars, may benefit from this topical fluoride. However, fluoride tablets are probably of greater benefit until the age of about 12 years because, in addition to having a topical effect while they are sucked or chewed, they have a systemic effect on the developing premolars and second molars. Mouthrinsing is most useful during the period of eruption of premolars and second molars, and may be continued until late adolescence, or into adulthood if caries activity remains high.

In common with fluoride tablet administration, a drawback to the use of the mouthrinsing method is that the child's and parent's interest must be maintained and the parent must be motivated enough to ensure that the child rinses conscientiously. The parent must also ensure that the stock bottle of solution is kept out of the child's reach. The 0.05 per cent solution is supplied in 500 ml bottles, and the 0.2 per cent solution in 150 ml bottles. Table 4.6 shows that gastro-intestinal symptoms may occur if, for example, a 5-year-old ingests about 30 ml of 0.2 per cent solution, or 130 ml of 0.05 per cent solution. However, lethal doses can only be reached by ingesting the contents of many bottles.

**Table 4.6** Volumes of mouthrinses required to cause gastrointestinal symptoms or lethal flouride poisoning: 0.05% NaF solution (0.23 mg F/ml) and 0.2% NaF solution (0.9 mg F/ml). Based on data given in Table 4.1

| Age (yrs) | Gast.-int. symptoms | | Lethal poisoning | |
|---|---|---|---|---|
| | 0.05% soln (ml) | 0.2% soln (ml) | 0.05% soln (ml) | 0.2% soln (ml) |
| 5 | 86 | 22 | 2783 | 711 |
| 10 | 130 | 33 | 4174 | 1067 |
| 15 | 196 | 50 | 6261 | 1660 |

### Gel

The effectiveness of frequent applications of fluoride gel to children's teeth in a non-fluoridated area was shown by Englander et al (1967). Children aged 11 to 14 years applied gel to their teeth in individually constructed trays under supervision at school for 6 minutes every school day for nearly 2 years. Children who used a sodium fluoride gel (0.5 per cent fluoride) developed, on average, 3.50 fewer carious surfaces than children in a control group, and children using an APF gel (0.5 per cent fluoride) developed 3.29 fewer carious surfaces; percentage reductions were 80 per cent and 75 per cent respectively, the highest reported for any topical fluoride method. However, less frequent applications (3 times weekly) by children in a fluoridated area reduced caries by only 29 per cent after 30 months (Englander et al, 1971).

### Selection of methods

The methods of using fluoride that are most commonly recommended in dental practice are topical applications of solution or gel, and home use of toothpaste, tablets or mouthrinses. The use of fluoride toothpaste may be recommended to all patients, but it must be decided which of the other methods to select for each patient. An obvious factor that affects this choice is the child's age; but another important factor that should be considered is the degree of risk that caries presents to the child. Patients may be classified either as 'high risk' or as 'low risk'. The 'high risk' patient may be described as having one or more of the following characteristics:

1. A high caries rate, as assessed by previous caries experience and present caries activity.

2. A medical condition (for example, congenital heart disease or a history of rheumatic fever) that may be complicated by bacteraemia resulting from infection or from some forms of dental treatment.
3. A medical condition (for example, a bleeding disorder) that makes certain forms of dental treatment hazardous.
4. Mental subnormality, which sometimes makes any treatment more than usually difficult.

The 'low risk' patient is one with a low caries rate and no complicating medical condition.

An outline for selecting appropriate methods is presented in Table 4.7. For pre-school children, systemic administration is the most effective and often the only practicable method. However, topical treatment should be given if possible for 'high risk' children. Pre-school children are too young to use mouthrinses.

From the age of 5 or 6 years to the eruption of premolars and second molars (age 12 to 14 years), tablet administration again is the most beneficial method. For the 'low risk' child taking fluoride tablets during this period (and, it may be assumed, using a fluoride toothpaste) the use of other methods cannot be justified (regime 1). It could be argued that every available method that might help to prevent caries should be used, but this must be considered against the time needed to apply topical fluoride and the expense incurred by the parents. However, proprietary mouthrinses are not expensive, and a keen parent may be encouraged to buy them for home use. For the 'low risk' child not taking fluoride tablets, mouthrinsing may be recommended more strongly (regime 2); if it is assessed that this is done conscientiously, there is little justification for topical applications. Some dentists would argue that topical treatment is not justified for the 'low risk' child even if mouthrinsing is not done, assuming that a fluoride toothpaste is used. On the other hand, full use of all available methods is strongly advocated for the 'high risk' child, for whom continued administration of tablets until premolars and second molars erupt should be encouraged.

After the age of 12 to 14 years, tablet administration should be stopped but topical methods may be continued, especially for the 'high-risk' child.

## METHODS FOR THE COMMUNITY

It is clear that child patients may receive the benefits of fluoride in various ways. However, there are many children who do not visit a dentist regularly and who therefore cannot benefit (except by using a fluoride-containing toothpaste); the national survey in the U.K. in 1983 (Todd and Dodd, 1985) showed that 42 per cent of 5-year-old children, 36 per cent of 8-year-olds and 34 per cent of 12-year-olds only attended a dentist occasionally or when in trouble. To reach these children, methods are required that can be applied to the community as a whole.

### Systemic administration

*Fluoridation of public water supplies*

The adjustment of the fluoride concentration of public water supplies to 1 part per million (ppm) is the most effective method now available of preventing dental caries. Over 150 million people in about 30 countries live in areas where water supplies are fluoridated, and a further 40 million live in areas naturally rich in fluoride. Over 100 million people in the U.S.A. drink fluoridated water (about 60 per cent of the population), but only about 3 million (6 per cent of the population) in the U.K. (Backer-Dirks, Kunzel and Carlos, 1978).

**Table 4.7** Selection of fluoride methods for the child patient.

| | age ranges (years) | | |
| | 0 to 6 | 6 to 12 | 12 to 18 |
|---|---|---|---|
| low-risk child | | | |
| regime 1 | drops-tablets | tablets | rinsing or topical |
| regime 2 | — | rinsing or topical | rinsing or topical |
| high-risk child | drops-tablets + topical | tablets + topical + rinsing | topical + rinsing |

Most commonly, fluoride is added in the form of hydrofluosilicic acid, but sodium silicofluoride and sodium fluoride have also been used. Fluoridation equipment delivers and maintains the level of fluoride between 0.9 and 1.1 ppm. The equipment cannot deliver much more than the desired amount, and automatic devices monitor the concentration of fluoride. In addition, daily records are kept of the amount of fluoride used and the volume of water pumped (from which the concentration of fluoride is calculated), and samples of water are analysed daily by waterworks staff and periodically by the Laboratory of the Government Chemist (Department of Health and Social Security, 1969). At a concentration of 1 ppm, hydrofluosilicic acid or other added fluoride compounds dissociate into their constituent ions, which have identical properties to those of fluoride, silicon and other ions naturally present in water.

The relationship between the concentration of fluoride in water supplies and the prevalence of dental caries was demonstrated in the U.S.A. by Dean, Arnold and Elvove (1942); their survey of over 7000 12- to 14-year-old children showed that children living in areas served by water supplies containing at least 1 ppm fluoride had about 50 per cent fewer carious teeth than children living in low-fluoride areas. This relationship has since been confirmed in a large number of studies throughout the world; moreover, the benefits of fluoride are life-long (Murray and Rugg-Gunn, 1982).

The safety of fluoridation has been extensively studied, and is beyond doubt (World Health Organisation, 1970; Royal College of Physicians, 1976). Water fluoridation is an ideal public health measure because its benefits are not dependent on the interest and cooperation of the recipients, and because it is cheap.

## Fluoride tablets

Fluoride tablets have been administered to children at school in many countries; in some countries this practice has become firmly established (for example, Austria, where a fluoride tablet scheme has been in operation in Vienna for more than 20 years). In the U.K. only one, small-scale study has been conducted, and another is in progress (Stephen, 1978).

Fluoride tablets (1 mg fluoride) are administered daily, usually by the school teachers. In some schemes, efforts are made also to involve the parents, so that tablets may be administered at home during school holidays. Since safe storage of tablets at school cannot be guaranteed, the tablets are supplied in limited quantities, for example 120 tablets, which is 1 week's supply for a class of 24 children. It is, of course, necessary to check that children are not already receiving systemic fluoride at home.

Studies of fluoride tablet administration to schoolchildren have shown reductions of dental caries in permanent teeth of between 20 and 40 per cent (Binder et al., 1978). However, the success of the method depends on the long-term cooperation of the teachers. Although little of the teachers' time is required, it is sometimes difficult to maintain their interest. Another disadvantage of the method is that it can only be started when children begin school, by which time the crowns of all permanent teeth (except third molars) are already well developed; for maximum benefit systemic fluoride should start soon after birth.

## Fluoridation of school water supplies

The fluoridation of school water supplies has been found to be feasible and effective. It has been tested in certain isolated rural schools in the U.S.A. that have independent water supplies. Since children at these schools drink fluoridated water only for a part of each day and not at weekends or during holidays, the amount of fluoride added is several times higher than the level that would be indicated for community water fluoridation in that area; thus, in Elk Lake, Pennsylvania, the school water is fluoridated to 5 ppm, and in Seagrave, North Carolina, to 6.3 ppm. Results after 12 years in Elk Lake (Horowitz, Heifetz and Law, 1972) and in Seagrave (Heifetz, Horowitz and Brunelle, 1983) indicate that the method is effective in reducing the prevalence of dental caries in children. It has the advantage over tablet administration that daily involvement of teachers is not necessary. However, the initial cost of the fluoridation equipment is a disadvantage.

*Fluoridated salt*

Fluoridated table salt was introduced in Switzerland in 1955. Much of the salt available in Switzerland today contains 90 ppm fluoride; in 2 cantons, salt containing 250 ppm fluoride is available. Studies conducted in Switzerland, Colombia, Spain and Hungary indicate that fluoridated salt is effective in preventing caries in children (Marthaler et al, 1978).

*Fluoridated milk*

Milk has been proposed as a suitable vehicle for fluoride, and equipment to fluoridate milk has been designed (Davis, 1972). A pilot study in the U.S.A., which gave promising results, was not followed up (Rusoff et al, 1962), but recent studies in Scotland (Stephen et al, 1981) and in Hungary (Banoczy et al, 1983) have confirmed the effectiveness of milk fluoridation; fluoridated milk given to children from the age of 3 or 4 years reduced caries incidence in first permanent molars.

Although the idea of fluoridating milk is attractive because milk is a natural food for children, the method is less precise than tablet administration because milk consumption by children varies greatly (even more than water consumption). This disadvantage could be overcome if the milk was given to children at school under supervision. However, the practical difficulties of obtaining the cooperation of dairies and of school authorities appear formidable.

## Topical application

*Mouthrinse*

Mouthrinsing by children with a fluoride solution, weekly or fortnightly at school, has been introduced in some countries, especially in Sweden. Generally, a 0.2 per cent neutral sodium fluoride solution is used. The procedure is very simple to administer. Each child is given a disposable cup containing 5 ml to 10 ml of solution and is instructed to retain and gently rinse the solution in the mouth for at least 1 minute, after which the solution is expectorated into the cup or into a bucket or sink. Although in fluoride tablet schemes the teachers dispense the tablets, supervising the

mouthrinsing procedure must be the responsibility of the authority that administers the scheme.

The disruption of normal school activities can be minimal if the procedure is carried out efficiently. However, it is essential for the dental team to establish and maintain good rapport with the school authorities.

*Solution, gel or prophylaxis paste*

Supervised 'brush-ins' at school, during which children brush their teeth with fluoride solution, gel or prophylaxis paste, is another method that has been investigated. This method has the advantage over mouthrinsing that it involves the children in toothbrushing, during which time oral hygiene instruction may be given and reinforced. However, the procedure is more difficult and time-consuming to administer and requires more highly trained staff.

Solutions containing 1 per cent sodium fluoride (0.4 per cent fluoride) have been tested in Sweden, APF solutions and gels (0.6 per cent fluoride and 1.23 per cent fluoride) in the U.S.A., Canada, and Brazil, and amine fluoride (1.25 per cent fluoride) in Switzerland. Caries reductions obtained with as few as 4 or 5 'brush-ins' a year have been comparable with those obtained with weekly or fortnightly mouthrinsing (Horowitz et al, 1974). 'Brush-ins' with prophylaxis pastes have mostly employed a 9 per cent stannous fluoride paste (2.18 per cent fluoride), but an APF paste (1.23 per cent fluoride) has also been tested. The results of either annual or semi-annual 'brush-ins' with these pastes have been inconclusive (Horowitz and Bixler, 1976).

## Selection of methods

Water fluoridation is not only the most effective method known at present for preventing dental caries but it is also the most cost-effective (Horowitz and Heifetz, 1979). It is widely believed that fluoridation should be the corner-stone for any local or national caries-preventive programme (Backer-Dirks, Kunzel and Carlos, 1978).

If water fluoridation is not feasible and a choice is to be made between other methods, the decision must be based, at least in part, on the relative cost-effectiveness of alternative methods. Calculating cost-effectiveness is complicated by a number of factors: for example, most of the information available about the effectiveness of different methods is based on clinical trials in which a method is tested on selected subjects for a limited number of years, under ideal conditions that do not necessarily apply in the community at large.

However, Horowitz and Heifetz (1979) have estimated the cost-effectiveness of various methods and concluded that fluoride tablet administration is more cost-effective than school water fluoridation and that weekly mouthrinsing with 0.2 per cent fluoride solution is the most cost-effective of topical methods.

## REFERENCES

American Dental Association Council on Dental Therapeutics 1982 Fluoride compounds: accepted dental therapeutics, 39th edn, p 344–368

American Academy of Pediatrics Committee on Nutrition 1979 Fluoride supplementation: revised dosage schedule. Pediatrics 63:150–152

Ashley F P, Mainwaring P J, Emslie R D, Naylor M N 1977 Clinical testing of a mouthrinse and a dentifrice containing fluoride: a 2-year supervised study in schools. British Dental Journal 143:333–338

Backer-Dirks O, Kunzel W, Carlos J P 1978 Caries-preventive water fluoridation. Caries Research 12 suppl 1:7–14

Barnhart W E, Hiller L K, Giles J L, Michaels S F 1974 Dentifrice usage and ingestion among four age groups. Journal of Dental Research 53:1317–1322

Banoczy J, Zimmerman P, Printer A, Hadas E, Bruszt V 1983 Effect of fluoridated milk on caries: 3-year results. Community Dentistry and Oral Epidemiology 11:81–00

Baxter P M 1980 Toothpaste ingestion during toothbrushing by school children. British Dental Journal 148:125–128

Bayless J M, Tinanoff N 1985 Diagnosis and treatment of acute fluoride toxicity. Journal of the American Dental Association 110:209–211

Binder K, Driscoll W S, Schutzmannsky G 1978 Caries-preventive fluoride tablet programmes. Caries Research 12 suppl 1:20–30

Birkeland J M, Torell P 1978 Caries-preventive fluoride mouthrinses. Caries Research 12 suppl 1:38–51

Blinkhorn A S, Holloway P J, Davies T G H 1983 Combined effects of a fluoride dentifrice and mouthrinse on the incidence of dental caries. Community Dentistry and Oral Epidemiology 11:7–11

Brudevold F, dePaola P F 1966 Studies on topically applied acidulated phosphate fluoride at Forsyth Dental Center. Dental Clinics of North America (July) 299–308

Brudevold F, Naujoks R 1978 Caries-preventive treatment of the individual. Caries Research 12 suppl 1:52–64

Bruun C, Stolze K 1978 In vivo uptake of fluoride by surface enamel of cleaned and plaque-covered teeth. Scandinavian Journal of Dental Research 84:268–275

Clark D C 1982 A review on fluoride varnishes: an alternative topical fluoride treatment. Community Dentistry and Oral Epidemiology 10:117–123

Davies J G 1972 Milk as a vehicle for fluoridation of the diet for children. In: The Fluoridation of Children's Milk: Proceedings of a Scientific Symposium, Kimpton, London p 34–40

Dean H T, Arnold F A, Elvove E 1942 Domestic water and dental caries V. Additional studies of the relation of fluoride domestic water to dental caries experience in 4425 white children aged 12–14 years of 13 cities in 4 States. Public Health Reports 57:1155–1179

Department of Health and Social Security 1969 Fluoridation studies in the United Kingdom and the results achieved after 11 years. Reports on Public Health and Medical Subjects, no. 22. Her Majesty's Stationery Office, London

Dowell T B, Joyston-Bechal S 1981 Fluoride supplements: age-related doses. British Dental Journal 150:273–275

Driscoll W S, Swango P A, Horowitz A M, Kingman A 1982 Caries-preventive effects of daily and weekly fluoride mouthrinsing in a fluoridated community: final results after 30 months. Journal of the American Dental Association 105:1010–1013

Ekstrand J, Koch G, Lindgren L E, Petersson L G 1981 Pharmacokinetics of fluoride gels in children and adults. Caries Research 15:213–220

Englander H R, Keyes P H, Gestwicki M, Sultz H A 1967 Clinical anticaries effect of repeated topical sodium fluoride applications by mouthpieces. Journal of the American Dental Association 75:638–645

Englander H R, Sherrill L T, Miller B G, Carlos T P, Mellberg J R, Senning R S 1971 Incremental rates of dental caries after repeated topical sodium fluoride applications in children with lifelong consumption of fluoridated water. Journal of the American Dental Association 82:354–358

Fehr F von der, Moller I 1978 Caries-preventive fluoride dentifrices. Caries Research 12 suppl 1:31–37

Forrest J O 1976 Preventive dentistry. Wright, Bristol, p 55

Gish C W, Muhler J C, Howell C L 1962 A new approach to the topical application of fluorides for the reduction of dental caries in children: results at the end of 5 years. Journal of Dentistry for Children 29:65–71

Hargreaves J A, Ingram G S, Wagg B J 1972 A gravimetric study of the ingestion of toothpaste by children. Caries Research 6:237–243

Heifetz S B, Horowitz H S 1984 The amounts of fluoride in current fluoride therapies: safety considerations for children. Journal of Dentistry for Children 51:257–269

Heifetz S B, Horowitz H S, Brunelle J A 1983 Effects of school water fluoridation on dental caries: results in Seagrave, N. C., after 12 years. Journal of the American Dental Association 106:333–337

Heifetz S B, Horowitz H S, Driscoll W S 1978 Effect of school water fluoridation on dental caries: results in Seagrave, North Carolina after 8 years. Journal of the American Dental Association 97:193–196

Hodge C, Smith F A 1965 Biological properties of inorganic fluorides. In: Simons J H (ed) Fluorine chemistry, vol 4. Academic Press, New York

Horowitz H S 1970 The current status of topical fluorides in preventive dentistry. Journal of the American Dental Association 81:166–177

Horowitz H S, Bixler D 1976 The effect of self-applied stannous fluoride-zirconium silicate prophylactic paste on dental caries in Santa Clara County, California. Journal of the American Dental Association 92:369–373

Horowitz H S, Heifetz S B 1979 Methods for assessing the cost-effectiveness of caries-preventive agents and procedures. International Dental Journal 29:106–117

Horowitz H S, Heifetz S B, Law F E 1972 Effect of school water fluoridation on dental caries: final results in Elk Lake, Pennsylvania, after 12 years. Journal of the American Dental Association 84:832–838

Horowitz H S, Heifetz S B, McClendon B J, Viegas A R, Guimaraes L O C, Lopes E S 1974 Evaluation of self-administered prophylaxis and supervised toothbrushing with acidulated phosphate fluoride. Caries Research 8:39–51

Houwink B, Wagg B J 1979 Effect of fluoride dentifrice usage during infancy upon mottling of the permanent teeth. Caries Research 13:231–237

Knutson J W 1948 Sodium fluoride solutions: technique for application to the teeth. Journal of the American Dental Association 36:37–39

LeCompte E J, Doyle T E 1985 Effects of suctioning devices on oral fluoride retention. Journal of the American Dental Association 110:357–369

McCall D R, Watkins T R, Stephen K W, Collins W J H, Smalls M J 1983 Fluoride ingestion following APF gel application. British Dental Journal 155:333–336

McCall D R, Watkins T R, Stephen K W, MacFarlane G J, Boyle P 1985 Distribution of APF gel on tooth surfaces. British Dental Journal 159:82–84

McDonald R E, Muhler J C 1957 The superiority of topical application of stannous fluoride on primary teeth. Journal of Dentistry for Children 24:84–86

Mainwaring P J, Naylor M N 1978 A 3-year clinical study to determine the separate and combined caries-inhibiting effects of sodium mono-fluorophosphate toothpaste and an acidulated phosphate fluoride gel. Caries Research 12:202–212

Marthaler T M 1969 Caries inhibiting effect of fluoride tablets. Helvetica Odontological Acta 13:1–12

Marthaler T M, Mejia R, Toth K, Vines J L 1978 Caries-preventive salt fluoridation. Caries Research 12 suppl 1:15–21

Mellberg J R, Ripa L W 1983 Fluoride in preventive dentistry. Quintessence, Chicago, ch 6

Modeer T, Twetman S, Bergstrand F 1984 Three-year study of the effect of fluoride varnish (Duraphat) on proximal caries progression in teenagers. Scandinavian Journal of Dental Research 92:400–407

Murray J J, Rugg-Gunn A J 1982 Fluorides in caries prevention 2nd edn. Wright, Bristol, ch 3

Ripa L W 1981 Professionally (operator) applied topical fluoride therapy: a critique. International Dental Journal 31:105–120

Ripa L W 1984 Need for prior toothcleaning when performing a professional topical fluoride application: review and recommendations for change. Journal of the American Dental Association 109:281–285

Rusoff L L, Konikoff B S, Frye J B, Johnston J E, Frye W W 1962 Fluoride addition to milk and its effects on dental caries in school children. American Journal of Clinical Nutrition 11:94–101

Silverstone L M 1978 Preventive dentistry. Update Books, London

Spoerke D G, Bennett D L, Gullekson D J K 1980 Toxicity related to acute low dose sodium fluoride ingestions. Journal of Family Practice 10: 139–140

Stephen K W 1978 Caries reduction and cost benefit after 3 years of sucking fluoride tablets daily at school. British Dental Journal 144:202–206

Stephen K W, Boyle I T, Campbell D, McNee S, Fyffe J A, Jenkins A S, Boyle P 1981 A 4-year double-blind fluoridated milk study in a vitamin D deficient area. British Dental Journal 151:287–292

Tyler J G, Andlaw R J 1987 Oral retention of fluoride after application of acidulated phosphate fluoride gel in air-cushion trays. British Dental Journal (In press)

World Health Organisation 1967 Fluorides and human health. World Health Organisation, Geneva, ch 8, p 273–322

RECOMMENDED READING

Mellberg J R, Ripa L W 1983. Fluoride in preventive dentistry: theory and clinical applications. Quintessence, Chicago

Murray J J, Rugg-Gunn A J 1982 Fluorides in caries prevention, 2nd edn. Wright, Bristol

Nikiforuk G 1985 Understanding dental caries: 2. Prevention: basic and clinical aspects. Karger, Basel, ch 2–6

# 5

# Pit and fissure sealants

The effect of systemic or topical fluorides in preventing dental caries is noted principally on the smooth surfaces of teeth; the effect on pit and fissure caries is relatively small. It is probable that the protected stagnation sites provided by pits and fissures offer such favourable conditions for the initiation of caries that fluoride is inadequate to combat it. Therefore there is a place in preventive dentistry for a method aimed specifically at preventing caries in these caries-prone sites.

The idea of sealing pits and fissures before they become carious is not new, but early attempts met with only limited success because the adhesion of tested materials to enamel was inadequate. The success of the current sealing technique is based on the discovery that adhesion of acrylic and composite resins to enamel is greatly increased if the enamel is first etched with acid (Buonocore, 1955).

Phosphoric acid, in the concentration range of 30–50 per cent, is normally used to etch enamel. A 1-minute application removes about 10 $\mu$m of surface enamel and etches the underlying surface to a depth of about 20 $\mu$m (Silverstone, 1974). Etching produces a porous layer of enamel into which resin can flow; the porosity provides a large surface area for adhesion of resin and also excellent mechanical retention.

The resins currently used as sealants are based on the 'Bis GMA' resin developed by Bowen (1963); 'Bis GMA' is the reaction product of bis (4-hydroxyphenyl) dimethylmethane and glycidyl methacrylate. Two types are available: those that polymerise after mixing catalyst and 'universal' components (autopolymerising types), and those that polymerise only after exposure to a suitable light source. Until recently, ultraviolet light (wavelength 365 nm) has been used, but this has been largely superceded by visible (blue) light (wavelength 430–490 nm).

Most of the resins that have been used as fissure sealants are 'unfilled', that is, they do not contain filler particles. Since the incorporation of filler into a resin increases its resistance to abrasion, there is some logic in using a filled resin for fissure sealing. A composite resin restorative material has been diluted 1:1 with unfilled resin and used successfully as a sealant (Ulvestad, 1976), but filled resins formulated specifically to be used as sealants have been introduced only recently; there

## Technique: fissure sealing

| Procedure | Method | Rationale | Notes |
|---|---|---|---|
| 1. Clean the tooth surface | Use a pumice-water slurry on a motor driven brush to clean the pit or fissure and surrounding tooth surface. | It is necessary to remove plaque and pellicle that might interfere with subsequent acid etching. Pumice is preferred to commercial prophylaxis pastes because the latter may contain fluoride and/or oily constituents that reduce the effectiveness of acid etching. | Fine debris may be dislodged from pits and fissures with a probe; some stain may similarly be removed. |
| | Wash the surface with an air/water spray. | Particles of pumice must be removed. | *(continued overleaf)* |

55

| Procedure | Method | Rationale | Notes |
|-----------|--------|-----------|-------|
| 2. Isolate and dry the tooth | Isolate the tooth, ideally with rubber dam, but otherwise with cotton wool rolls and/or absorbent pads. Use a saliva ejector. When treating a mandibular tooth, use a flanged saliva ejector (Figs 5.1a and 7.1). | For successful bonding of resin to enamel to occur, it is essential that the tooth is kept isolated from saliva. | Ideally, fissure sealing is done early, when teeth are only partially erupted; rubber dam application often is difficult in these cases. |
| | Dry the tooth surface with compressed air. | Water or saliva on the tooth surface would dilute the acid etchant. | It is essential to have an oil-free air line. |
| | With one hand, carefully maintain the position of saliva ejector, cotton wool rolls and/or absorbent pads until the treatment is completed. Do not attempt to isolate teeth in more than 1 quadrant at a time. | Close control is necessary because any movement of the tongue or cheeks may displace the saliva ejector, cotton rolls or absorbent pads. | Since this task immobilises one hand, it is essential to have assistance with the procedures that follow. |
| 3. Etch the enamel | Apply 30–50% phosphoric acid with a small cotton wool pledget or sponge pad, or with a small brush. | 30–50% phosphoric acid produces the optimum degree of etching to ensure good bonding of resin. | The etchant or 'conditioner' supplied with commercial products is phosphoric acid in the concentration range of 30–50%. Since these are strong acids, care must be taken to avoid dripping them on to the patient — the eyes are particularly at risk. |
| | Extend the area of etching beyond the fissures up to the tips of the cusps (Fig. 5.1b) (or to a radius of 3–4 mm around a pit). | Adequate extension of the etched area is essential to ensure that the margin of the sealant is placed on etched enamel | |
| | Keep the enamel wet with acid for 1 minute. | A 1-minute application produces an etching pattern that ensures a strong bond with resin. | A deciduous tooth requires a 2-minute, rather than a 1-minute, etch. |
| 4. Wash and dry the enamel surface | With an assistant holding the tip of a high-volume aspirator tube close to the tooth, wash the acid off with a stream of water directed at the etched surface for 15 seconds (Fig. 5.1c) Do not allow the patient to rinse. | Efficient aspiration is important; if the considerable volume of water that is used is not removed, the patient may be forced to swallow and, in so doing, may displace saliva on to the etched surface. | Aspiration also spares the patient the unpleasant taste of acid washed from the tooth. |
| | Holding the cheek away from the tooth, remove wet cotton wool rolls and replace with dry ones. | Inadequate washing, or contamination of the etched surface by saliva, prevents resin from bonding to enamel. | Essential requirements for strong bonding of resin to enamel are:- i) to etch enamel adequately ii) to wash and dry the etched surface thoroughly iii) to keep the etched surface absolutely free of any contaminants. If the etched surface does become contaminated, a further 1-minute etch is recommended. |
| | Dry the etched surface thoroughly with oil-free compressed air for 30 seconds. | Inadequate drying, or contamination by oil, also reduces the resin-enamel bond strength. | When the etched surface is dried it should appear 'chalky'. If it does not, it should be re-etched. |
| 5. Apply the resin | Apply the resin (mixed according to the manufacturer's instructions) with any convenient dental instrument (e.g. a small excavator), or with the applicator provided with the commercial product. | The manufacturer's instructions must be followed precisely to ensure a predictable setting time. | The type of applicator used is not important provided that the resin can be placed with precision. The outline of the sealant should resemble that of a Class I restoration |

| Procedure | Method | Rationale | Notes |
|---|---|---|---|
| | Place the resin at one end of the fissure (or pit) and encourage it to flow into and over the entire length of the fissure. Add further increments if required until the fissure is covered and the margin of the resin is about 2 mm up the incline planes of the cusps (Fig 5.1b); the margin must be within the periphery of the etched area. | Resin is retained principally on etched enamel of the cuspal incline planes. The margin must be firmly based on etched enamel to prevent marginal leakage. | The outline of the sealant is dictated by the morphology of the fissure (Fig. 5.1d).<br><br>Etched enamel remaining uncovered by resin soon remineralises because saliva is supersaturated with calcium salts. |
| 6. Allow the resin to polymerise | Maintain careful isolation for the polymerisation time recommended by the manufacturer or, if using a light-cured resin, apply the polymerisation light for the recommended time period. | | The time required to polymerise a light-sensitive resin varies according to the light source used, but any of the currently available visible light sources will polymerise any of the resins within 60 seconds (Stephen and Strang, 1985). |
| 7. Check the sealant | Pass a blunt probe gently over the surface of the resin to check that it covers the entire fissure. If any part of the fissure is not sealed, add further resin immediately and allow it to polymerise (this addition may only be made if isolation has been maintained and the surface is therefore uncontaminated).<br>Wipe away the thin, sticky surface film of unpolymerised resin with a cotton wood pledget. | Removal of the surface film is optional, but spares the patient its unpleasant taste. | |

**Fig. 5.1a**

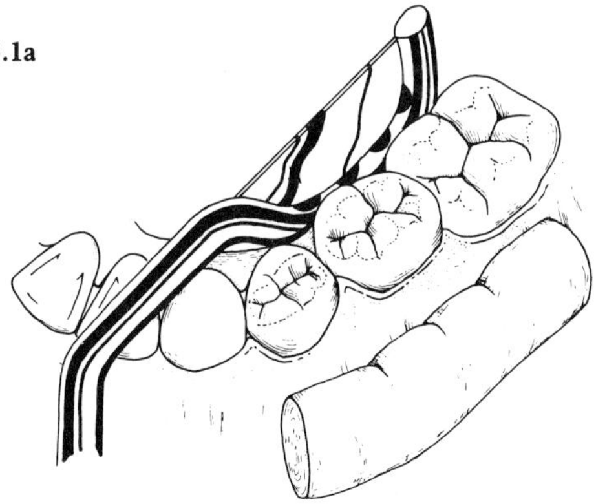

**Fig. 5.1c**

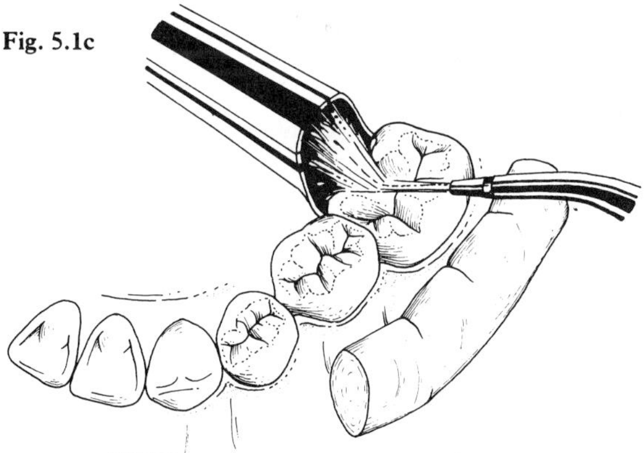

**Fig. 5.1b**

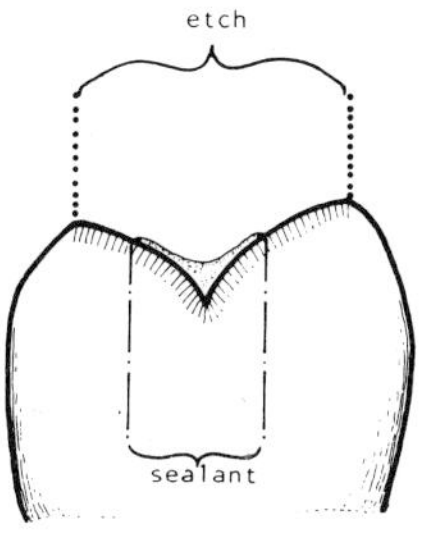

**Fig. 5.1d**

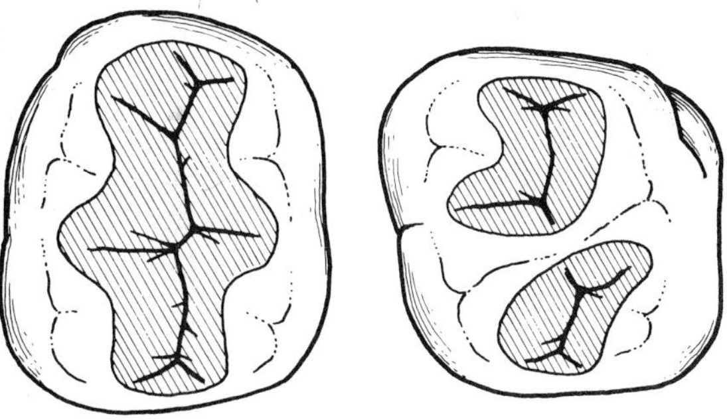

are, therefore, few clinical studies of their use, but those that have been conducted indicate that the retention of filled resins is comparable to that of unfilled resins (Stephen and Strang, 1985).

Clinical trials of pit and fissure sealants have been reviewed recently (Ripa, 1980; Gordon, 1983; Mertz-Fairhurst, 1984; Rock, 1984; Stephen and Strang, 1985). Although some trials have given disappointing results, the great majority have shown that sealants are well retained if applied correctly, and that they are highly effective in preventing dental caries.

In view of the high susceptibility to caries of the occlusal surfaces of first and second permanent molars, fissure sealing is the ideal preventive treatment for these teeth. Other surfaces that may be sealed are occlusal fissures of premolars and of primary molars, buccal grooves of mandibular molars, palatal grooves of maxillary molars, and palatal pits of maxillary incisors. Sealing is especially indicated for teeth that have marked pits or fissures, and for 'high-risk' patients (see p. 49). Teeth should be sealed as soon as possible after they erupt.

Sealing of all caries-susceptible pits and fissures in all patients may be considered to be ideal treatment. However, when financial constraints limit the use of sealants, priorities must be established. The highest priority may be given to sealing first permanent molars of children between the ages of 6 and 8 years, and second permanent molars of children between the ages of 11 and 13 years; a high priority may also be given to sealing premolars and primary molars in high-risk children (National Institutes of Health, 1984). Fissure sealing should always be done as part of comprehensive preventive treatment, which includes diet counselling, oral hygiene instruction and the use of fluorides.

Ideally, sealant is placed over pits and fissures that are diagnosed as caries-free. However, if sealant is inadvertently placed over a carious lesion, it is reassuring to know that the lesion probably will not progress; the evidence on this topic has been reviewed by Going (1984). If a small lesion is diagnosed, a preventive resin restoration may be placed (see p. 113).

## REFERENCES

Bowen R L 1963 Properties of a silica-reinforced polymer for dental restorations. Journal of the American Dental Association 66:57–64

Buonocore M G 1955 A simple method of increasing the adhesion of acrylic filling material to enamel. Journal of Dental Research 34:849–853

Going R E 1984 Sealant effect on incipient caries, enamel maturation, and future caries susceptibility. Journal of Dental Education 48:35–41

Gordon P H 1983 Fissure sealants. In: Murray J J (ed) The prevention of dental disease. Oxford University Press, Oxford, ch 5

Mertz-Fairhurst E J 1984 Current status of sealant retention and caries prevention. Journal of Dental Education 48:18–26

National Institutes of Health 1984 Consensus development conference statement on dental sealants in the prevention of tooth decay. Journal of the American Dental Association 108: 233–236

Ripa L W 1980 Occlusal sealants: rationale and review of clinical trials. International Dental Journal 30:127–139

Rock W P 1984 The effectiveness of fissure sealant resins. Journal of Dental Education 48:27–31

Silverstone L M 1974 Fissure sealants — laboratory studies. Caries Research 8:2–26

Stephen K W, Strang R 1985 Fissure sealants: a review. Community Dental Health 2:149–156

Ulvestad H 1976 Evaluation of fissure sealing with a diluted composite sealant and an uv-light polymerised sealant after 36 months' observation. Scandinavian Journal of Dental Research 84:401–403

## RECOMMENDED READING

Murray J J, Bennett T G 1985 A colour atlas of acid etch technique. Wolfe, London

Nikiforuk G 1985 Understanding dental caries: 2. Prevention: basic and clinical aspects. Karger, Basel, ch 7

Simonsen R J 1978 Clinical applications of the acid etch technique. Quintessence, Chicago, ch 2

# PART THREE

# Treatment of dental caries
# — operative methods

# 6

# Local analgesia

Equipment  
Infiltration  
Modified posterior superior alveolar nerve block  
Inferior dental nerve block  

Intraligamentary  
Intrapillary  
Jet injection

It is the dentist's responsibility not only to provide treatment but also to ensure that the patient remains comfortable and relaxed. The elimination of pain is essential, particularly with children; whereas adults may tolerate discomfort and remain cooperative, many children become frightened if they are hurt and will not cooperate further. Not only is the elimination of pain important to the patient: it also allows the dentist to proceed with treatment relaxed in the knowledge that the patient will not be hurt. Only when the dentist and patient are relaxed can treatment proceed smoothly and be performed efficiently.

Although most people dislike injections of any kind, the great majority accept local analgesia for dental treatment if it is introduced properly. The technique of administration to a child patient is crucially important. If done carefully the procedure can be painless and therefore acceptable; if done carelessly it may be so unpleasant and frightening that the child may refuse to accept it again, with serious consequences for future dental treatment.

Before introducing local analgesia, it is essential to be aware of the child's attitudes towards it; gathering this information is an important part of history-taking (Ch. 1). The child who has had previous experience of injections and whose attitudes are favourable, or the child with no previous experience but whose behaviour is cooperative, may be introduced to local analgesia at any time (although it is always preferable, especially in the latter case, not to introduce local analgesia at the first visit). On the other hand, the frightened child must be approached in a different way: the first objective must be to allay the child's fears. A series of three or four short introductory appoint-

ments may be arranged (Hill and O'Mullane, 1976), after which a decision is made either to proceed with the administration of local analgesia or, if the child remains apprehensive, to introduce some form of sedation or even general anaesthesia. If there is greater urgency to begin treatment, sedation or general anaesthesia may be introduced at an earlier stage. The important point is that the dentist must first know the child's attitudes towards local analgesia and then plan its introduction accordingly. An injection should be administered only to a cooperative child; to give it carelessly to a frightened child is bad practice: to force it on the child can only be condemned as barbaric.

Local analgesia is not always essential for conservative dentistry. Although pain thresholds vary greatly, the general statement may be made that local analgesia is desirable if sound dentine needs to be cut in cavity preparation. However, it is a strong clinical impression, albeit unsupported by scientific evidence, that primary teeth are less sensitive to cavity preparation than permanent teeth. Certainly, small occlusal cavities in primary teeth can often be prepared without local analgesia, as can some large cavities that need little further extension; on the other hand, it is almost always essential if cavity preparation involves considerable cutting of sound dentine.

Local analgesia presents a special problem with preschool children because they are, in general, less tolerant of pain and discomfort than older children. With care and skill a painless injection can be given, but the strange sensations of local analgesia cannot be avoided and these cause some children considerable anxiety. Reassurances and explanations may not be understood or may be inadequate to allay this anxiety. Therefore, for pre-school children it is often preferable, and justifiable, to attempt simple treatment first without local analgesia.

## EQUIPMENT

It is good practice to use an aspirating syringe routinely. A possible hazard with any injection is the penetration of a blood vessel and intravascular injection of solution, which might have toxic effects. Only by the use of an aspirating syringe can this hazard be eliminated. Although the risk of intravascular injection exists primarily when giving deep injections (e.g. inferior dental nerve block), and is minimal when giving infiltrations, the use of an aspirating syringe for all injections is recommended. After the needle is inserted, slight retraction of the plunger aspirates a small volume of fluid into the cartridge; if this fluid is blood, the needle must be repositioned before injecting.

The use of disposable needles avoids any risk of conveying infection from one patient to another.

'Short' needles are used for most injections; these are 2 cm or 2.5 cm in length. 'Long' needles (3.0 cm) are used for inferior dental nerve blocks. Fine needles (gauge 30) are recommended for infiltrations, and thicker (gauge 27) needles for all other injections.

The solution most commonly used is 2 per cent lignocaine with 1:80 000 adrenaline. Prilocaine (3 per cent) with felypressin (0.31 i.u./ml) is also commonly used and is the solution of choice when there are reasons for avoiding the injection of adrenaline.

## INFILTRATION

A solution deposited supraperiostally infiltrates through the alveolar bone to reach the root apex. Since alveolar bone in children is more permeable that it is in adults, less local analgesic solution suffices to produce analgesia of primary teeth, and analgesia of mandibular primary molars may usually be achieved by infiltration in children up to the age of about 5 years.

## Technique: maxillary infiltration

| Procedure | Method | Rationale | Notes |
|---|---|---|---|
| 1. Organise equipment and materials | Have all the necessary equipment and materials ready for use *before* the patient enters the surgery. | For a successful technique it is important to be able to proceed smoothly from start to finish, without interruptions to prepare equipment. | |
| | Place these on a clean surface *behind* the dental chair; it is especially important to keep the syringe out of sight. | The sight of a needle causes some anxiety to most patients (adults as well as children). | |
| 2. Establish a good operating position | Adjust the chair and headrest position so that the child's line of vision is at least 45° from the horizontal. | Control of the child's field of vision is important so that the syringe will not be seen by the child. | |
| | Sit or stand in *front* of and facing the child (8 o'clock position). Adjust the height of the chair to allow the injection site to be seen easily and comfortably. | Correct positioning of the dentist is important to provide optimal access and visibility. | Some dentists prefer to work from behind the patient (11 o'clock position) when injecting on the left side. |

| Procedure | Method | Rationale | Notes |
|-----------|--------|-----------|-------|
| 3. Inform the child | Tell the child, clearly but casually, that to 'clean decay' from his tooth it is best to 'make the tooth go to sleep'. Stress that *he* will not go to sleep, only the tooth, and that it will 'wake up' later. | Lengthy, detailed explanations are unnecessary and may arouse anxiety in the child. Proper selection of words is imperative. Avoid the use of 'needle', 'injection', 'prick', 'hurt', unless the child mentions them. 'Make it go to sleep' is better than 'put to sleep' — the latter may have unpleasant connotations in relation to pets or farm animals. | The precise method of informing the child will be influenced by the child's age and stage of psychological development, and also by his attitudes to previous injections, evident from the dental history. |
| 4. Apply topical analgesic | Show the child a cotton roll on one end of which has been placed topical analgesic cream solution, and let him smell its 'fruity' smell. Tell him that this will start to make his tooth go to sleep. | The use of topical analgesics, while not essential, increases the chance of giving a completely painless injection, and is therefore strongly recommended. Suggestions of generally-acceptable fruity smells reduces the risk of objections to their taste. | If topical analgesic cream is used, care should be taken not to place too much on the end of the cotton roll, because it can be squeezed out when applied to the tissues, and run back into the throat. To minimise this problem, one end of the cotton roll may be pulled out, so forming a cupshaped depression at the other end in which the cream is better localised when placed against the tissues. |
| | After checking that the child's seating and head positions are correct, retract the cheek with the left hand and dry the tissue at the muco-buccal fold above the tooth to be treated, using the dry end of the cotton roll. Then turn the roll around and hold the topical analgesic against the tissue for 2 minutes; distract the child during this period. Maintain the child's head position during this period (and indeed until the end of the injection procedure) by continuing to hold the cheek with the left hand. | The surface analgesic will be most effective if applied to dry tissue, and allowed to act for at least 2 minutes. | Some dentists prefer to apply topical analgesic on a cotton pledget held in tweezers, especially for posterior teeth when access for cotton rolls is difficult. Jet injection also produces excellent topical analgesia. |
| 5. Prepare to give the injection | While still maintaining control of the child's head position with the left hand, remove the cotton roll after 2 minutes and receive the syringe from an assistant in the right hand. If the injection is to be given in the maxillary *left* quadrant, receive the syringe over the child's left shoulder. If the injection is for a maxillary *right* tooth, the assistant should pass the syringe from behind the patient, over his right shoulder. The assistant should first carefully place the syringe in the dentist's hand, so that it can be used immediately, and then remove the needle guard. | Maintenance of the correct line of vision is essential at this stage. It should not be necessary to hide the syringe — good technique ensures that it is not displayed. Receiving the syringe in this manner avoids passing it in front of the patient. Unnecessary movement and noise in transferring the syringe to the dentist might attract the child's attention. The dentist should not need to change his grip on the syringe before using it. | If the child becomes anxious at this stage and cannot be quickly reassured, it is usually better to return the syringe to the assistant, release control of the child's head and attempt, through further explanation, to obtain the child's consent to proceed. Forcing an injection on an unwilling child may succeed in obtaining analgesia but can only damage the good relationship on which further cooperation rests. If consent is not obtained quickly, it may be preferable to proceed without analgesia or to consider introducing some form of sedation. |

(continued overleaf)

| Procedure | Method | Rationale | Notes |
|---|---|---|---|
| 6. Give the injection | With the left hand, pull the cheek outwards so that the mucous membrane is made taut (Fig. 6.1a). Position the tip of the needle at the muco-buccal fold just above the tooth to be treated, supporting the syringe against the left hand, which is stabilised by resting free fingers on the patient's face. | A needle penetrates taut tissue more easily.<br><br>Supporting the syringe against a stable left hand gives better control in positioning and directing the needle. | When producing analgesia of first permanent molars, infiltrations are given mesial and distal to the tooth (i.e. over the 2nd molar and 2nd premolar), because the dense zygomatic arch lies over the 1st molar root apex. Alternatively, a Maxillary Molar Nerve Block may be given (p. 67). |
|  | Gently insert the tip of the needle into the tissue, or draw the taut tissue over the needle (Fig. 6.1b). Immediately inject a few drops of solution, pause for a few seconds, then advance the needle carefully about 1 cm, 45° to the long axis of the tooth, to bring its tip close to the root apex. | A few drops of solution quickly produces analgesia of the soft tissue, thus reducing or eliminating pain during further penetration of the needle. |  |
|  | Inject slowly. | Fast injection invariably causes pain. |  |
|  | For primary teeth in children under about 6 years of age, about 1 ml of solution is sufficient. In older children, use a full cartridge. | The buccal plate of bone is more permeable in young children. |  |
|  | Take about 30 seconds to give the injection. While injecting, casually inform the child that as the tooth 'goes to sleep' it will 'feel funny', and reassure him that it will 'wake up later'. | The child's anxiety may be aroused by strange sensations that have not been explained. |  |
| 7. Withdraw the syringe and give post-operative instructions | When the solution has been injected, withdraw the needle but continue to maintain the child's head position with the left hand until the syringe has been passed to the assistant, *below* the child's field of vision, and the needle guard replaced on it. | A successful technique may be spoilt by careless manipulation of the syringe at this stage. |  |
|  | Ask the child to rinse. | Rinsing is not necessary, but by doing so the child's attention is distracted while the analgesic is taking effect, and the freedom of movement may be appreciated following the previous few minutes' restriction. |  |
|  | Warn the child (and parent) about the danger of cheek or lip biting. Reinforce the child's good behaviour. | A child may 'play' with an insensitive cheek or lip by biting it, sometimes causing severe trauma. |  |

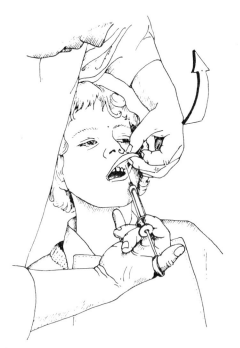 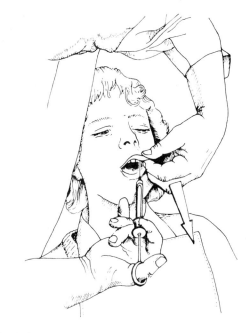

**Fig. 6.1a**                    **Fig. 6.1b**

## Technique: mandibular infiltration

| Procedure | Method | Rationale | Notes |
|-----------|--------|-----------|-------|
| 1. Organise equipment and materials | | | |
| 2. Establish a good operating position | See 'maxillary infiltration' | | |
| 3. Inform the child | | | |
| 4. Apply topical analgesic | | | |
| 5. Prepare to give the injection | For left or right mandibular infiltrations, receive the syringe from an assistant in the same way as for left or right maxillary infiltrations. | | |
| 6. Give the injection | With the left hand, pull the cheek outwards so that the mucous membrane is made taut. | | |

(continued overleaf)

| Procedure | Method | Rationale | Notes |
|---|---|---|---|
| | Holding the syringe in a horizontal position, take it carefully to the patient's mouth (Fig. 6.2). Position the tip of the needle at the muco-buccal fold just below the tooth to be treated. Proceed as outlined under 'maxillary infiltration' *except* that the syringe should be kept approximately parallel to the occlusal plane rather than being brought in line with the long axis of the tooth. | The child is least likely to see the syringe if it is kept horizontal. To give the injection in the same way as a maxillary infiltration, with the syringe 45° to the long axis of the tooth, would necessitate raising the syringe into the patient's line of vision; this is unnecessary. | |
| 7. Withdraw the syringe and give post-operative instructions | See 'maxillary infiltration' | | |

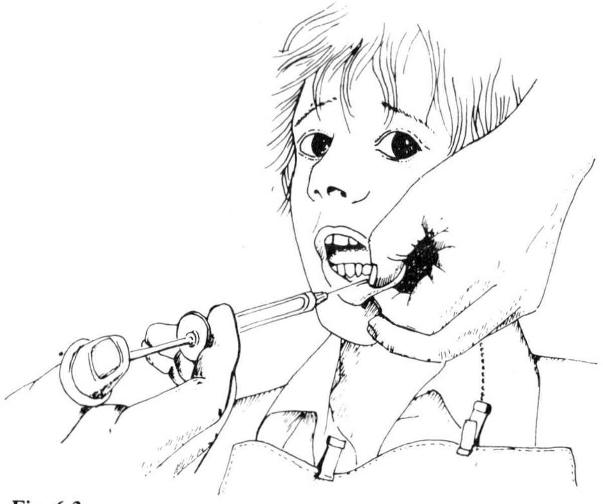

**Fig. 6.2**

## MODIFIED POSTERIOR SUPERIOR ALVEOLAR NERVE BLOCK (MAXILLARY MOLAR NERVE BLOCK)

It is sometimes difficult to achieve analgesia of maxillary first molars by infiltration because solution does not easily penetrate the dense zygomatic bone over the first molar roots. Moreover, attempts to give a supraperiosteal injection in that region often cause pain because the needle contacts the prominent zygomatic process. These problems may be overcome by giving the infiltration distal to the zygomatic process, that is, over the second molar; but an additional injection may be required over the second premolar (or second primary molar) because the mesio-buccal root of the maxillary first molar is sometimes innervated by the middle or anterior superior alveolar nerve.

An alternative approach is to block the main trunk of the posterior superior alveolar nerve. However, the conventional technique for the posterior superior alveolar nerve block requires a deep injection into a region containing a venous plexus, and therefore carries the danger of intra-vascular injection and of causing a haematoma; these dangers can be avoided by using the maxillary molar nerve block (Adatia, 1976).

## INFERIOR DENTAL NERVE BLOCK

The inferior dental nerve block is used to produce analgesia of mandibular teeth. However, for restorative dentistry, satisfactory analgesia of mandibular anterior teeth and, in young children, of mandibular primary molars, can usually be produced by infiltration, thus avoiding the need for the potentially more unpleasant block injection.

## Technique: maxillary molar nerve block (modified posterior superior alveolar nerve block)

| Procedure | Method | Rationale |
|---|---|---|
| 1. Organise equipment and materials | | |
| 2. Establish a good operating position | See 'maxillary infiltration' | |
| 3. Inform the child | | |
| 4. Locate anatomical landmarks | Palpate the zygomatic process and note its relationship to the teeth. Note the position of the distal root of the second molar (in a young child estimate this position).<br>Pass the finger posteriorly along the muco-buccal fold towards the maxillary tuberosity. | The injection will be given in line with the distal root of the second molar. |
| 5. Apply topical analgesic | | |
| 6. Prepare to give the injection | See 'maxillary infiltration' | |
| 7. Give the injection | If injecting on the right side, retract the cheek with the left index or middle finger. If injecting on the left side, retract with the left thumb.<br>Place the tip of the finger or thumb on the tuberosity.<br>Insert the needle between the tip of the retracting finger and the distal surface of the zygomatic process, in line with the distal root of the second molar (Fig. 6.3). Inject a few drops of solution. | A few drops of solution produces analgesia of soft tissue, thus reducing or eliminating pain during further penetration of the needle. |
| | Advance the needle upwards and backwards about 1.5 cm, towards the alveolar bone. | Penetrating about 1.5 cm takes the tip of the needle into the space above the attachment of the buccinator muscle. |
| | Aspirate and, if no blood is aspirated, slowly inject 1.5–2 ml of solution. | Injection of solution into a blood vessel may cause toxic reactions or may result in poor analgesia. |
| | While injecting, apply pressure to the alveolar mucosa with the finger or thumb; as solution accumulates it causes a bulge in the tissues anterior to the finger. | Finger pressure localises the solution, which facilitates the next step in the procedure. |
| 8. Withdraw the syringe and massage the solution towards the posterior superior alveolar foramen | Withdraw the syringe as described previously (p. 64).<br>Place a finger over the bulge at the injection site, ask the patient to close the mouth a little, and push the solution upwards, backwards and inwards towards the posterior superior alveolar foramen. | This method avoids the risk of causing a haematoma, which exists when a conventional posterior superior alveolar nerve block is given. |

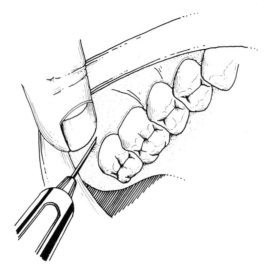

**Fig. 6.3**

## Technique: inferior dental nerve block

| Procedure | Method | Rationale | Notes |
|---|---|---|---|
| 1. Organise equipment and materials | See 'maxillary infiltration' | | Ideally, an inferior dental block should be given to a child who previously has accepted a simple infiltration injection. Even with an excellent technique, a block injection possibly may be painful. Together with the unpleasant numbness of face and tongue, this might cause a child to refuse any type of injection in the future, with far-reaching consequences to his dental treatment. |
| 2. Inform the child | | | |
| 3. Establish a good operating position | Adjust the chair and headrest so that the child's line of vision is about 45° to the horizontal. | Although when giving an inferior dental block it is more difficult to keep the syringe out of the patient's line of vision than when giving a maxillary infiltration, it is helpful to recline the patient to some extent. | |
| | If treating the mandibular *left* quadrant, sit or stand either behind the patient (11 o'clock position) or facing the patient (8 o'clock position). If treating the mandibular *right* quadrant, sit or stand facing the patient (8 o'clock position). Adjust the chair height to permit a comfortable view of the injection site. | Access to the injection site is obtained equally well from either position. | |

| Procedure | Method | Rationale | Notes |
|---|---|---|---|
| 4. Locate the anatomical landmarks | Palpate the internal oblique ridge of the anterior border of the ramus, and note the pterygomandibular raphe and pterygomandibular triangle. The injection site is within the pterygomandibular triangle level with the occlusal surfaces of the molar teeth. | | |
| 5. Apply topical analgesic | Introduce the topical analgesic to the child as suggested under 'maxillary infiltration'. Ask the child to open his mouth wide, dry the injection site and apply the analgesic agent with a cotton roll or with a pledget held in tweezers. Attempt to keep the analgesic in place for 2 minutes without saliva contamination. If this is not practicable, prepare to give the injection sooner. | Effective surface analgesia is not usually produced in less than 2 minutes. | Some dentists omit the use of topical analgesic when giving an inferior dental nerve block because it often becomes quickly diluted and washed away by saliva, and patients may react to its unpleasant taste. Jet injection is very effective. |
| 6. Prepare to give the injection | LEFT QUADRANT<br>If positioned behind the patient, place the index or middle finger of the left hand on the internal oblique ridge at the level of the occlusal surfaces of the molar teeth, and support the mandible by placing the thumb on the posterior border of the ramus.<br>If facing the patient, place the thumb on the internal oblique ridge and support the mandible posteriorly with the index finger. Receive the syringe from an assistant over the patient's left shoulder.<br><br>RIGHT QUADRANT<br>Place the thumb of the left hand on the internal oblique ridge and support the mandible posteriorly with the index finger.<br>The assistant should pass the syringe behind the patient and hand it to the dentist under his left arm, over the patient's right shoulder.<br>　As in the infiltration technique, the transfer of syringe should be done quietly and efficiently. | The position of the index finger or thumb is an important guide to the injection site (see below).<br><br>Receiving the syringe as described avoids passing it within the patient's line of vision. | |

(continued overleaf)

| Procedure | Method | Rationale | Notes |
|---|---|---|---|
| 7. Give the injection | INDIRECT TECHNIQUE<br>Ask the patient to help by keeping his mouth open as wide as possible. Direct the needle towards the injection site, holding the syringe parallel to the occlusal plane and in line with the premolar and molar teeth. Insert the needle just medial to the thumb or index finger positioned on the internal oblique ridge, at the level of the occlusal surfaces of the molar teeth (Fig. 6.4a).<br>Immediately on penetrating the tissue (a few millimetres only), inject a few drops of solution. Slowly advance the needle about 1.5 cm, then, keeping the tip of the needle in the same position, swing the syringe across the midline of the mouth, to lie over the opposite first primary molar (or first premolar) region (Fig. 6.4b).<br>Then advance the needle *gently* for about another 1 cm when it should contact bone.<br>If bone is not contacted, do not insert the needle down to the hub of the syringe. Instead, withdraw it partly or completely, and reposition.<br>When bone is contacted, aspirate; if blood is aspirated, withdraw the needle slightly and reposition. | | The use of the indirect or direct technique is dictated by the dentist's personal preference. |
| | | A few drops of solution quickly produces analgesia of soft tissue, thus reducing pain during further penetration of the needle. | Some dentists inject small increments while advancing the needle gradually, thus moving the needle behind injected solution. |
| | | Contacting bone with any force causes pain. | |
| | | Inserting the needle to the hub of the syringe is bad practice because should the needle break it would be difficult to recover. | Breakage of a needle is, fortunately, a very rare occurrence. |
| | | Aspiration of blood indicates that the needle has penetrated a blood vessel. | |
| | If no blood is aspirated, inject about ¾ of the cartridge *slowly*, over a period of about 30 seconds. Then withdraw the syringe slowly. If analgesia of lingual soft tissues is required, inject the remainder of the cartridge after withdrawing the syringe about half way.<br>Inform and reassure the child about the 'funny feeling' he will soon note.<br><br>DIRECT TECHNIQUE<br>The technique is the same as the indirect technique except that the needle is directed towards the injection site while holding the syringe over the first primary molar (or first premolar) region of the opposite side of the mandible. | Fast injection is painful. | |
| 8. Withdraw the syringe and give post-operative instructions | See 'maxillary infiltration' | | |

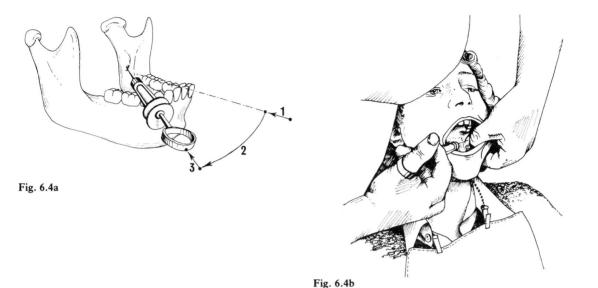

Fig. 6.4a

Fig. 6.4b

## INTRALIGAMENTARY INJECTION

The intraligamentary injection is given into the periodontal ligament. This injection has become more popular in recent years following the introduction of syringes specially designed for the purpose (Fig. 6.5a). Intraligamentary injections can be given with a conventional needle and syringe, but the special syringes are preferred because they more easily produce the pressure that is required to inject into the periodontal ligament. As a safety feature, the barrel of the special syringe completely encloses the anaesthetic cartridge, in case the pressure should cause the glass to break.

A short or ultra-short 30 gauge needle is usually used, and the syringes accept standard 1.8 or 2.2 ml cartridges of anaesthetic solution. To minimise the risk of tissue damage due to vasoconstriction, it is recommended that solutions containing adrenaline are not used (Brännström et al, 1982), because the pressure under which the solution is injected itself produces vasoconstriction in the periodontal ligament. One complete pull of the trigger delivers 0.2 ml of solution.

### Technique

1. Remove any calculus from the injection site,

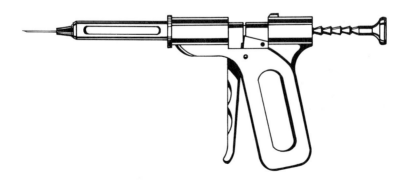

Fig. 6.5a

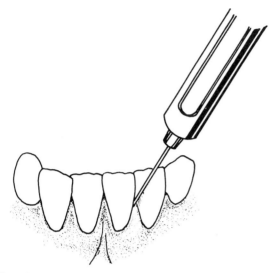

**Fig. 6.5b**

clean the gingival crevice with a rubber cup and prophylaxis paste, and apply hibitane or other disinfectant with a small cotton wool pledget. A surface anaesthetic paste or solution may be used instead of disinfectant solution, but the effectiveness of surface anaesthesia in this technique is uncertain.

2. Introduce the needle into the gingival crevice down the mesial or distal surface of the tooth, with the bevel of the needle facing away from the tooth (Fig. 6.5b).

3. Squeeze a few drops of solution into the gingival crevice to anaesthetise tissues ahead of the needle.

4. Move the needle apically until it becomes wedged between the tooth and the alveolar crest — usually about 2 mm.

5. Squeeze the trigger slowly. If the needle is correctly placed there should be definite resistance to injection and the tissues around the needle should blanch. If resistance is not felt the needle is probably incorrectly place, and injected solution will flow into the mouth.

If a conventional syringe is being used, support the needle with fingers of the free hand before and during the injection.

6. Inject slowly. The injection of 0.2 ml should take at least 20 seconds.

7. For a posterior tooth, give an injection around each root.

8. Injections on the mesial and distal sides of a root may be given, but it is recommended that not more than 0.4 ml of solution is injected per root.

9. Despite the small volume of solution used, the cartridge must be discarded — it must not be used for another patient.

The intraligamentary injection has several advantages over conventional methods. It is usually considered to be less uncomfortable than either an inferior dental block injection, or a palatal injection, or a buccal infiltration in the premaxilla; analgesia is obtained very quickly and surrounding soft tissues are less affected. Since analgesia of mandibular teeth can be obtained, it is a useful injection when an inferior dental block injection must be avoided (e.g. for patients with bleeding disorders) or when a patient finds the block injection unacceptable.

The intraligamentary injection may be given to produce analgesia for restorative dentistry or for tooth extraction. However, after-pain has sometimes been reported following its use for restorative treatment. This pain is usually minor and subsides within a day or two, but can nevertheless be distressing to the patient.

Histological studies have shown that tissue damage caused by the pressure of injection is minor and resolves within a few weeks (Brännström et al, 1982). Concern has been expressed about the possibility of forcing infected material from the gingival crevice into the periodontal tissues and (when the injection is given around a deciduous tooth) of the pressure damaging the developing permanent tooth, but there is no published evidence that these undesirable effects have actually occurred. However, because of these possible hazards and because of the lack of scientific knowledge concerning the mode of action of the injection, the American Dental Association has recommended that the injection should be used only to supplement conventional methods when the latter fail, or in circumstances when an inferior dental block is impracticable or to be avoided (American Dental Association, 1983).

## INTRAPAPILLARY

The intrapapillary injection may be given to produce analgesia of palatal or lingual tissues, to avoid the need for the more painful injections directly into palatal or lingual tissues.

1. Give a submucosal injection buccally.
2. After about 1 minute, when soft tissue analgesia will have been obtained, inject into the interdental papilla mesial and distal to the tooth to be treated.
3. Pass the needle horizontally through the papilla from buccal to lingual.
4. Inject a small volume of solution.

## JET INJECTION

It is possible to inject local analgesic solution into oral tissues without using a hypodermic needle, by using an instrument that propels solution at high velocity through a fine orifice. Such instruments were first used to inject through skin, and later became available for oral use.

Early jet injection instruments were investigated by Stephens and Kramer (1964) and by Whitehead and Young (1968). A more satisfactory instrument currently available is the 'Syrijet' (Mizzy Inc., New York) (Fig. 6.6); this incorporates a compressible spring which generates a pressure of 2000 pounds per square inch when released, injecting solution through mucous membrane and into bone to a depth of about 1 cm. The instrument accepts standard 1.8 ml cartridges, and is calibrated to deliver volumes of between 0.05 and 0.2 ml.

Jet injection may be used not only to provide excellent soft tissue analgesia prior to hypodermic injection but also to produce analgesia for dental procedures for which infiltrations are normally used. Blocks of the greater palatine, nasopalatine, long buccal and mental nerves also may be achieved,

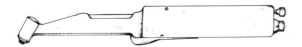

**Fig. 6.6** The 'Syrijet'.

but not of the inferior dental, posterior superior alveolar or incisive nerves (Bennett and Monheim, 1971).

Jet injection is particularly useful for producing soft tissue analgesia before those hypodermic injections that normally tend to be painful even after application of topical analgesic, for example, inferior dental nerve block, infiltration in the maxillary incisor region, and palatal injections. It is also useful for producing analgesia for extraction of loose primary teeth, minor oral surgery, and the application of rubber dam clamps. Despite its useful applications in paedodontics, jet injection is not widely used; no doubt the cost of the instrument is a factor limiting its use.

### Technique

1. Explain to the child that a 'spray' is to be used 'to make the gum (or tooth) go to sleep', and demonstrate by spraying a small volume into the air.
2. Clean the injection site with antiseptic solution and then dry with cotton wool or gauze.
3. Fit the detachable rubber sleeve, which is provided, over the nozzle of the instrument (except for palatal injections, when the rubber sleeve is not used).
4. Cock the spring mechanism.
5. Set the dosage.
   For analgesia of teeth: 0.1 ml for maxillary anterior teeth and premolars. 0.15 ml for mandibular incisors. For analgesia of soft tissues (prior to hypodermic injection): 0.05 ml.
6. Grasp the instrument firmly, with the base of the index finger under the trigger.
7. Place the nozzle of the instrument at the injection site.
   For analgesia of teeth: direct the long axis of the nozzle at right angles to the underlying bone, on attached gingiva near the root apex (Fig. 6.7). For soft tissue analgesia: direct the long axis of the nozzle in the direction of the proposed needle insertion. The risk of causing slight trauma to the mucosa is greater when injecting into loose tissue than when injecting into attached gingiva, but is minimal if the

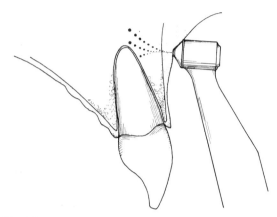

**Fig. 6.7**

volume injected is not more than 0.05 ml.
Keep the tip of the nozzle in gentle contact
with the tissue; do not exert pressure.

8. Warn the child that he may 'feel the spray a
   little'.
9. Hold the instrument immobile while squeez-
   ing the trigger. If it is moved the jet may
   traumatise the mucosa; although this is slight

and quickly resolves, it should be avoided if
possible.
10. If analgesia of a tooth is found to be inad-
    equate during cavity preparation, give a second
    jet injection or a hypodermic injection. Soft
    tissue analgesia is almost instantaneous; hy-
    podermic injection may follow immediately.

Unlike some previous jet injection instruments,
the 'Syrijet', when fired, is quiet and has little
perceptible recoil. However, it is inevitable that
patients should feel something at the moment of
injection; this may be described as a 'tap' or a
'bump', or sometimes as pain. Therefore, jet injection offers no advantage when a painless hypodermic injection can be given (for example, to
produce analgesia of maxillary premolars), except
with a patient who has a phobia of needles. However, when using jet injection prior to potentially
painful hypodermic injections, it may be anticipated that the minor discomfort caused by the jet
injection, followed by a painless hypodermic injection, will be accepted better than the hypodermic
injection alone.

## REFERENCES

Adatia A K 1976 Regional nerve block for maxillary permanent
  molars. British Dental Journal 140:87–92
American Dental Association 1983 Status report: the
  periodontal ligament injection. Journal of the American
  Dental Association 106:224–224
Bennett C R, Monheim L M 1971 Production of local
  anaesthesia by jet injection. Oral Surgery, Oral Medicine,
  Oral Pathology 32:526–530
Brännström M, Nordenvall KJ, Hedström G 1982 Periodontal
  tissue changes after intraligamentary anesthesia. Journal of
  Dentistry for Children 49:417–423
Hill F J, O'Mullane D M 1976 Preventive programme for the
  dental management of frightened children. Journal of
  Dentistry for Children 43:30–36
Stephens R R, Kramer I R H 1964 Intra-oral injections by high
  pressure jet. British Dental Journal 117:465–481

Whitehead F I H, Young I 1968 An intra-oral jet injection
  instrument. British Dental Journal 125:437–440


## RECOMMENDED READING

Bennett C R 1984 Monheim's local anesthesia and pain control
  in dental practice, 7th edn. Mosby, St. Louis
Howe G L, Whitehead F I H 1981 Local anaesthesia in
  dentistry, 2nd edn. Wright, Bristol
Mink J R, Spedding R H 1966 An injection procedure for the
  child dental patient. Dental Clinics of North America (July)
  309–325
Roberts D H, Sowray J H 1979 Local analgesia in dentistry,
  2nd edn. Wright, Bristol

# 7

# Isolation of teeth

Saliva ejectors
Cotton wool rolls
Absorbent pads
Rubber dam

A prerequisite for successful restorative dentistry is that the teeth under treatment be adequately isolated from the cheeks, tongue and saliva. Isolation from the cheeks and tongue is necessary to permit good access to, and a clear view of, the teeth; isolation from saliva is important because moisture affects the setting reactions and the physical properties of amalgam and other restorative materials, and reduces the adhesion of lining materials to dentine. In addition, contamination by salivary bacteria must be avoided when pulp treatment is being performed.

## SALIVA EJECTORS

Common types of saliva ejectors are illustrated in Figure 7.1. To ensure maximum patient comfort it is sensible to select the smallest saliva ejector that will suffice. For example, for treatment of a maxillary tooth, a flange-type ejector is not required and a simple tube ejector may be used; for treatment of a mandibular tooth of a preschool child, the small rather than the large coil ejector should be selected.

The suction sources to which saliva ejectors are connected provide either low-volume or high-volume suction. Many dental units provide only low-volume suction and special units are then required for high-volume suction. Low-volume suction is adequate for patients with average saliva flow when a slow-speed handpiece is used without water coolant. However, for patients who salivate profusely, or when high-speed cutting instruments are used with water coolant, connection to a high-volume suction source is essential, especially if the patient is supine. When high-volume suction is

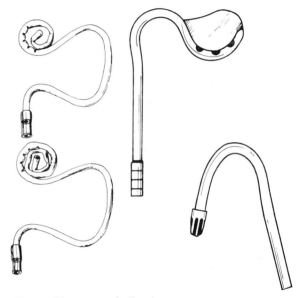

**Fig. 7.1** Three types of saliva ejectors.

used, the saliva ejector may be supplemented or replaced by a suction tube; if an assistant holds its tip close to the tooth under treatment, efficient evacuation of water and saliva is possible. Suction tubes are available in various diameters, and some incorporate a mirror head to combine the functions of mouth mirror and suction device.

## COTTON WOOL ROLLS

Cotton wool rolls of various diameters are available, the smaller sizes being particularly useful for young children. Long cotton rolls are also available that can be placed either buccal and lingual to mandibular teeth, or buccal to both maxillary and mandibular teeth. One type has a flexible central core that maintains the shape of the roll after it has been bent.

## ABSORBENT PADS

Thin absorbent pads are available that may be used instead of, or in addition to, cotton wool rolls (Fig. 7.2). Usually they are used in the buccal sulcus, but they may also be placed lingually. They are particularly effective when treating maxillary molar teeth.

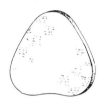 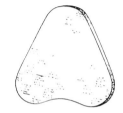

**Fig. 7.2** Absorbent pads.

The edges of the pads are sometimes rather rough; therefore they should be checked before use and trimmed with scissors if necessary. The pad must be placed properly, with its apex high in the sulcus posterior to the tooth to be treated. Since, when dry, it adheres to mucosa, it must be placed directly into the correct position; bending it slightly, so that it is convex on the cheek side, helps in placing it. When treatment is complete the pad must be moistened so that its removal does not damage the mucosa.

## RUBBER DAM

The ideal method of isolating teeth is by the use of rubber dam. In the U.K. rubber dam is rarely used except to isolate teeth for endodontic treatment; in some other countries (for example, the U.S.A.) it is widely used in routine restorative dentistry.

Those who do not use rubber dam claim that it is awkward and time-consuming to place, that patients do not like it and that it is unnecessary. On the other hand, those who use it regularly claim that it is easy and quick to place, that patients accept it happily (assuming that they

accept other dental procedures) and that, although not essential, its use is a great help in performing most restorative procedures (Elderton, 1971; Curzon and Barenie, 1973; Reuter, 1983).

The principal advantages of using rubber dam are (a) that it greatly improves visibility of posterior teeth by isolating them from the cheeks and tongue (this advantage is, of course, minimal in the front of the mouth where visibility is always good); (b) that it provides a dry operating field by isolating the teeth from saliva, and (c) that it protects the patient from the risk of swallowing or inhaling instruments or materials that may be inadvertently dropped into the mouth. In addition, many patients appreciate the fact that tooth debris, water, dental materials and instruments are all excluded from their mouths. Rubber dam provides ideal working conditions which help the dentist to carry out treatment more efficiently and more safely.

### Isolation of posterior teeth with rubber dam

Various techniques may be used to apply rubber dam to posterior teeth. The techniques described are those that the authors have found most satisfactory.

*Clamps:* The large variety of clamps available

**Table 7.1** Recommended rubber dam clamps

|  | New range[+] | Clamp numbers[++] |
|---|---|---|
| *First choices* |  |  |
| For permanent molars |  |  |
| partially erupted | AW* | 14 |
| fully erupted | BW | 27A, UW4 |
| For permanent incisors or canines | C | 6, 9 |
| For second primary molars | DW | 27 |
| For premolars | E, EW |  |
| *Alternatives* |  |  |
| For partially erupted permanent molars | FW | 14A |
| For premolars | G, GW | 1 |
| For partially erupted permanent molars | H | 14LH |
| For large permanent molars | JW K | UW5, 26 |

[+] Ash Instruments, Dentsply
[++] Clamp numbers given in 1st edition of this book
* 'W' denotes a wingless clamp

and the wide range of numbers by which they are identified often cause confusion. In an attempt to simplify the selection of clamps, a new set has recently been introduced which are identified by letters ranging from A to K (Ash Instruments, Dentsply). The recommended clamps are listed in Table 7.1.

*Rubber dam frame*    : Young
*Rubber dam punch*    : Ainsworth
*Clamp forceps*    : Stokes

*Wedges and floss*
*Rubber dam material*    : Squares 6 × 6 in or 5 × 5 in. 'Heavy' or 'extra heavy' thickness.

## Technique: rubber dam application

| Procedure | Method | Rationale | Notes |
|---|---|---|---|
| 1. Prepare the dam | Mark a horizontal line across the middle of the dam and mark the line about 5 cm from the right border. Punch holes (the largest hole on the punch) about 5 mm apart (Fig. 7.3a). METHOD 1 — Slit dam. With scissors, join holes 1, 2 and 3. The prepared dam now has a slit and a hole (Fig. 7.3b). METHOD 2 — Separate holes. Punch a hole overlapping hole 1, to produce a larger hole. The prepared dam now has 1 large hole and three smaller ones (Fig. 7.3c). | Enlarging the hole makes it easier to pass the dam over the clamp at stage 8. | Methods 1 and 2 both provide excellent isolation of teeth from cheeks and tongue. Saliva control is less efficient with Method 1, but this is compensated by the easier application of the slit dam over the clamp (at stage 8), and by the absence of rubber interdentally when preparing deep Class II cavities. In addition, the slit technique is useful when preparing a tooth for a crown. Since dams prepared as described can be used in any quadrant, chairside time can be saved if some are always available. Use of a polythene or thin cardboard template ensures that all dams are the same. Some dentists claim that the matt side of the dam is more comfortable to the patient than the shiny side. A dam prepared as described, with shiny side up, would then only be used on lower left and upper right quadrants. |
| | METHOD 3 — 1 hole only. Punch one hole only and enlarge it by overlapping with a second hole. | | Method 3 is sometimes suitable when only the clamped tooth is to be treated (see stage 3 below). |
| 2. Attach the dam to the frame. | Place the dam on a flat surface and position it according to the quadrant to be worked on (e.g. as in Fig. 7.3b for the lower left quadrant). Place the frame over the dam, with its transverse part towards the lower edge of the dam and with its convexity upwards (Fig. 7.3d). Attach the dam to the pegs at the corners of the frame (not to the other pegs). Do not stretch the dam tight between the pegs; keep it as loose as possible. | Attaching the dam loosely at this stage allows it to be stretched easily into the mouth when applying it at stage 8. | |

| Procedure | Method | Rationale | Notes |
|---|---|---|---|
| 3. Decide which tooth to clamp. | Clamp second primary molars or first permanent molars only (premolars or second molars may be chosen in older patients). The decision on which tooth to clamp depends on the treatment to be done: | The morphology of second primary molars and first permanent molars enables clamps to be applied easily and securely. | |
| | *restoration*    *tooth to clamp*<br>occlusal    second primary<br>   first or      molar<br>   second<br>   primary<br>   molar | | |
| | Class II    second primary<br>   first primary    molar<br>   molar | For Class II restorations it is preferable to clamp the tooth distal to the one being restored, as the clamp interferes with the placement of most types of matrix band. | |
| | Class II    first permanent<br>   second      molar<br>   primary<br>   molar | | |
| | occlusal    first permanent<br>   first       molar<br>   permanent<br>   molar | | |
| | Class II    first permanent<br>   first       molar<br>   permanent<br>   molar | | |
| 4. Select a clamp. | Recommended first choice clamps are given in Table 7.1 | | |
| 5. Introduce to the child. | Explain that the dam is 'a sort of raincoat'. 'It helps me to clean your teeth better and more quickly.' | If good rapport exists between child and dentist, the child will want to help. | The form of introduction will, of course, depend on the age of the child. |
| 6. Tie a length of floss to the clamp. | Attach a length of floss (about 40 cm) to the arch of the clamp and slide it down the side that will be on the buccal of the tooth. The child's help may be enlisted in holding the clamp while the floss is attached. The clamp may be described as the 'clip' or 'button' that will hold the 'raincoat'. | The floss will be held while placing the clamp on the tooth, as a precaution in case it should spring off the tooth. Attaching it to the buccal side of the clamp ensures that it will not be in the way later on.<br>It is desirable to allow the child to familiarize himself with an object that is to be placed in his mouth. | Although attachment of floss as shown in Fig. 7.3e is satisfactory to hold a clamp until it is firmly seated on the tooth, the method described by Reuter (1983), illustrated in Fig. 7.3f, can be recommended because it also secures the clamp should it fracture (though this is a very rare occurrence). |

| Procedure | Method | Rationale | Notes |
|---|---|---|---|
| 7. Place the clamp. | Use clamp forceps to take the clamp to the tooth, holding the floss in the left hand (Fig. 7.3e) Place the clamp carefully just away from the gingival margin, releasing the forceps gradually. Still holding on to the floss with one hand, check the stability of the clamp with your fingers, making sure that it cannot be pulled off the tooth | With care, the clamp can be placed without causing discomfort to the child, even when a local analgesic has not been used. When a local analgesic has been given, pain could still be caused on the buccal gingival margin of a lower molar (innervated by the long buccal nerve), or on the palatal gingival margin of an upper tooth. Topical analgesia could be used but should not be necessary. | In other methods of applying rubber dam, the dam is placed on the teeth first, or the dam is supported on a winged clamp which is then placed on the tooth. The advantage of placing the clamp first is that this can be done more easily, and therefore with less risk of causing discomfort, because there is a clear view of the tooth. |
| | Ask the child to close his mouth gently. Explain that he cannot close completely, but that he can 'rest' his teeth on the clamp. | It is important for the child to accept this limitation of jaw movement before proceeding to the next stage. | |
| 8. Apply the dam. | Sit (or stand) behind the patient's head and bring the dam, attached to the frame and in the correct position, to the mouth. Place the index fingers of both hands at the back of the slit or of the most distal hole in the dam, and open it up widely. Holding the dam in this way, extend into the mouth with the index fingers, reaching for the clamp. When the arch of the clamp can be seen through the opening in the dam, carry the dam over and behind it (Fig. 7.3g). Then slide the dam under the wings of the clamp. *In method 1*, slip the front end of the slit over any convenient tooth in the arch, and the hole over the next tooth (Fig. 7.3h) *In method 2*, slide each hole in the dam over the appropriate tooth. If necessary, place a small saliva ejector under the dam, placing its tip in the lingual sulcus near the isolated teeth to be treated. Use a high-volume aspirator to remove water and debris during cavity preparation. To remove the dam, remove the clamp first; the dam can then easily be lifted off. | The hole is used to hold the dam in place anteriorly; a wedge can also be used if necessary.<br><br>The smallest possible saliva ejector should be used, to give the patient the greatest comfort and freedom of tongue movement. A flanged type is not required because the tongue is retracted by the dam. | A saliva ejector may not be required, especially when treating maxillary teeth; the patient can swallow when necessary with the dam in place. |

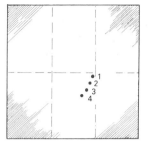

**Fig. 7.3a**

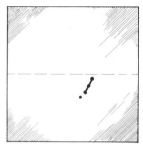

**Fig. 7.3b**

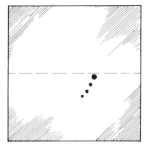

**Fig. 7.3c**

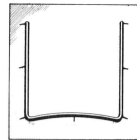

**Fig. 7.3d**

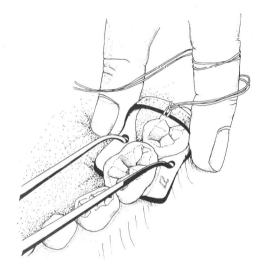

**Fig. 7.3e**

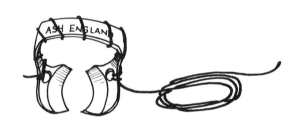

**Fig. 7.3f**

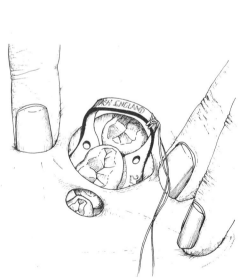

**Fig. 7.3g**

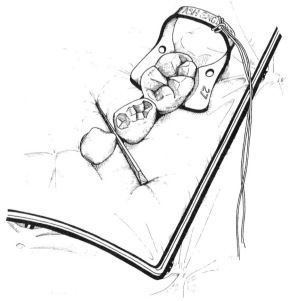

**Fig. 7.3h**

## Isolation of anterior teeth with rubber dam

Anterior teeth are isolated with rubber dam principally to control saliva, which adversely affects the setting reactions of restorative materials and which is a source of bacterial contamination during endodontic treatment. The dam is also an effective barrier during endodontic treatment should a reamer or other small hand instrument be dropped accidentally into the mouth.

To isolate several anterior teeth, a premolar on one or both sides of the mouth may be clamped; a No. 27 (wingless) or No. 1 (Ivory) is usually suitable. However, if only one tooth is to be treated, it is often preferable to isolate that tooth only by using an incisor clamp, for example, a No. 6 or 9 (Ivory). Because of the large wings on these clamps, it is necessary either to apply the dam to the tooth and then fit the clamp over it, or to support the dam on the wings of the clamp before placing the clamp on the tooth.

REFERENCES

Curzon M E J, Barenie J T 1973 A simplified rubber dam technique for children's dentistry. British Dental Journal 135:532–536

Elderton R J 1971 A modern approach to the use of rubber dam. Dental Practitioner 21:187–193, 226–232, 267–273

Reuter J E 1983 The isolation of teeth and the protection of the patient during endodontic treatment. International Endodontic Journal 16:173–181

# 8

# Restoration of carious primary teeth

During the last 10–15 years, a marked decrease in the prevalence of dental caries in children has been noted in the U.K. and many other countries. For example, two surveys of child dental health carried out in England and Wales in 1973 and 1983 have shown that the proportion of 5-year-old children affected by caries has decreased from 71 per cent to 48 per cent (Todd and Dodd, 1985a). This finding confirmed the results of previous local surveys; for example in Somerset, where 54 per cent of 5-year-old children were found to be caries-free in 1979 compared to 40 per cent in 1975 (Palmer, 1980). However, by the age of 9 years, nearly 70 per cent of children in England and about 80 per cent of children in Scotland and Northern Ireland have experienced caries of primary teeth (Todd and Dodd, 1985b). In addition to regional variations in caries experience there are considerable social class differences, children from lower social class families having higher caries experience (Bradnock, Marchment and Anderson, 1984; Todd and Dodd, 1985c).

The principal reasons for restoring carious primary teeth are:

1. To eradicate disease and restore health. Disease of primary teeth should no more be ignored than disease of permanent teeth or, indeed, disease of any other part of the body.
2. To give the child the simplest form of treatment. When caries is treated early, a minimal restoration suffices; if, however, it is allowed to progress, treatment is likely to be more complex (e.g. pulpotomy) or more unpleasant (e.g. extraction).
3. To prevent the child suffering pain. Although untreated caries does not always cause pain, it is more likely to do so as it nears the pulp and,

especially, if a pulpal or periradicular abscess is formed.

4. To avoid the infection that follows carious exposure of the pulp. Exposure of the pulp permits oral bacteria to gain access to the pulp chamber, root canals and periradicular tissues.
5. To preserve space that is required for the eruption of permanent teeth. However, retention of primary teeth until their normal exfoliation does not guarantee that the permanent teeth will erupt in good alignment.
6. To ensure comfortable and efficient mastication. Even the little mastication required by the soft diet of Western society can be painful and difficult if teeth are unhealthy.

During the primary dentition period, restoration of carious teeth is always desirable because the anterior teeth are important for aesthetic reasons and the posterior teeth are important for mastication and space maintenance. After the primary incisors are shed, space maintenance is the principal function of primary teeth; their function in mastication is diminished because first permanent molars are present. The benefit of restoring carious primary molars depends on the importance of maintaining space, and this varies greatly in different dentitions (Chapter 17).

## PRINCIPLES OF CAVITY PREPARATION

The principles governing cavity preparation in primary teeth are similar to those that are applied in the treatment of permanent teeth. These may be summarised as follows:

1. The cavity outline should include the carious lesion and contiguous caries-susceptible pits

and fissures. This principle should be followed with discretion; it is most important to avoid unnecessary destruction of sound tissue.

2. Whenever possible, but not when it necessitates excessive destruction of tooth substance, cavity margins should be placed where they are accessible to cleaning with a toothbrush and where they are least exposed to occlusal forces.
3. The cavity shape should be designed to provide the restoration with good resistance to masticatory forces and adequate retention against dislodgement.

Cavity preparations in primary teeth differ principally in their size and depth, because primary teeth have relatively thin enamel (about 1 mm thick) and relatively large pulps.

## CLASS I, II AND V AMALGAM RESTORATIONS

Amalgam has long been the material of choice for restoring primary and permanent posterior teeth. Composite resin and glass ionomer cement have been gaining popularity in recent years, particularly for the restoration of primary teeth, but amalgam is still the material most commonly used. High copper alloys have been introduced which produce restorations that have been shown in

## Technique: Class I amalgam restoration

| Procedure | Method | Rationale | Notes |
|---|---|---|---|
| 1. Select a bur | Recommended burs are:<br>*for high-speed handpiece* — pear-shaped diamond No. 525 straight diamond No. 541 or 544 straight tungsten carbide No. 1.<br>*for slow-speed handpiece* — round steel or tungsten carbide No. ½ or 1. | A small bur conserves tooth substance | The choice of working with a high- or slow-speed handpiece is based on the preferences of clinician and patient. Miniature head handpieces have obvious advantages in small mouths. |
| 2. Gain access and establish cavity depth | Penetrate the occlusal surface within the carious area to a depth of about 1½ mm (i.e. about ½ mm into dentine) (Fig. 8.1a) The depth may be judged against the bur. | The enamel is penetrated most easily through the soft carious area. Penetrating deeper than 1½ mm would risk exposure of the pulp when the cavity is later extended laterally. | The depth of penetration is most easily judged when using the pear-shaped diamond because its head is 1½ mm long. |
| 3. Prepare the cavity outline | If using a high-speed handpiece, continue with the same bur. If using slow-speed, change to a No. ½ or 1 flat fissure bur (Fig. 8.1b). Maintain the bur at the established cavity depth and, using intermittent strokes, move it through the fissures of the occlusal surface. Hold the pear-shaped bur parallel to the long axis of the tooth, or the straight bur at a slight angle. In maxillary second molars and mandibular first molars, do not extend across the oblique ridges unless they are undermined by caries (Fig. 8.1c).<br>If a fissure extends near to the mesial or distal marginal ridge, do not undercut the mesial or distal wall. | In preparing the cavity outline, the aims are to remove superficial caries and to eradicate caries-susceptible fissures. The prepared cavity should have a flat or slightly concave floor, and walls diverging from the occlusal to provide retention for the restoration.<br><br>The oblique ridges are not caries-susceptible areas and should therefore be conserved if possible.<br><br>Undercutting a wall near a marginal ridge would weaken the ridge and risk subsequent fracture. | The pear-shaped diamond produces a slightly concave floor and rounded cavity wall angles, which some authorities claim improve the mechanical properties of the restoration, (Guard *et al.*, 1958). |
| 4. Remove any remaining caries | Use a sharp excavator (Fig. 8.1d) or a medium-sized round bur in a slow-speed handpiece (Fig. 8.1e) to remove caries first from the walls and then from the floor of the cavity. | Excavators or burs are equally effective in removing caries. It is important to remove peripheral caries first, before pursuing deeper caries. | After caries removal, the cavity floor may be irregular in depth, but a flat floor will later be restored by lining material. |

*(continued overleaf)*

| Procedure | Method | Rationale | Notes |
|---|---|---|---|
| | If a bur is chosen, use it at slow speed and with light pressure. If enamel of the cavity walls become undermined (Fig. 8.1f) it must be taken back to sound dentine with the fissure bur (Fig. 8.1g). If the cavity becomes deep, proceed very gently with an excavator; a decision regarding pulp treatment may have to be made (Ch. 9). | Excessive bur speed or pressure might endanger the pulp. Undermined enamel would probably fracture and leave a defect at the margin of the restoration. | |
| 5. Wash, dry and assess the cavity preparation | Wash the cavity with water (Fig. 8.1h) and dry with compressed air. Using a probe, confirm that caries has been removed and that the cavity shape conforms with the accepted principles of cavity design (Fig. 8.1i) | | |
| 6. Line the cavity (if necessary) | No lining is required in minimal depth cavities (i.e. just into dentine). | Clinical experience has shown no undesirable after-effects when shallow cavities in primary teeth are not lined. | A layer of copal resin varnish may be applied to the cavity floor and walls; there is some evidence that it reduces marginal leakage around freshly inserted amalgam (Barber et al., 1964). |
| | In deeper cavities apply a hard-setting calcium hydroxide lining to the dried dentine on the floor of the cavity (Fig. 8.1j). After the material has set, remove any excess from the enamel walls of the cavity with an excavator. | Calcium hydroxide is a thermal insulator protecting the pulp. In deep cavities it stimulates the formation of secondary dentine. | Various calcium hydroxide preparations are available. After lining, copal resin varnish may be applied to the walls and cavo-surface margin, to reduce marginal leakage (Silva et al, 1985). |
| 7. Condense amalgam into the cavity | Mix amalgam according to the manufacturer's instructions and carry it to the cavity in an amalgam carrier. Eject not more than about one third of the amount required to fill the cavity, and condense it firmly with an amalgam plugger into the deepest parts of the cavity (Fig. 8.1k). Add further similar-sized increments and condense each with overlapping strokes covering the entire surface, until the cavity is overfilled by about 1 mm (Fig. 8.1m). Condense the overfilled amalgam over the margin of the cavity. | Adding amalgam in small increments allows for efficient condensation. Overlapping strokes help to ensure good condensation. Overfilling allows carving to the original tooth contour and permits removal of the mercury-rich surface layer of amalgam. Strong amalgam at the cavity margins is essential to prevent breakdown and leakage. | A small plugger should be used; pluggers suitable for permanent teeth are often too large. Mechanical condensers are available that ensure consistently efficient condensation, but many children find the vibration unpleasant. The strength of amalgam is markedly reduced when its mercury content exceeds 55% (Nadal, 1961). |
| 8. Carve the amalgam | With a carver (e.g. Ward's or Hollenbach), remove excess amalgam from the margin of the restoration by sweeping the instrument along the margin, supporting it on the adjacent enamel (Fig. 8.1n). Produce a contour similar to that of the original tooth surface, but do not attempt to reproduce deep fissures. | Supporting the carver on enamel prevents over-carving, which would leave a thin, weak edge of amalgam at the margin. | |

| Procedure | Method | Rationale | Notes |
|---|---|---|---|
| 9. Lightly burnish the amalgam margin | Run a burnisher lightly over the margin of the amalgam, again supporting the instrument on the adjacent enamel (Fig. 8.1p). | Light burnishing of the margin of an amalgam improves its adaptation to the cavity walls. Heavy burnishing would tend to bring mercury into the surface amalgam, thus weakening it. | Although there is evidence that light burnishing improves the marginal seal and reduces corrosion of amalgam restorations (Kato & Fusayama, 1968; Svare & Chan, 1972), the procedure is not universally adopted. |
| 10. Smoothe the restoration | Pass the burnisher lightly over the surface of the restoration. Finally, smoothe the surface with a cotton pledget (Fig. 8.1q). | | |
| 11. Check the occlusion | Remove the rubber dam (if used) and ask the patient to tap the teeth together gently 'on the back teeth' Check the surface for any shiny 'high' spots; if present, remove them with the carver and re-check the occlusion. | Premature contacts could cause fracture of the restoration. | |
| 12. Finish the restoration | Delay finishing for at least 24 hrs. Pass a probe carefully around the entire margin of the restoration to detect any edges that may exist. Pass the probe alternately from amalgam to enamel and from enamel to amalgam, to detect either amalgam or enamel edges. Check also for marginal voids, when both enamel and amalgam edges would be detected. Use a pear-shaped finishing bur to remove amalgam or small enamel edges (Fig. 8.1r). Move the bur along the margin, resting on adjacent enamel. Use the same bur, or a stone, to make minor modifications to the surface contour of the restoration, if necessary. Polish the restoration using a rubber cup or bristle brush mounted in a slow-speed handpiece (Fig. 8.1s). Use a slurry of pumice and water or a proprietary prophylaxis paste. For a final polish use a slurry of zinc oxide powder in water or alcohol. | Amalgam does not attain its final hardness until about 24 hrs. after mixing. The detection and removal of edges is important because they encourage the accumulation of plaque and recurrence of caries at the margin. Polishing reduces surface corrosion and tarnish, and produces a smooth surface that discourages the retention of food debris and that is easy to clean. | An amalgam edge indicates that carving was inadequate. An enamel edge indicates that the cavity was under-filled or that carving was excessive. A marginal void suggests that the amalgam was underpacked or poorly condensed. Gross enamel edges or marginal voids cannot be corrected, except by replacement of the restoration. Various types of abrasive stones are available that may be used for trimming and polishing amalgam. |

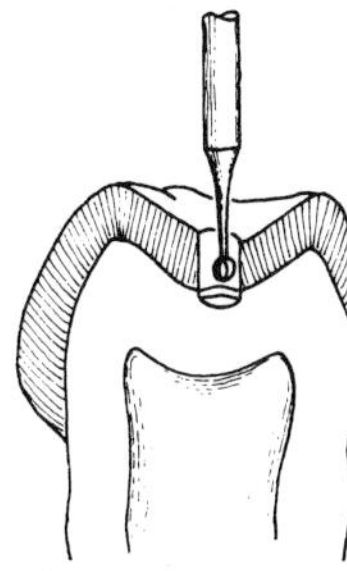

Fig. 8.1a

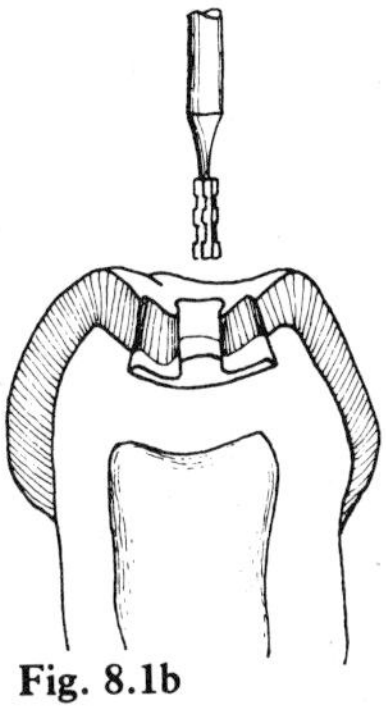

Fig. 8.1b

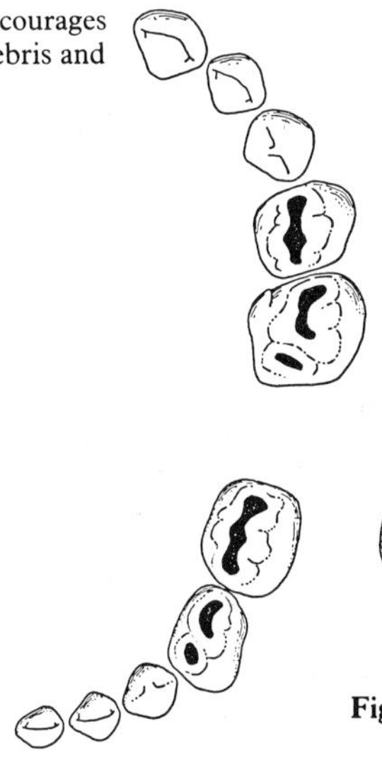

Fig. 8.1c

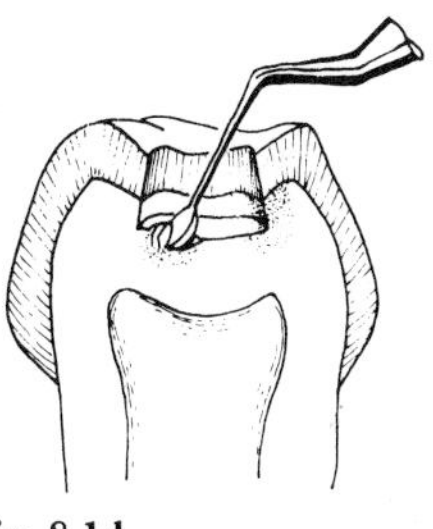

Fig. 8.1d

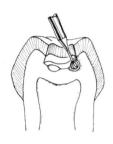

Fig. 8.1e

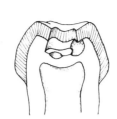

Fig. 8.1f

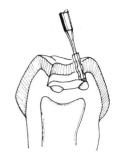

Fig. 8.1g

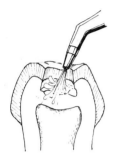

Fig. 8.1h

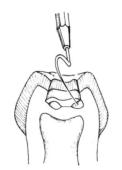

Fig. 8.1i

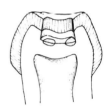

Fig. 8.1j

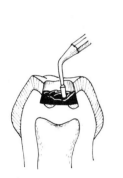

Fig. 8.1k

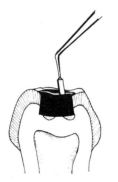

Fig. 8.1m

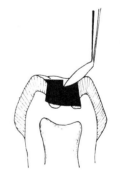

Fig. 8.1n

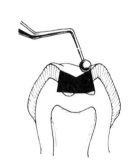

Fig. 8.1p

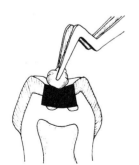

Fig. 8.1q

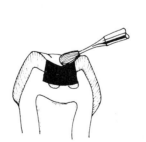

Fig. 8.1r

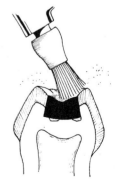

Fig. 8.1s

## Technique: Class II amalgam restoration

| Procedure | Method | Rationale | Notes |
|---|---|---|---|
| 1. Select a bur. | | | |
| 2. Gain access and establish occlusal cavity depth. | See 'Class I amalgam restoration'. | | |
| 3. Prepare the occlusal cavity outline. | | | |
| 4. Establish the isthmus. | Extend the occlusal cavity outline towards the approximal surface above the centre of the contact area (Fig. 8.2a). If the approximal surface has not already been destroyed by caries, try not to break it down at this stage; ideally leave a thin enamel wall (Fig. 8.2b). Make the width of the isthmus about ⅓ of that between the buccal and lingual cusps. | Maintaining the approximal wall intact diminishes the risk of damaging the adjacent tooth. If the approximal wall does break down, great care should be taken to avoid damage to the adjacent tooth. Restorations are liable to fracture at the isthmus; to reduce this risk, the cavity must be prepared to allow sufficient bulk of amalgam in this region. | The isthmus is that part of the cavity between the occlusal dovetail and the approximal box; it lies above what will be the axial wall of the box. Widening the isthmus would also produce more bulk of amalgam but is not advocated because it would weaken adjacent cusps. |
| | From the isthmus, direct the buccal and lingual walls in turn towards the approximal surface such that, when they are later carried through the approximal wall, they will be just detectable with a probe in the buccal and lingual embrasures, and form angles of about 90° with the enamel surface (Fig. 8.2c). Again, if the approximal surface is still intact try to retain a thin enamel wall. | The buccal and lingual margins of the approximal box should be placed so that the margins of the restoration will be accessible to toothbrush bristles. A cavo-surface angle of 90° ensures that there are no unsupported enamel prisms at the margin and that the amalgam margin is strong. The cavo-surface angle must not exceed 110° because an amalgam margin angle of less than 70° is very weak. | Care must be taken to avoid excessive destruction of buccal or lingual walls. |
| 5. Prepare the approximal 'box'. | First establish the level of the gingival floor of the box by moving the bur gingivally 1-2 mm (if using a slow-speed handpiece, this is more easily achieved with a No. 1 round bur (Fig. 8.2d) than with the No. 1 flat fissure bur used for preparing the occlusal outline — then change back to the fissure bur) | Extending gingivally by 1–2 mm places the floor of the box gingival to the contact area with the adjacent tooth, which allows a matrix band to be passed between the teeth and which places the gingival margin of the restoration in a less caries-susceptible area. | When there is more than minimal caries, the level of the gingival floor is dictated by the extent of caries. When the floor must be carried subgingivally, problems arise because of the cervical constriction characteristic of deciduous molars. Having established an adequate width of floor, great care must be taken to avoid the pulp, especially at the buccal and lingual walls. |

*(continued overleaf)*

| Procedure | Method | Rationale | Notes |
|---|---|---|---|
| | Maintaining the tip of the bur at this level, move it buccally and lingually in turn to place the walls of the box in line with the previously-prepared coronal part (Fig. 8.2e). The walls should converge towards the occlusal. The axial wall of the box should be just in dentine and be parallel to the convexity of the tooth surface. If the approximal enamel wall is still intact (Fig. 8.2f), break it away by gently twisting or levering against the wall with an excavator or chisel (Fig. 8.2g). Then use the chisel to plane the walls of the box. | The convergent walls provide retention for the amalgam restoration. | Retention grooves may be placed at the junctions of buccal and axial walls, of lingual and axial walls, and of axial wall and gingival floor. However, this is not normal practice, especially in primary teeth. |
| | The enamel at the gingival margin of the box need not be bevelled. | The enamel prisms in the cervical region of primary molars slope occlusally from the amelo-dentinal junction; therefore none are left unsupported at the gingival margin of the box. | In permanent teeth the enamel prisms slope cervically from the amelo-dentinal junction, and therefore the gingival margin should be bevelled. |
| | Deepen the central part of the pulpo-axial line angle by about 1 mm (Fig. 8.2h). | Deepening the cavity at this point produces a restoration with greater strength at the isthmus, which is a common site of amalgam fracture. This deepening must be restricted to the central part because extending laterally would endanger the pulp horns. | |
| 6. Remove any remaining caries. | | | |
| 7. Wash, dry and assess the cavity preparation. | See 'Class I amalgam restoration.' | | |
| 8. Line the cavity. | | | |
| 9. Fit a matrix. | Adjust the diameter of the matrix band to approximately the size of the tooth crown. Slide the band down the crown until it passes the gingival margin of the cavity, then tighten the band firmly. Place a wedge either from the buccal or lingual to press against the band at the gingival margin of the cavity — the wedge must not push the band into the approximal box. | If the band is too large, gingiva may be trapped between it and the tooth when the band is tightened; this might prevent close adaptation of the band and also cause discomfort to the patient. Since primary molars have marked constrictions at their cervical margins, wedging is desirable to prevent amalgam from being pushed past the gingival floor of the cavity. | Several types of matrix band holders are available. Alternatively, individual matrix bands may be used without a holder (Winstanley, 1977). |

| Procedure | Method | Rationale | Notes |
|---|---|---|---|
| 10. Condense amalgam into the cavity. | See 'Class I amalgam restoration'. Place the first small increment into the approximal box and condense it firmly into the corners (Fig. 8.2i). Build up with several additional increments and overfill by about 1 mm. Pay particular attention to condensing the area next to the matrix band which will form the marginal ridge of the restoration (Fig. 8.2j). | It is important to obtain close adaptation of amalgam to the cervical margins of the box.<br><br>Inadequate condensation of the amalgam close to the matrix band may result in its fracture when the band is removed. | |
| 11. Carve the amalgam. | Establish the level of the marginal ridge by directing the tip of a probe against the matrix band at the desired level, and moving the probe buccally and lingually to remove excess amalgam.<br>Start carving with the matrix band in place.<br>Remove the wedge, loosen the matrix band and carefully remove it. Trim excess amalgam from the buccal and lingual margins of the box with a sharp carver, supporting the instrument on the adjacent enamel. Complete carving as described for Class I amalgam restoration. | Delaying the removal of the matrix band allows the amalgam to harden; this reduces the risk of fracture when the band is removed. | |
| 12. Lightly burnish the amalgam margin.<br><br>13. Smooth the restoration.<br><br>14. Check the occlusion.<br><br>15. Finish the restoration. | See 'Class I amalgam restoration'. | | |

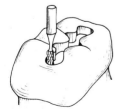

Fig. 8.2a

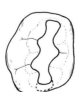

Fig. 8.2b

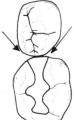

Fig. 8.2c

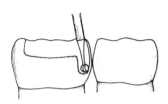

Fig. 8.2d

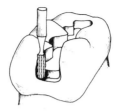

Fig. 8.2e

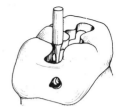

Fig. 8.2f

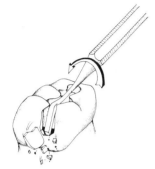

Fig. 8.2g

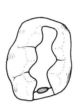

Fig. 8.2h

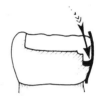

Fig. 8.2i

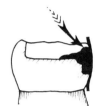

Fig. 8.2j

## Technique: Class V amalgam restoration

| Procedure | Method | Rationale | Notes |
|---|---|---|---|
| 1. Select a bur | | | |
| 2. Gain access and establish cavity depth | See 'Class I amalgam restoration'. | | |
| 3. Prepare the cavity outline | If using a high-speed handpiece, continue with the same bur. If using slow speed, change to a No. 1 flat fissure bur. Holding the bur at the established cavity depth and approximately perpendicular to the tooth surface, prepare the cavity outline (Fig. 8.3a). Place the occlusal margin just occlusal to the gingival ⅓ of the buccal or lingual surface.<br>Place the cervical margin of the cavity just short of the gingival margin.<br>Extend mesially and distally just enough to eliminate the caries and to place the cavity margin in sound enamel. | The occlusal margin is placed in a less caries-susceptible area, i.e. just outside the gingival ⅓ of the buccal or lingual surface.<br>Laceration of the gingival margin should be avoided.<br><br>There is not scope for placing the mesial or distal margins in less caries-susceptible areas. | Where there is extensive caries, the position of the cavity margin is dictated by the carious area. |

| Procedure | Method | Rationale | Notes |
|---|---|---|---|
| | Check that the walls of the cavity are slightly undercut but meeting the surface at nearly 90°. If the extent of caries dictates that the mesial or distal wall of the cavity must be placed near the mesial or distal tooth surface, do not undercut this wall (Fig. 8.3b); instead, increase the retention in the occlusal and cervical walls, using an inverted cone bur. Finally, use a small chisel or cervical margin trimmer to place the cervical margin of the cavity just below the free gingival margin, and also to smooth the entire cavity margin. | Undercutting walls on the mesial or distal corners of the tooth would leave undermined enamel that might chip off and leave a marginal defect.<br><br>Caries is less likely to recur if the margin is placed subgingivally. | |
| 4. Remove any remaining caries<br>5. Wash, dry and assess the cavity preparation<br>6. Line the cavity (if necessary)<br>7. Condense amalgam into the cavity<br>8. Carve the amalgam<br>9. Burnish the amalgam margin<br>10. Smooth the restoration<br>11. Finish the restoration | See 'Class I amalgam restoration'. | | |

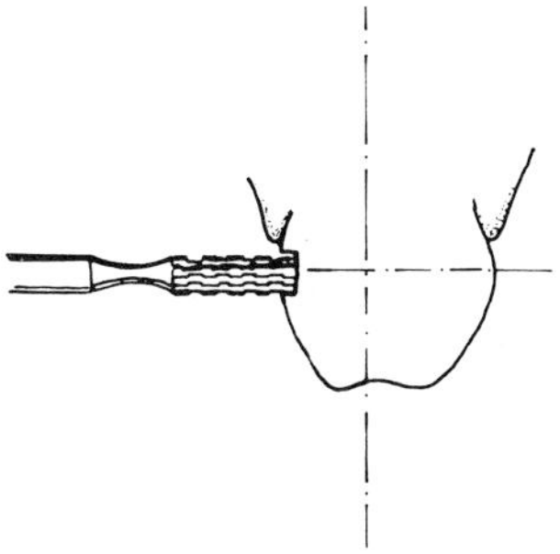

Fig. 8.3a

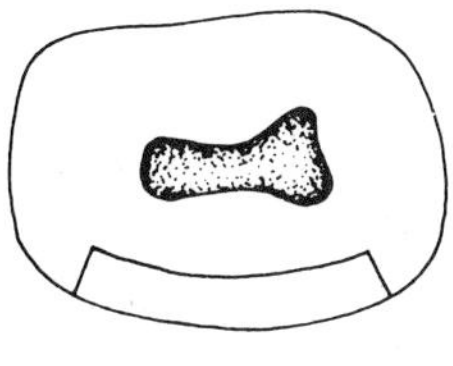

Fig. 8.3b

clinical trials to suffer less marginal breakdown and surface corrosion than previous types of amalgam (Fan and Leinfelder, 1983).

## CLASS I AND II COMPOSITE RESIN RESTORATIONS

Much research has been conducted in recent years in efforts to develop a composite resin that is suitable for restoring posterior teeth, and several manufacturers have introduced materials for this purpose. Studies of composite resin restorations in primary molars have shown that the material can be used successfully for Class I and II restorations (Roberts, Moffa and Broring, 1985). Composite resins are more subject to wear than amalgam and it has been concluded that they cannot yet be considered acceptable substitutes for amalgam. However, occlusal wear only becomes significant after 2 years (Nelson et al, 1980), and restoration for this time period is often all that is required in primary teeth.

Modifications of conventional cavity preparations have been tested (Oldenburg, Vann and Dilley, 1985). One simple modification was to bevel the enamel margin of the conventional amalgam cavity. Another, more radical, modification was to remove only enough enamel and dentine to eliminate caries, and to bevel the enamel margin: no attempt was made to provide resistance or retention form as is done in conventional cavity preparation. However, composite restorations placed in the latter type of cavity were less successful than those placed in conventional or enamel-bevel cavities.

### Technique: Class II composite resin restoration

| Procedure | Method | Rationale | Notes |
|---|---|---|---|
| 1. Prepare a conventional cavity | See pages 87–90 | Modified cavity preparations that have been tested have not proved successful. | The enamel margin of the cavity may be bevelled. |
| 2. Line the cavity | Use a quick-setting calcium hydroxide material to line the floor of the cavity. | | Alternatively, glass ionomer cement may be used as a base (p. 94), using calcium hydroxide only to line very deep parts of the cavity. |
| 3. Place a matrix | Use a thin metal matrix material (e.g. Softrix, Espe), contour it with a burnisher so that it contacts the adjacent tooth, and place a wedge at the cervical margin, (Fig. 8.4a). Alternatively, use a polyester matrix (e.g. Contact Band, Vivadent). | The pressure exerted on the matrix when condensing composite resin is not sufficient to shape the matrix, as it is when condensing amalgam. | The difficulty of obtaining a satisfactory approximal surface contour and a good contact with the adjacent tooth is one of the disadvantages of using composite resin rather than amalgam. |
| 4. Etch the enamel at the margin of the cavity | Apply 30–50% phosphoric acid to the enamel with a cotton pledget, foam pad or small brush, and keep the enamel wet for 1½–2 minutes. Wash for 15 seconds and dry for 30 seconds. | Etching is required to ensure bonding of the composite resin to enamel. Primary tooth enamel requires a longer etching period than does enamel of permanent teeth. | It is preferable to use etchant in gel form to avoid the risk of solution flowing into the cavity and possibly irritating the pulp. |
| 5. Apply unfilled resin to the etched enamel | Use a small brush to apply unfilled resin (bonding agent) to the etched enamel (Fig. 8.4b). Alternatively, use a dentine adhesive, and apply it in the same manner to the dentine wall of the cavity and to the enamel margin. Allow the resin to polymerise, or polymerise with a light source. | The low-viscosity unfilled resin penetrates into the etched enamel. | Although use of unfilled resin has not been shown to be essential, it is generally used. Both autopolymerising and light-sensitive composite resin materials are available. |

| Procedure | Method | Rationale | Notes |
|---|---|---|---|
| 6. Insert composite resin restorative material | Mix the material according to the manufacturer's instructions (if using an autopolymerising material)<br><br>Carry the first increment into the deepest part of the cavity on the tip of a small hand instrument, or by using a special syringe (Fig. 8.4c).<br><br>Condense with an amalgam plugger (Fig. 8.4d). Add further increments and condense.<br><br>If using a light-sensitive material polymerise each increment before adding further material. | | Several syringes are available for delivering composite or other materials: for example, the Composite Syringe (S. S. White), and the Centrix Syringe (Centrix) |
| 7. Remove the matrix, trim excess and polish | After the material has polymerised, remove the matrix, trim excess and polish the restoration with fine diamond and tungsten carbide burs, and abrasive discs. | | |

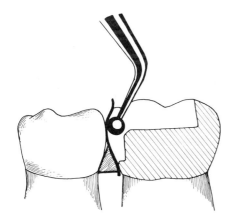

Fig. 8.4a

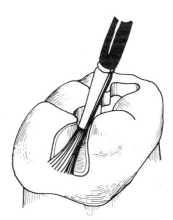

Fig. 8.4b

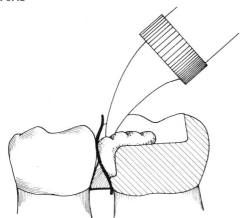

Fig. 8.4c

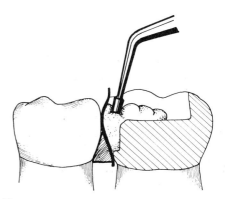

Fig. 8.4d

## CLASS I AND II GLASS IONOMER RESTORATIONS

Glass ionomer cement was developed from poly-carboxylate cement. The most important property of both materials is adhesion to enamel and dentine, which ensures a good seal at the margins of restorations. In addition, the cements leache fluoride, which may help prevent caries should the marginal seal be defective.

Since the introduction of glass ionomer cement about 10 years ago, one of the suggested uses has been the restoration of primary teeth, including molars. However, only one controlled clinical study appears to have been carried out, with disappointing results (Fuks, Shapira and Bielak, 1984): nearly a third of 101 Class II restorations were either fractured or lost within 6 months. Although the restorations were placed in conventional Class II cavities, all the cavities were lined with calcium hydroxide, which, of course, reduced the area of dentine to which the cement could adhere; it is generally accepted that only very deep cavities need be lined before restoring with glass ionomer cement. Another reason suggested for the poor results is the low shearing strength of the material.

To improve the mechanical properties and the resistance to abrasion of glass ionomer cement, silver powder has been incorporated; the silver is sintered to the glass at high temperature to form a glass-cermet cement (McLean and Gasser, 1985). A commercial product is now available (Ketac Silver, Espe), either in capsule form for mechanical mixing or in powder-and-liquid form for hand mixing. No reports have yet been published on the use of these materials in the restoration of primary teeth.

The manufacturers of glass ionomer cements claim that, because of the adhesive properties of the cements, it is not necessary to prepare retentive cavities, but this has not been tested in a controlled clinical study. However, glass ionomer cement is a useful material to use when poor patient cooperation makes it difficult to prepare a conventional cavity.

It has recently been suggested that glass ionomer cement makes an ideal base under composite restorations (McLean, Prosser and Wilson, 1985). Not only does the cement bond to dentine and release fluoride but, after etching with phosphoric acid, composite resin bonds to it. A material is marketed specifically for this purpose (Ketac Bond, Espe).

### Technique: Class II glass ionomer restoration

| Procedure | Method | Rationale | Notes |
|---|---|---|---|
| 1. Prepare a conventional cavity | See pages 87–90 | Although glass ionomer cement adheres to enamel and dentine, a conventional cavity provides optimal retention. | |
| 2. Line the cavity only if it is deep | Place calcium hydroxide over the deep part of the cavity only. | It is desirable to cover the minimum area of dentine consistent with protecting the pulp, to provide the greatest possible dentine area for adhesion of cement. | |
| 3. Place a matrix | See Class II composite resin restoration page 92. | | |
| 4. Clean the cavity walls | Use 10% polyacrylic acid or 25% tannic acid, applying it with a cotton wool pledget to the cavity walls for about 30 seconds, followed by washing with water and drying. | The surface of enamel and dentine cut during cavity preparation is covered by fine debris, which is removed by the acid cleanser, enhancing adhesion. | Since glass ionomer cement adheres satisfactorily to freshly cut enamel and dentine, this procedure may be considered optional. It is however mandatory when applying glass ionomer cement to dentine surfaces previously exposed to the oral environment (for example erosion or abrasion cavities in adults). |

| Procedure | Method | Rationale | Notes |
|-----------|--------|-----------|-------|
| 5. Insert the glass ionomer cement | Mix the material according to the manufacturer's instructions. Carry the first increment into the deepest part of the cavity on the tip of a small hand instrument, or by using a special syringe. Condense with an amalgam plugger. | | In addition to the syringes mentioned on page 93, a special syringe is supplied for dispensing Ketac Silver. |
| | Add further increments quickly, and condense. | The working time of the materials is only 1½ to 2 minutes. | |
| 6. Apply varnish | When the cavity is filled, apply a layer of varnish over the restoration. | Varnish protects the cement from moisture contamination during the setting period. | |
| 7. Remove the matrix and trim excess | After the material has set (a further 2 to 3 minutes), remove the matrix and trim excess with a sharp carver. Apply further varnish over newly exposed material. | | |
| 8. Polish the restoration | Delay polishing for another 4 minutes (Chemfil II) or 10 minutes (Ketac Fil). Polish with abrasive stones and discs lubricated with vaseline. | | Ketac Silver may be polished, and also burnished, immediately. |

## STAINLESS STEEL CROWNS FOR MOLARS

When a primary molar has such extensive caries that it is not possible to prepare a satisfactory cavity for amalgam, a stainless steel crown may be the ideal restoration (Mink and Bennett, 1968; Full, Walker and Pinkham, 1974). Two types of crown are currently available in the U.K.: Unitek (Unitek crown, Unitek) and 3M (Nichrome crown, 3M). Six sizes are made for each primary molar, and the crowns are shaped to conform with the gingival contour of the teeth. In addition, the 3M crowns are contoured inwards at the gingival margins, which is an advantage (see stage 6 below).

## CLASS III AND IV RESTORATIONS

Caries of anterior primary teeth is less common than caries of posterior teeth. When it occurs, it is often associated with rampant caries in the dentition as a whole. In young infants this is related to the frequent and prolonged consumption of sweet drinks from a feeding bottle or reservoir-type pacifier (Winter, 1980). In such cases, caries progresses very rapidly, starting on the labial surfaces of maxillary anterior teeth and quickly involving all surfaces; often it is impossible to prepare conventional cavities to restore these teeth.

In children over 3 or 4 years of age, new lesions of primary incisors are not usually associated with the use of pacifiers and do not progress so rapidly, although they are, nevertheless, indicative of high caries activity. In these children, it is feasible to prepare Class III or Class IV cavities. However, these lesions are less common in primary teeth than in permanent teeth, and therefore techniques for cavity preparation and tooth restoration are described in Chapter 11.

Glass ionomer cement or composite resin may be used to restore Class III lesions in anterior primary teeth. Glass ionomer lacks the translucency of composite resin, but has the useful advantages of being adhesive and of not requiring a lining unless the cavity is very deep. For Class IV lesions, the greater strength of composite resin makes it the material of choice.

## Technique: stainless steel crown

| Procedure | Method | Rationale | Notes |
|---|---|---|---|
| 1. Prepare equipment. | Fine tapered diamond, e.g. No. 582. Straight diamond, e.g. No. 541. Dividers or Boley gauge. Contouring pliers — Johnson No. 114. Curved crown scissors. Large stone on long mandrel. Rubber wheel on long mandrel. Wooden tongue blade. | | |
| 2. Remove caries. | Administer local analgesia and, ideally, place rubber dam using the slit dam method. | Although the preparation of a tooth for a crown is fairly superficial, use of local analgesia is usually preferred because caries may be extensive, and because gingival trauma may be caused during tooth preparation and when fitting the crown. Use of rubber dam is ideal, especially if caries is deep and pulp exposure is possible. | Local analgesia is not required if the tooth has previously received pulpotomy treatment. Discomfort from gingival trauma can be minimised by using a topical analgesic. |
| | Remove caries using excavators or a large round bur at slow speed. If caries is superficial the shape of the resulting cavity is not important. If caries is deep and a pulp exposure possible, prepare a retentive cavity first before proceeding to remove deep caries. | The cavity left after excavating superficial caries is later filled with the material used to cement the crown. If pulpotomy is required, a retentive cavity is needed to seal medicaments in the pulp chamber. | If pulpotomy is required, preparation of the tooth for a crown may proceed directly after treatment by the 1-visit formocresol technique but must be postponed if a 2-visit technique is chosen. |
| 3. Prepare the tooth. | Use a high-speed handpiece with water coolant. Occlusal surface: Penetrate the occlusal fissure with the straight diamond to a depth of 1.0–1.5 mm. Extend through the pits and fissures at this depth, passing through any oblique ridges and extending to the buccal, lingual and approximal surfaces (Fig. 8.5a). Then reduce the cusps also by 1.0–1.5 mm (Fig. 8.5b). Check the occlusion to check that there is sufficient clearance. | A reduction of 1.0–1.5 mm is required to allow placement of the crown without opening the bite. | The order in which the tooth surfaces are prepared is not important. If a rubber dam has been placed, checking the occlusion may be deferred till later. |

| Procedure | Method | Rationale | Notes |
|---|---|---|---|
| | *Approximal surfaces*: Place the tapered diamond in contact with the tooth at the buccal or lingual embrasure, angled about 20° from vertical and with its tip at the gingival margin (Fig. 8.5c). Keep the instrument in this position while slicing across the tooth. After progressing about 2 mm, check that the cut is satisfactory and that a shoulder is not being produced (Fig. 8.5d). | Angling the diamond reduces the risk of damaging the adjacent tooth. It is better to slice from lingual to buccal (or vice versa) than from occlusal to gingival; the latter is more likely to produce a shoulder which might prevent the proper seating of the crown. | The retention of a stainless steel crown depends primarily on a tight fit at the gingival margin. Since, unlike a cast gold crown, it need not fit the tooth closely elsewhere, the shape of the preparation is relatively unimportant. |
| | *Buccal and lingual surfaces*: With the tapered diamond, reduce the buccal and lingual surfaces, to the level of the gingival margin, by about 1 mm, and round off the angles between these surfaces and the approximal surfaces (Fig. 8.5e). It is not essential to eradicate all undercuts at the gingival margin. | Some undercut may be useful in retaining the crown, e.g. mesiobuccally in a mandibular first molar. | |
| | Do not smooth the preparation as is recommended in finishing a preparation for a cast gold crown. | Smoothing is not necessary because the technique does not involve taking an impression of the preparation. | |
| 4. Select the crown. | Place the points of the dividers or gauge on the mesial and distal surfaces of the tooth at the level of the gingival margin. From the six sizes available, select a crown with the same mesio-distal dimension as that indicated by the dividers or gauge. Try the crown on the tooth to confirm that it is a close fit. | Use of dividers or gauge helps in the selection of the correct size of crown. | It is possible to select a crown by trial and error. |
| | If no crown fits exactly, choose one that is slightly large. | A slightly large crown can be made to fit well by crimping its edge (see below). | |
| 5. Fit the crown. | Try the selected crown on the tooth. With a probe, check that the edge of the crown is within the gingival crevice; if it is resting on the gingival margin, crimp the edge of the crown with the No. 114 plier (Fig. 8.5f). Gently press the crown into place. If the crown is over-extended the gingiva will blanch; if so cut the crown in that area with crown scissors or reduce it with a stone, and try it in again. (If the crown was cut with scissors, smooth with the stone before replacing it on the tooth). When the crown appears to be seated satisfactorily, check the occlusion (rubber dam, | | When trying in the crown, care should be taken to avoid the possibility of it being swallowed or inhaled should it slip from the fingers. A piece of gauze may be held behind the tooth. (These precautions are unnecessary if rubber dam has been placed). |
| | | | Since commercially-available crowns are manufactured with occluso-gingival dimensions equal to average clinical tooth crown heights, reduction of the crown often is not required. |

*(continued overleaf)*

| Procedure | Method | Rationale | Notes |
|-----------|--------|-----------|-------|
| | if used, must be removed at this stage). If the crown is still high, remove it and re-check that there is sufficient clearance when the teeth are in occlusion. Further reduce either the occlusal surface of the tooth or the periphery of the crown to permit the crown to be seated properly. | | Many crowns are fitted with margins over-extended sub-gingivally (Spedding, 1984). |
| 6. Contour the crown. | Contour the gingival third of the crown with the Johnson No. 114 plier, placing the convex beak inside and the concave beak outside the crown (Fig. 8.5g). Move the plier around the margin of the crown, squeezing and releasing repeatedly. | The margin of the crown is crimped to produce a tight fit on the tooth. | A 3M crown may need no, or only minimal, contouring. |
| | Try the crown on the tooth again and check that it is a tight fit. Check the margin with a probe, and eliminate any edges by further crimping. Use an excavator or scaler to remove the well-fitting crown. Check the contacts of the crown with adjacent teeth. If necessary, use an Abel No. 112 plier (Fig. 8.5h) to expand the crown and produce better contacts. | Ideally the crown should snap into place and not be too easy to remove. | Sometimes it is difficult to place a well-fitting crown directly from the occlusal; it may be easier to place the lingual margin first and then rotate the crown buccally until it is fully seated. |
| 7. Polish the crown. | Polish the margin of the crown with a stone or rubber wheel. | A rough surface will irritate the gingiva and favour the accumulation of plaque. | |
| 8. Cement the crown. | Wash and dry the tooth and the crown, and isolate the tooth with saliva ejector and cotton rolls. Use an adhesive cement (e.g. polycarboxylate), mixing to a creamy consistency and flowing it down the inside walls of the crown until the crown is almost full. Seat the crown on the tooth from lingual to buccal (Fig. 8.5i) and press it firmly into place first with finger pressure and then by inserting a wooden tongue blade and asking the patient to bite firmly on it. When the cement is set, remove all excess, particularly from the gingival crevice and from interdental areas, using a probe and dental floss respectively. | The tooth and crown must be clean and dry for good adhesion of cement.<br><br>Flowing cement down the walls of the crown reduces the risk of trapping air in it.<br><br>Seating the crown from lingual to buccal allows excess cement to flow out buccally | |

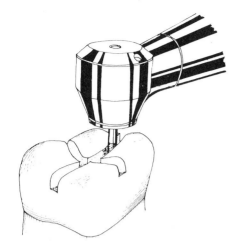

Fig. 8.5a

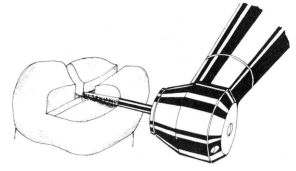

Fig. 8.5b

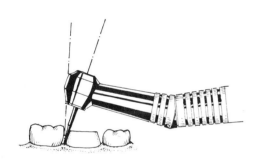

Fig. 8.5c

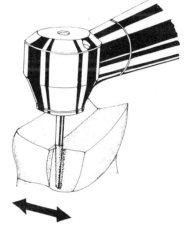

Fig. 8.5d

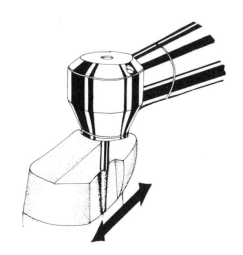

Fig. 8.5e

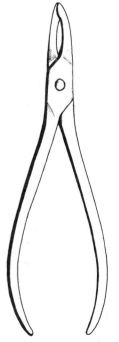

Fig. 8.5f

(*illustrations overleaf*)

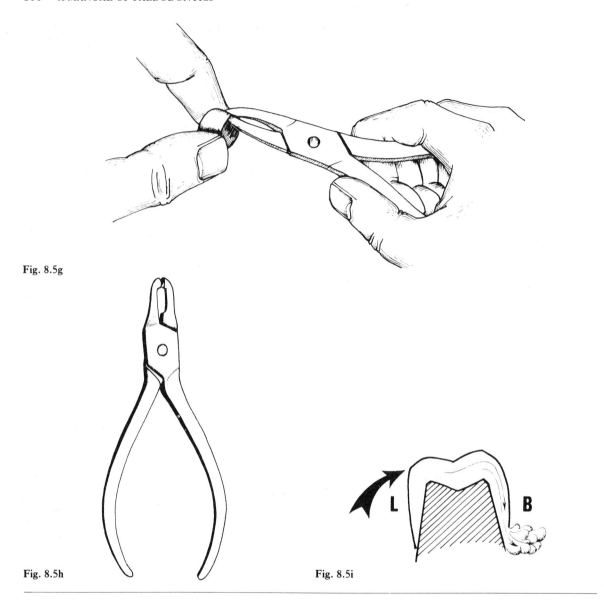

Fig. 8.5g

Fig. 8.5h

Fig. 8.5i

---

## CROWNS FOR ANTERIOR TEETH

Several types of crown may be considered for the restoration of anterior primary teeth: stainless steel, acrylic, epimine or composite resin, and polycarbonate crowns.

### Stainless steel crown

Stainless steel crowns provide strong, durable restorations for primary incisors. No tooth prepara-

tion is required other than for the removal of caries. Their poor appearance can be improved by cutting out the labial surface and replacing with acrylic or composite resin (Hartmann, 1983; Helpin, 1983).

### Acrylic, epimine or composite resin crown

More aesthetic restorations may be made with acrylic, epimine or composite resin. This method has the disadvantage that some tooth reduction is required to provide space for the restorative material, but the reduction is minimal in a tooth with gross caries.

## Technique

1. Use a fine tapered diamond in a high-speed handpiece to reduce the incisal edge and all tooth surfaces, finishing the preparation in a chamfer below the gingival margin.
2. Make a groove with a small round bur on the labial surface, near the gingival margin; this provides additional retention.
3. Remove any remaining caries.
4. Line dentine with hard-setting calcium hydroxide.
5. Trim a crown form so that it fits accurately around the gingival margin.
6. Isolate the tooth, etch enamel for 1½–2 minutes, wash and dry.
7. Fill the crown form with acrylic, epimine or composite resin, and place it on the tooth.
8. Remove excess resin that extrudes beyond the crown.
9. After the resin has set, smooth the margin with fine diamonds or stones.

If several teeth are to be crowned, chairside time may be reduced by preparing the crown forms beforehand on a model of the child's dentition.

## Alternative technique

A disadvantage of the technique described above is the need to trim and smooth the gingival margin of the crown after the material has polymerised in the mouth. An alternative method is to apply the restorative material in the crown form to the tooth (which has been moistened and not etched), to remove the crown before it has completely polymerised, to allow the resin to polymerise, to trim and smooth the gingival margin, and then to cement the crown. If this method is used the tooth preparation must not be grooved or otherwise undercut.

## Polycarbonate crown

Polycarbonate crowns are made in a range of sizes and make aesthetic restorations for primary incisors (Mink and Hill, 1973; Stewart, Luke and Pike, 1974).

## Technique

1. Prepare the tooth, remove caries and line dentine.
2. Try a selected crown on the tooth and reduce the margin as necessary with a stone.
3. Roughen the inside of the crown with a bur to increase the adhesion of the acrylic resin that will be used to cement it.
4. Drill a hole through the palatal surface of the crown with a small round bur; this will allow excess resin to escape and will probably also increase the retention to the crown.
5. Fill the crown with acrylic resin and place it on the tooth.
6. Remove excess resin that extrudes beyond the crown.
7. After the resin has set, smooth the margin.

## Alternative technique

Some problems have been encountered with the retention of polycarbonate crowns, and it has been suggested that best results are obtained using the alternative technique described above for acrylic, epimine or composite crowns, that is inserting acrylic resin into the polycarbonate crown and removing it from the tooth before the acrylic has completely polymerised (Wiggins, Caputo and Jedrychowski, 1978).

REFERENCES

Barber D, Lyell J, Massler M 1964 Effectiveness of copal resin varnish under amalgam restorations. Journal of Prosthetic Dentistry 14:533–536
Fan P L, Leinfelder K F 1983 High copper content amalgam alloys. Journal of the American Dental Association 105:1077–1079
Full C A, Walker J D, Pinkham J R 1974 Stainless steel crowns for deciduous molars. Journal of the American Dental Association 89:360–364
Fuks A B 1984 Clinical evaluation of a glass ionomer cement used as Class II restorative material in primary molars. Journal of Pedodontics 8:393–399
Guard W F, Haack D C, Ireland R L 1958 Photoelastic stress analysis of buccolingual sections of Class II cavity

Hartmann C R 1983 The open face stainless steel crown: an esthetic technique. Journal of Dentistry for Children 50:31–33

Helpin M L 1983 The open face steel crown restoration in children. Journal of Dentistry for Children 50:34–36

Kato S, Fusayama T 1968 The effect of burnishing on the marginal seal of amalgam restorations. Journal of Prosthetic Dentistry 19:393–398

McLean J W, Gasser O 1985 Glass-cermet cements. Quintessence International 5:333–343

McLean J W, Prosser H J, Wilson A D 1985 The use of glass ionomer cements in bonding composite resins to dentine. British Dental Journal 158:410–414

Mink J R, Bennett I C 1968 The stainless steel crown. Journal of Dentistry 35:186–196

Mink J R, Hill C J 1973 Crowns for anterior primary teeth. Dental Clinics of North America 17:85–92

Nadal R, Phillips R W, Swartz M L 1961 Clinical investigation of the relation of mercury to the amalgam restoration. Journal of the American Dental Association 63:488–496

Nelson G V, Osborne J W, Gale E N, Norman R D, Phillips R W 1980 A three-year clinical evaluation of composite resin and a high-copper amalgam in posterior primary teeth. Journal of Dentistry for Children 47:414–418

Oldenburg T R, Vann W F, Dilley D C 1985 Composite restorations for primary molars: two-year results. Pediatric Dentistry 7:96–103

Palmer J D 1980 Dental health in children: an improving picture? British Dental Journal 149:48–50

Roberts M W, Moffa J P, Broring C L 1985 Two-year clinical evaluation of a proprietary composite resin for the restoration of primary posterior teeth. Pediatric Dentistry 7:14–18

Silva M, Messer L B, Douglas W, Weinberg R 1985 Base-varnish interactions around amalgam restorations: spectrophotometric and microscopic assessment of leakage. Australian Dental Journal 30:89–95

Spedding R M 1984 Two principles for improving the adaption of stainless steel crowns to primary molars. Dental Clinics of North America 28:157–175

Stewart R E, Luke L S, Pike A R 1974 Preformed polycarbonate crowns for the restoration of anterior teeth. Journal of the American Dental Association 88:103–107

Svare C W, Chan K L 1972 Effect of surface treatment on the corrodibility of dental amalgam. Journal of Dental Research 51:44–47

Todd J E, Dodd T 1985a Children's dental health in the United Kingdom 1983. Her Majesty's Stationery Office, London, p 6

Todd J E, Dodd T 1985b Children's dental health in the United Kingdom 1983. Her Majesty's Stationery Office, London, p 22

Todd J E, Dodd T 1985c Children's dental health in the United Kingdom 1983. Her Majesty's Stationery Office, London, p 52

Wiggins C E, Caputo A A, Jedrychowski J R 1978 An investigation of bonding systems for the polycarbonate crown restoration. Journal of the American Dental Association 96:823–826

Winstanley R B 1977 The individual matrix band. Quintessence International No 1 report no. 1459 p 73–80

Winter G B 1980 Problems involved with the use of comforters. International Dental Journal 30:28–38

RECOMMENDED READING

Van Beek G C 1983 Dental morphology: an illustrated guide, 2nd edn. Wright, Bristol

Kennedy D B 1983 Paediatric operative dentistry, 3rd edn. Wright, Bristol

Davis J M, Law D B, Lewis T M 1981 An atlas of pedodontics, Saunders, Philadelphia

# Pulp treatment of primary teeth

Exposure of the pulp is caused most commonly by caries, but may also be caused by trauma from a blow or during cavity preparation. Pulp exposures caused by caries occur more frequently in primary than in permanent teeth because the former have relatively large pulp chambers, more prominent pulp horns, and thinner enamel and dentine.

Exposure of the pulp by caries is invariably accompanied by infection of the pulp, and traumatic exposure is followed by infection if the exposed pulp becomes contaminated by saliva. The infected pulp becomes inflamed, and necrosis of the pulp may result; if the infection spreads to the alveolar bone the developing permanent tooth may be affected. Furthermore, although the inflammation may remain sub-acute or chronic and therefore give the patient little or no pain, the process may become acute by any time. For these reasons, a primary tooth with a pulp exposure should not be left untreated; a choice must be made between conservation by some form of pulp treatment, or extraction, perhaps accompanied either by a 'balancing' extraction or by space maintenance (Ch. 17).

Primary molars require pulp treatment much more commonly than do primary anterior teeth. The methods of treatment include pulp capping and pulpotomy, but pulpectomy is generally considered to be impracticable because of the difficulty of obtaining adequate access to the root canals in the small mouths of children, and because of the complexity of root canals in primary molars. The canals are ribbon-shaped (narrow mesio-distally and wide bucco-lingually) and their complexity increases as physiological root resorption progresses; when root calcification ends at about the age of 3 years there is usually only one canal in each root, but later each root may have several intercommunicating canals (Hibbard and Ireland, 1957). Thus, when the canals are least complex the patients are young and least likely to tolerate root canal treatment; in older patients the canals are too complex to be cleaned adequately. Because of these difficulties, a pulpotomy technique is generally used even for a tooth with a necrotic pulp, though the ideal pulpectomy treatment may be attempted if conditions are favourable.

These difficulties do not exist with primary anterior teeth, and pulpectomy presents no technical problems. The canal may be filed, or cleaned with a small straight excavator, and filled with a resorbable material (eg calcium hydroxide paste).

## PULP CAPPING

The aim of pulp capping is to maintain the vitality of the pulp by placing a suitable dressing either directly on the exposed pulp or on a thin residual layer of slightly soft dentine; in the later case the method is known as indirect pulp capping (Shovelton, 1972).

Calcium hydroxide is usually used for pulp capping because it stimulates the formation of secondary dentine more effectively than do other materials (Glass and Zander, 1949). Clinical studies have shown that the technique is successful when strict criteria are applied in selecting cases for treatment (Jeppeson, 1971). Pulp capping is not recommended if the diameter of the exposure is greater than a pin-point, if there is more than gentle bleeding from the exposure site, or if there is a history of spontaneous pain.

Less commonly, preparations containing anti-biotic and anti-inflammatory drugs are used instead of calcium hydroxide. The rationale of using these materials is that they suppress infection and inflammation. Clinical success has been reported in the treatment of small, symptomless pulp exposures in permanent teeth (Cowan, 1966) and in primary teeth (Hargreaves, 1969). However, slow pulp necrosis and abscess formation tend to occur in teeth treated with these materials, without causing symptoms. Because these changes develop slowly the use of these materials in primary teeth is not contra-indicated, but in permanent teeth it is recommended that they are used only temporarily, to alleviate symptoms before treating by pulpectomy (F.D.I., 1968).

## Technique: pulp capping

| Procedure | Method | Rationale | Notes |
|---|---|---|---|
| 1. Prepare instruments and materials | Ideally, use a sterile, pre-packed tray containing cotton wool pledgets, burs and hand instruments required for pulpotomy. | | Before starting to treat a tooth with a large carious lesion, it is important to prepare for pulp treatment so that it can be given without delay should the need arise. |
| 2. Isolate the tooth | Apply rubber dam. If rubber dam cannot be used, isolate with cotton rolls and a saliva ejector, and maintain them in position throughout the treatment. | An essential condition for successful pulp treatment is that the pulp should not become contaminated by saliva. | Rubber dam also protects the patient should materials or instruments be inadvertently dropped into the mouth. |
| 3. Prepare the cavity | Prepare a cavity in the normal way (Ch. 8). | It is important to complete the cavity preparation before removing deep caries so that the tooth can be quickly restored after pulp treatment, thus reducing the risk of contamination. | Before commencing treatment of a vital tooth suspected of having a pulp exposure, adequate local analgesia must be provided. |
| 4. Excavate deep caries | Gently remove caries with an excavator, first removing peripheral caries, then proceeding towards the pulp. If, in a very deep cavity, it is assessed that the pulp is nearly exposed, and the overlying dentine is only very slightly soft, do not proceed to expose the pulp. If caries is more advanced, it must be removed. If the pulp is vital and the exposure is not more than pin-point in diameter, pulp capping may be performed. | The prognosis of indirect pulp capping is good.<br><br>The prognosis for pulp capping is poor unless the exposure is very small. | Some dentists consider that the prognosis for pulp capping is too uncertain, and prefer to treat all pulp exposures in primary teeth by pulpotomy. |
| 5. Apply calcium hydroxide | Dry the cavity with a cotton pledget.<br><br>Cover the deep parts of the cavity, including the pulp exposure (if present), with hard-setting calcium hydroxide paste. | The capping material will not adhere to a wet surface.<br><br>Calcium hydroxide stimulates the formation of secondary dentine. A hard-setting material is more convenient to use than a non-setting type. | Compressed air should not be used to dry the cavity because this might irritate the pulp. Many calcium hydroxide preparations are available. If a non-setting paste is used it must be covered with a cement base before restoring the tooth with amalgam. A cement base should also be placed over hard-setting calcium hydroxide if the exposure is on the floor of the cavity, subject to direct pressure during condensation of amalgam. |
| 6. Restore the tooth | (see Ch. 8) | | |

## PULPOTOMY (PARTIAL PULPECTOMY)

Pulpotomy is a procedure in which the entire coronal pulp is removed, with the aim of removing all infected pulp tissue; the radicular pulp is then treated in different ways, according to the technique employed. Pulpotomy is performed mainly in vital teeth with pulp exposures larger than those considered suitable for pulp capping.

In permanent teeth, the classical pulpotomy technique involves placing calcium hydroxide in the base of the pulp chamber after having removed the coronal pulp. This technique has been used with success in the treatment of vital pulps in premolars and molars (Masterton, 1966; Santini, 1983). However, in primary teeth this method has been found to be relatively unsuccessful, often being accompanied by internal resorption of the roots (Magnusson, 1970; Schroder, 1978). Therefore, other pulpotomy methods have been developed for primary molars: *vital pulpotomy* using formocresol, and *devitalisation pulpotomy*. These are alternative methods for teeth with vital pulps; guidelines for deciding which method to use are given on page 110.

For non-vital pulps, pulpectomy and root canal therapy is the ideal treatment, but since this is not usually practicable for primary molars, a pulpotomy method is advocated; this is called mortal pulpotomy.

### Vital pulpotomy (formocresol pulpotomy)

After removal of coronal pulp, formocresol solution is applied to the radicular pulp for 4 or 5 minutes, after which an antiseptic dressing containing formocresol is placed over the radicular pulp stumps before restoring the tooth (Redig, 1968). The use of this technique has been reviewed recently (Teplitsky and Grieman, 1984).

The formocresol solution that has been used most commonly has the following composition:

| | |
|---|---|
| Formalin (37%) | 19 ml |
| Cresol | 35 ml |
| Glycerin | 25 ml |
| Water | 21 ml |

However, successful results have also been obtained using a 1 to 5 dilution of this solution (Morawa et al, 1975), and this solution is now widely used.

Formaldehyde diffuses through the pulp and, by combining with cellular protein, fixes the tissues. Histological and histochemical studies have shown that the pulp closest to the pulp chamber becomes well fixed; more apically, fixation may not be complete, and the most apical tissue may remain vital (Berger, 1965; Mejare, Hasselgren and Hammarstrom, 1976; Rolling and Lambjerg-Hansen, 1978). The fixed pulp tissue may later become replaced by vital granulation tissue. It is not known whether the strongly antiseptic properties of cresol play an essential part in the success of the method.

The effectiveness of the method, judged by clinical criteria, is high; after 5 years, success rates of 89 per cent and 98 per cent have been reported (Law and Lewis, 1964; Morawa et al., 1975). Judged by histological criteria, however, the technique cannot be considered ideal because it does not promote pulp healing (Magnusson, 1978).

Because formaldehyde is potentially mutagenic and carcinogenic, its use in dentistry has been questioned (Lewis and Chestner, 1981), but it has been concluded that formocresol presents no health hazard in the quantities used in pulpotomy techniques (Ranly, 1984).

### Technique: vital pulpotomy (formocresol)

| Procedure | Method | Rationale | Notes |
|---|---|---|---|
| 1. Prepare instruments and materials | See 'pulp capping'. | | |
| 2. Isolate the tooth | To provide easy access to the pulp chamber for pulpotomy, it is important to extend the occlusal part of the cavity across the whole of the occlusal surface, extending across the oblique ridges in maxillary second molars and mandibular first molars. | | |
| 3. Prepare the cavity | | | |
| 4. Excavate deep caries | | | |

(continued overleaf)

| Procedure | Method | Rationale | Notes |
|---|---|---|---|
| 5. Remove roof of pulp chamber | Use a sterile fissure bur (about No. 2) in a slow-speed handpiece. Insert it into the exposure and move it mesially and distally as required to remove the roof of the pulp chamber (Fig. 9.1a). Remove any over-hanging ledges of destine. | Pulp tissue under ledges may not be easy to remove. | Opening the pulp chamber with a bur at slow speed is simple since only a thin shelf of dentine needs to be removed (assuming a normal cavity has been prepared previously). Some dentists prefer to use a high-speed handpiece. Care must be taken not to perforate the base of the pulp chamber. |
| 6. Remove the coronal pulp | Remove the coronal pulp with a large excavator (Fig. 9.1b) or with a slowly rotating round bur. | | |
| 7. Wash and dry the pulp chamber | Syringe the pulp chamber with sterile water or saline; a disposable syringe with a sterile needle is ideal for this purpose (Fig. 9.1c). Dry and control bleeding with sterile cotton wool pledgets. | Syringing washes debris and pulp remnants from the pulp chamber. | |
| 8. Apply formo-cresol | Dip a cotton pledget in formocresol solution, remove excess by dabbing on a cotton roll, and place it in the pulp chamber, covering the radicular pulp stumps, for 4–5 minutes (Fig. 9.1d). Do not allow solution to leak on to the gingiva. | It is undesirable to fix gingival tissues. | |
| 9. Apply antiseptic dressing | Prepare an antiseptic paste by mixing equal parts of eugenol and formocresol with zinc oxide. Remove the pledget containing formocresol and place just enough paste to cover the radicular pulp stumps (Fig. 9.1e). Dab the paste lightly into place with a moist cotton pledget. | The antiseptic dressing is used to combat any residual infection. Pressure on the vital radicular pulp should be avoided. | Other antiseptic pastes are probably equally effective. |
| 10. Restore the tooth | Place quick-setting cement base before restoring with amalgam (Fig. 9.1f), or fill with cement before preparing the tooth for a stainless steel crown. | Since the antiseptic paste sets slowly, a cement base is required before restoring the tooth. | A stainless steel crown is the ideal restoration because the crown of a tooth treated by pulpotomy is weak and may fracture. |

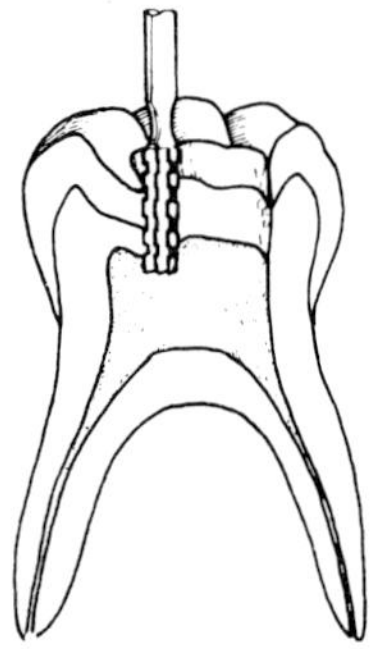

Fig. 9.1a

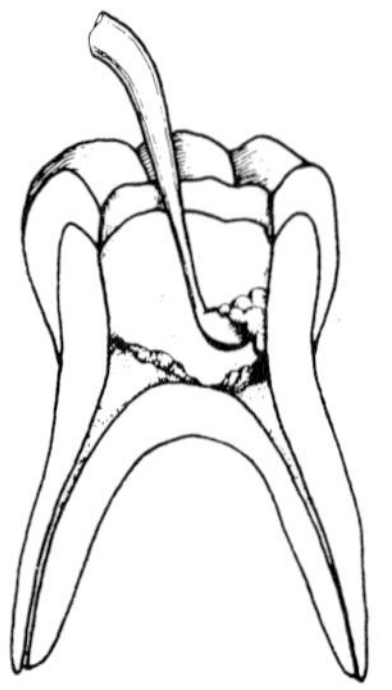

Fig. 9.1b

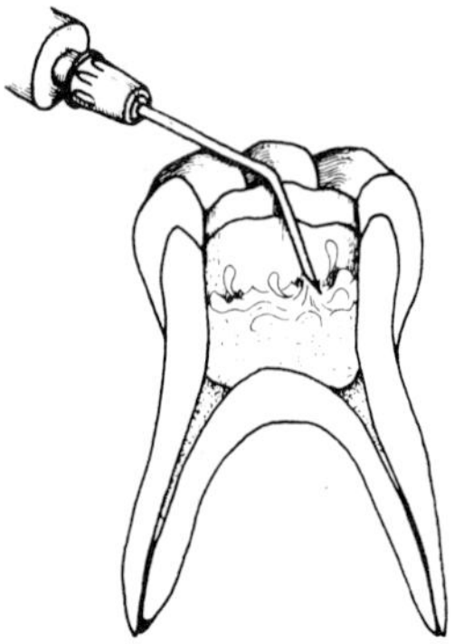

Fig. 9.1c

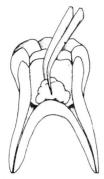

**Fig. 9.1d**

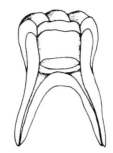

**Fig. 9.1e**

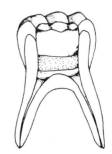

**Fig. 9.1f**

## Devitalisation pulpotomy

This is a two-stage procedure involving the use of paraformaldehyde to fix the entire coronal and radicular pulp tissue. The paraformaldehyde paste that is usually used has the following composition (Hobson, 1970):

| | | |
|---|---|---|
| Paraformaldehyde | 1.0 | g |
| Lignocaine | 0.06 | g |
| Carmine (colour) | 0.01 | g |
| Carbowax 1500 | 1.3 | g |
| Propylene glycol | 0.5 | ml |

The paste is placed over the exposure and sealed in the tooth for 1 to 2 weeks. Formaldehyde gas liberated from the paraformaldehyde permeates through the coronal and radicular pulp, fixing the tissues. On the second visit, the pulpotomy is carried out (without the need for local analgesia) and an antiseptic paste is placed over the radicular pulp before restoring the tooth. Hobson (1970) reported a success rate of 77 per cent after 3 years.

An alternative method is to perform a vital pulpotomy at the first visit, devitalise the radicular pulp with paraformaldehyde paste for 1 or 2 weeks and, at the second visit, replace the paste with an antiseptic paste and restore the tooth.

A related method employs a different paraformaldehyde-containing material in a one-stage procedure. Following vital pulpotomy, the paste is placed over the radicular pulp stumps and the tooth restored (Hannah and Rowe, 1971).

## Technique: devitalisation pulpotomy

| Procedure | Method | Rationale | Notes |
|---|---|---|---|
| 1. Prepare instruments and materials<br>2. Isolate the tooth<br>3. Prepare the cavity<br>4. Excavate deep caries | See 'pulp capping'.<br>To provide easy access to the pulp chamber for pulpotomy, it is important to extend the occlusal part of the cavity across the whole of the occlusal surface, extending across the oblique ridges in maxillary second molars and mandibular first molars. | | |
| 5. Apply paraformaldehyde paste | Ensure that the exposure site is free of debris. Ideally, enlarge the exposure with a round bur. Prepare a cotton pledget large enough to cover the exposure but small enough to be clear of cavity margins. Incorporate paraformaldehyde paste into the pledget, pick it up on the tip of a probe and place it gently over the exposure (Fig. 9.2a). | Adequate exposure of the pulp is essential for the devitalising paste to be effective; formaldehyde gas liberated from paraformaldehyde permeates the pulp tissue and fixes it. Leakage from the cavity would cause fixation of adjacent gingival tissues. | Paraformaldehyde paste may be applied to the exposure directly rather than on a cotton pledget. However, use of a pledget will minimise pressure on the pulp and reduce the risk of after-pain. |

*(continued overleaf)*

| Procedure | Method | Rationale | Notes |
|---|---|---|---|
| 6. Seal the cavity with temporay dressing | Seal the paraformaldehyde paste into the cavity with a thin mix of quick-setting zinc oxide-eugenol (Fig. 9.2b). | A thin mix avoids causing pressure on the pulp. | The child and parent should be warned of the possibility of temporary discomfort, and advised to take an analgesic if necessary. |
| *SECOND VISIT*: 1–2 weeks later | | | |
| 7. Remove temporary dressing | Do not produce local analgesia. Isolate the tooth. Remove temporary dressing and paraformaldehyde paste. Probe the pulp at the exposure site — it should not bleed or be sensitive. If vital pulp is found, either re-dress with paraformaldehyde paste for a further 1–2 weeks, or perform a vital pulpotomy under local analgesia. | The pulp should be non-vital if the paste has been effective. | |
| 8. Remove roof of pulp chamber<br>9. Remove the coronal pulp<br>10. Wash and dry the pulp chamber<br>11. Apply antiseptic dressing<br>12. Restore the tooth | See 'vital pulpotomy'. | | The pulpotomy procedure is relatively simple compared with vital pulpotomy because there is no bleeding. |

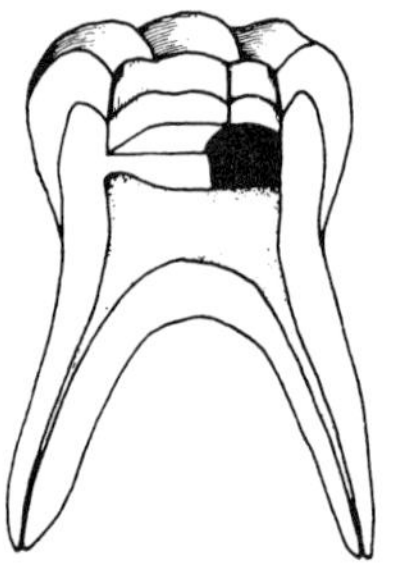

Fig. 9.2a 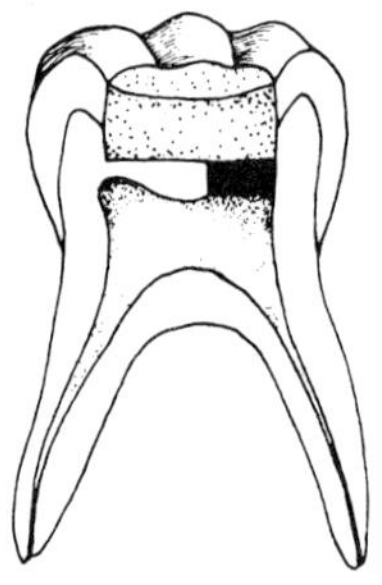          Fig. 9.2b

## Mortal pulpotomy (non-vital pulpotomy)

Ideally, a non-vital tooth should be treated by pulpectomy and root canal filling (Retief, 1980; Coll, Josell and Casper, 1985). However, pulpectomy of a primary molar is often impracticable (p. 103), and a two-stage pulpotomy technique is therefore more commonly used. Necrotic coronal pulp is first removed and the infected radicular pulp is treated with a strong antiseptic solution, which is applied on a cotton pledget and sealed in the pulp chamber for 1 or 2 weeks. Beechwood creosote is usually used (Hobson, 1970), but formocresol (Droter, 1963) or camphorated monochlorophenol (Palmer, 1971) may also be used. Beechwood creosote is a mixture of cresol, guaicol

and other phenols which is less irritant to the tissues than phenol itself. At the second visit, the antiseptic solution is replaced by an antiseptic paste that is placed over the radicular pulp remnants before restoring the tooth. Hobson (1970) found that the 3-year success rate of this method was 66 per cent.

The presence of a sinus associated with a chronic abscess, or of some degree of tooth mobility, is not necessarily a contra-indication for this method; a sinus is expected to disappear following control of the infection, and a mobile tooth becomes firm as periapical bone reforms. A tooth with an acute abscess may be treated by this method, after draining the pus and controlling the infection.

## Technique: mortal pulpotomy

| Procedure | Method | Rationale | Notes |
|---|---|---|---|
| 1. Prepare instruments and materials | | | |
| 2. Isolate the tooth | See 'pulp capping'. | | Since the pulp is necrotic, local analgesia is not required. |
| 3. Prepare the cavity | | | |
| 4. Excavate deep caries | | | |
| 5. Remove roof of pulp chamber | | | If access to the root canals is good, some radicular pulp may be removed with a small excavator. If vital pulp is encountered at any stage, treatment should be changed to devitalisation pulpotomy or to a two-visit formocresol treatment. |
| 6. Remove the coronal pulp | See 'vital pulpotomy (formocresol)' | | |
| 7. Wash and dry the pulp | | | |
| 8. Apply beechwood creosote | Prepare a cotton pledget that will fit into the pulp chamber. Dip the pledget in beechwood creosote solution, remove excess by dabbing on a sterile cotton roll and place it in the pulp chamber over the radicular pulp (Fig. 9.3a). | The strong antiseptic action of beechwood creosote combats infection in the radicular pulp | |
| 9. Seal the cavity with a temporary dressing | Seal the beechwood creosote into the cavity with any temporary cement (Fig. 9.3b). | Since the radicular pulp is necrotic, no precautions need be taken to avoid pressure. | |

*SECOND VISIT*: 1–2 weeks later

| Procedure | Method | Rationale | Notes |
|---|---|---|---|
| 10. Remove temporary dressing | Isolate the tooth. Remove the temporary dressing and the pledget containing beechwood creosote. | | If symptoms persist, or if there are no signs of resolution of a sinus, a decision must be made either to repeat the treatment or to extract the tooth. |
| 11. Apply antiseptic dressing | As in vital pulpotomy — but press the antiseptic paste firmly into the root canals with a cotton pledget (Fig. 9.3c). | Pressure forces the paste down the root canals, compressing the pulp tissue apically where residual infection is more accessible to the periapical blood supply. | |
| 12. Restore the tooth | | | |

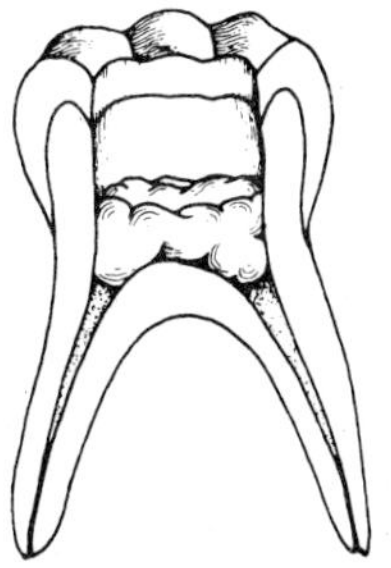

Fig. 9.3a 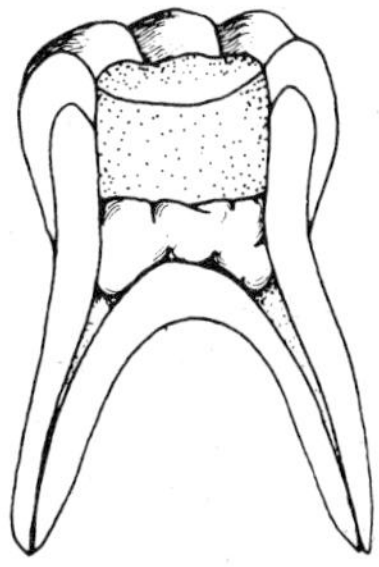    Fig. 9.3b 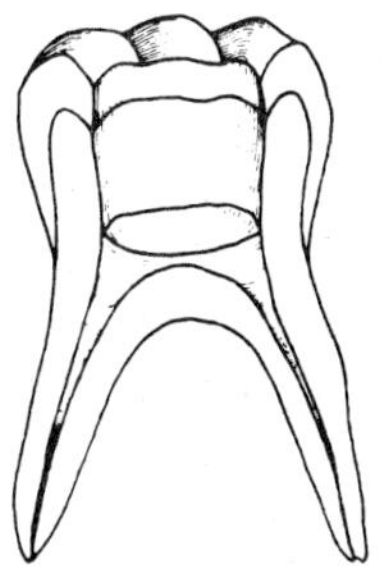    Fig. 9.3c

**Table 9.1** Factors in the selection of pulp treatment method.

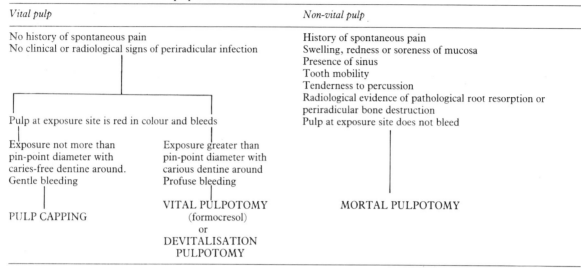

| Vital pulp | Non-vital pulp |
|---|---|
| No history of spontaneous pain<br>No clinical or radiological signs of periradicular infection | History of spontaneous pain<br>Swelling, redness or soreness of mucosa<br>Presence of sinus<br>Tooth mobility<br>Tenderness to percussion<br>Radiological evidence of pathological root resorption or periradicular bone destruction |
| Pulp at exposure site is red in colour and bleeds | Pulp at exposure site does not bleed |
| Exposure not more than pin-point diameter with caries-free dentine around. Gentle bleeding | Exposure greater than pin-point diameter with carious dentine around Profuse bleeding | |
| PULP CAPPING | VITAL PULPOTOMY (formocresol) or DEVITALISATION PULPOTOMY | MORTAL PULPOTOMY |

## SELECTION OF METHOD

The decision about which method to use is based mainly on the assessment of whether the pulp is vital or non-vital, and this is based on preoperative signs and symptoms and on the appearance of the pulp at the exposure site. Factors that should be considered, and their influence on the selection of treatment method, are outlined in Table 9.1.

Vital pulpotomy and devitalisation pulpotomy are alternative methods of treatment. Normally, if local analgesia is adequate, the one-stage vital pulpotomy is preferred but, if analgesia is inadequate or if the necessary time is not available, the two-stage devitalisation method may be chosen.

## INDICATIONS AND CONTRAINDICATIONS FOR PULPOTOMY

The indications and contraindications for pulpotomy may be summarised as follows:

### Indications

*General*

1. A cooperative patient.
2. A patient with a bleeding abnormality (e.g.

haemophilia) for whom extraction would require hospitalisation. Any bleeding accompanying the pulpotomy treatment can easily be controlled.
3. A patient with an unhappy previous experience of extraction; pulpotomy may be preferable to extraction for psychological reasons, and may be justified even if there is no dental indication for conserving the tooth.

*Dental*

1. A primary dentition in which all molars are present, or in which the effects of previous extractions have been controlled by either balancing extraction or space maintenance.
2. A mixed dentition in which it is assessed that there is just enough space for the eruption of permanent canines and premolars. Space maintenance is very important in these cases (p. 156), and the primary tooth is preferable to an artificial space maintainer.
3. A mixed dentition in which it is assessed that there is a gross shortage of space for the eruption of permanent canines and premolars. Again, space maintenance is very important in these cases (p. 156).

## Contraindications

### General

1. A patient from a family having unfavourable attitudes towards dental health and the conservation of teeth (unless these attitudes can be changed).
2. A patient with inadequate cooperation for pulp treatment (unless this can be improved by successful behaviour management).
3. A patient with congenital heart disease or a history of rheumatic fever. Although the pulp treatment could be performed under antibiotic cover, it is not certain that infection is eliminated during treatment; any residual infection is a potential source of bacteraemia that might be a hazard to the patient in the future.
4. A patient in poor general health (e.g. diabetes, chronic kidney disease, leukaemia); these patients have poor resistance to infection and poor healing qualities.

### Dental

1. A dentition in which the effects of previous extractions have not been controlled. Extraction is usually preferable to pulp treatment if the contralateral tooth is missing.
2. A mixed dentition in which it is assessed that there is mild shortage of space for the eruption of permanent canines and premolars. In these cases, space maintenance is not critical and there is no benefit in conserving first primary molars. Extraction of a permanent tooth unit will be required later, which will provide more than enough space. Extraction of first primary molars often allows crowded permanent incisors to align, and the small amount of mesial drift of posterior teeth that can be expected to occur is acceptable, and often advantageous. Second primary molars, however, should be conserved, because of the greater amount of space loss that generally follows their extraction.
3. A tooth with an acute abscess. However, in some cases it is possible to drain the pus and then treat as a chronic abscess. If the swelling points into the buccal mucosa, incision with a scalpel blade will obtain drainage; otherwise, drainage may be obtained by making as large an opening as possible into the pulp chamber and by passing a blunt probe down the gingival crevice to the root furcation where the abscess is usually located.
4. A dentition in which more than 2 or 3 teeth have pulp exposures. Such a dentition is probably neglected and does not justify pulp treatment unless the prognosis for improving home care is good.
5. A tooth with such gross coronal breakdown that restoration would be impossible following pulp treatment.
6. A tooth with caries penetrating the floor of the pulp chamber.
7. A tooth close to natural exfoliation.
8. A tooth with advanced pathological root resorption.

REFERENCES

Berger J E 1965 Pulp tissue reaction to formocresol and zinc oxide-eugenol. Journal of Dentistry for Children, 32:13–27
Coll J A, Josell S, Casper J S 1985 Evaluation of a one-appointment formocresol pulpectomy technique for primary molars. Pediatric Dentistry 7:123–129
Cowan A 1966 Treatment of exposed vital pulps with a corticosteroid antibiotic agent. British Dental Journal 120:521–532
Droter J A 1963 Formocresol in vital and non-vital teeth: a clinical study. Journal of Dentistry for Children 30:239–242
Federation Dentaire Internationale 1968 The use of corticosteroids in endodontic therapy. International Dental Journal 18:471–472

Glass R L, Zander H A 1949 Pulp healing. Journal of Dental Research 28:97–107
Hannah D R, Rowe A H R 1971 Vital pulpotomy of deciduous molars using N$_2$ and other materials. British Dental Journal 130:99–107
Hargreaves J A 1969 Maintenance of exposed deciduous teeth with Ledermix. In: Odontoiatria Infantile: Proceedings of the 2nd international symposium of the international association of dentistry for children. Italian Society of Dentistry for Children, Rome p 279–289
Hibbard E D, Ireland R L 1957 Morphology of the root canals of the primary molar teeth. Journal of Dentistry for Children 24:250–257

Hobson P 1970 Pulp treatment of deciduous teeth. Part 2: clinical investigation British Dental Journal 128:275–283

Jeppesen K 1971 Direct pulp capping on primary teeth: a long term investigation. Journal of the International Association of Dentistry for Children 2:10–19

Law D B, Lewis T M 1964 Formocresol pulpotomy in deciduous teeth. Journal of the American Dental Association 69:601–607

Lewis B B, Chestner S B 1981 Formaldelyde in dentistry: a review of mutagenic and carcinogenic potential. Journal of the American Dental Association 103:489–434

Magnusson B 1970 Therapeutic pulpotomy in primary molars: a clinical and histological follow-up. Odontologisk Revy 21:415–431

Magnusson B O 1978 Therapeutic pulpotomies in primary molars with the formocresol technique. Acta Odontologica Scandinavica 36:137–165

Masterton J B 1966 The healing of wounds of the dental pulp of Man: a clinical and histological study. British Dental Journal 120:213–224

Mcjare I, Hasselgren G, Hammarstrom L E 1976 Effect of formaldehyde-containing drugs on human dental pulp evaluated by enzyme histochemical technique. Scandinavian Journal of Dental Research 84:29–36

Morowa A P, Straffon L H, Han S S, Corpron R E 1975 Clinical evaluation of pulpotomies using dilute formocresol. Journal of Dentistry for Children 42:360–363

Palmer J 1971 Treatment of non-vital deciduous teeth in general practice. Dental Practitioner 21:150–152

Ranly D M 1984 Formocresol toxicity: current knowledge. Acta Odontologica Pediatrica 5:93–98

Redig D F 1968 A comparison and evaluation of two formocresol pulpotomy techniques using 'Buckley's' formocresol. Journal of Dentistry for Children 35:22–32

Rifkin A 1980 A simple, effective, safe technique for the root canal treatment of abscessed primary teeth. Journal of Dentistry for Children 47:435–441

Rolling I, Lambjerg-Hausen H 1978 Pulp condition of successfully formocresol-treated primary molars. Scandinavian Journal of Dental Research 80:267–272

Santini A 1983 Assessment of the pulpotomy technique in human first permanent mandibular molars. British Dental Journal 155:151-154

Schroder 1978 A two-year follow-up of primary molars pulpotomized with a gentle technique and capped with calcium hydroxide. Scandinavian Journal of Dental Research 83:273–278

Shovelton D S 1972 The maintenance of pulp vitality. British Dental Journal 133:95–101

Teplitsky P E, Grieman R 1984 History of formocresol pulpotomy. Journal of the Canadian Dental Association 50:629–634

# 10

# Restoration of carious permanent teeth

Preventive resin restoration (sealant restoration)
Class I, II and V restorations for posterior teeth
Class III, IV and V restorations for anterior teeth
Stainless steel crowns for first permanent molars

In the U.K. in 1983, caries affected the permanent teeth of 17 per cent of 6-year-old children, 65 per cent of 10-year-olds and 93 per cent of 15-year-olds (Todd and Dodd, 1985). However, the prevalence of dental caries appears to have decreased in recent years: in Somerset, the mean caries experience of 12-year-old children in 1978 was 35 per cent less than in 1963 (Anderson, 1981), and in Bristol, a difference of 36 per cent was noted in the caries experience of 11-year-old children between 1970 and 1979, and of 30 per cent in 14-year-olds between 1973 and 1979 (Andlaw, Burchell and Tucker, 1982).

## PREVENTIVE RESIN RESTORATION (SEALANT RESTORATION)

The ideal preventive treatment for the occlusal surfaces of molars and premolars, as well as for other pits and fissures on these and other teeth, is pit and fissure sealing (Ch. 5). Sealing is especially indicated for deep pits and fissures, which are particularly caries-susceptible. However, it is not uncommon when probing a pit or fissure to remain uncertain about whether it is caries-free. Also, it is not uncommon to detect a small, discrete carious lesion in an otherwise sound surface. Although sealing over an early lesion may be a justifiable form of treatment, because the lesion will probably become arrested under the sealant (Going, 1984), the preferred treatment is to open up, very conservatively with a bur, the part of the fissure where diagnosis is uncertain or where early caries exists, to fill the resulting small cavity with composite resin and to seal the adjacent fissures. This type of restoration was originally called a sealant restoration (Simonsen and Stallard, 1977) but is now generally referred to as a preventive resin restoration (Simonsen, 1985). It is more conservative than a Class I amalgam, and has been shown in clinical trials to be effective (Raadal, 1978; Simonsen, 1980; Houpt et al, 1985).

## Technique: composite resin sealant restoration

| Procedure | Method | Rationale | Notes |
| --- | --- | --- | --- |
| 1. Investigate the 'sticky' part of the fissure, or the small carious lesion | With a small round bur (e.g. No. 2) in a slow-speed or high-speed handpiece, penetrate the 'sticky' part of the fissure, or the carious lesion, to a depth of about 1 mm (Fig. 10.1a and b). Open out the fissure so that its base can easily be probed. If it is assessed as caries-free proceed to 2 below. | Removal of about 1 mm of enamel allows a better assessment to be made of the state of the fissure base. | Local analgesia is not required because only enamel is penetrated. |

(continued overleaf)

| Procedure | Method | Rationale | Notes |
|---|---|---|---|
| | If doubt persists, or if caries remains, proceed deeper with a slightly larger bur. | As the cavity becomes deeper it must be widened so that its base can be seen and probed. | If caries is deeper than originally expected and involves the dentine, a decision must be made whether to proceed with this technique or to prepare a Class I cavity for restoration with amalgam. |
| | When the cavity is caries free, undercut its walls slightly with an inverted cone bur. | It is not essential to produce a retentive cavity, but it is a simple procedure which increases the retention of the restoration. | The sealant restoration is retained primarily by the bonding of composite resin to acid-etched enamel. |
| | If dentine has been exposed, line with hard-setting calcium hydroxide. | Since it is planned to use acid to etch the enamel, any exposed dentine should be lined. | |
| 2. Isolate the tooth<br>3. Etch<br>4. Wash<br>5. Dry | See 'fissure sealing' (Ch. 5). | | |
| 6. Place the sealant restoration | If the cavity produced in enamel was minimal, apply resin as described for fissure sealing (Fig 10.1c and d). If a deeper cavity was made, fill the cavity first with a mix of composite paste (i.e. filled resin); then cover it and the adjacent fissures with resin (Fig. 10.1e and f, g and h). | Composite paste is more resistant to abrasion than the unfilled resin and is therefore more appropriate to fill the cavity. | |

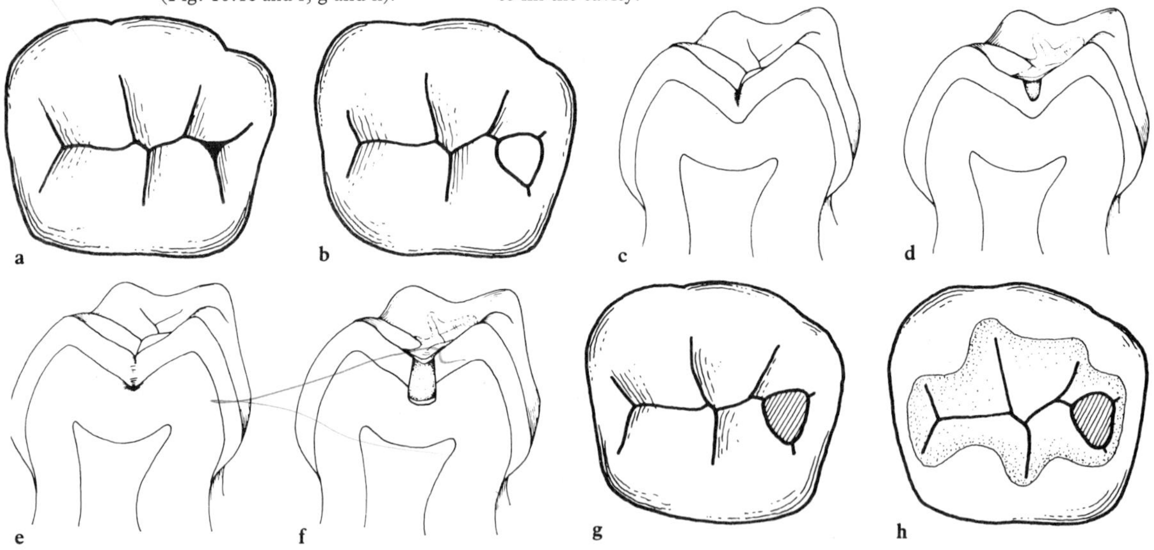

Fig. 10.1

# CLASS I, II AND V RESTORATIONS FOR POSTERIOR TEETH

Amalgam is still the material most commonly used for the restoration of Class I, II and V cavities in permanent teeth, but the continual development of composite resins suggests that these materials may provide an acceptable alternative to amalgam. The techniques for cavity preparation and restoration with amalgam will not be described here; they are similar to those described for primary teeth in Chapter 8, and further details may be obtained from textbooks on operative dentistry.

## CLASS III AND V RESTORATIONS FOR ANTERIOR TEETH

The most common sites for carious attack in anterior permanent teeth are the approximal and labial surfaces; these lesions are treated by the preparation of Class III and V cavities respectively which, most commonly, are filled with composite resin.

When approximal lesions undermine and cause fracture of incisal corners, Class IV restorations are required.

The Class V cavity preparation in an anterior tooth is the same as that described for a primary

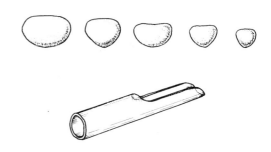

**Fig. 10.2** Matrices for Class V restorations

molar in Chapter 8. Restoration of a Class V cavity in an anterior tooth with composite resin requires the use of a suitable matrix (Fig. 10.2).

## Technique: Class III composite resin restoration

| Procedure | Method | Rationale | Notes |
|---|---|---|---|
| 1. Select a bur | Recommended burs are: *for high-speed handpiece* — small round diamond No. 520, small round tungsten carbide No. 1. *for slow-speed handpiece* — round steel No. ½ or 1 | | The choice of working with a high- or slow-speed handpiece is based on the preferences of the clinician and patient. |
| 2. Gain access | Whenever possible, gain access to the cavity from the palatal/lingual aspect (Fig. 10.3a). If the cavity is large, enter through the surface most destroyed by caries. Penetrate the enamel as close as possible to the interdental space without risking damage to the adjacent tooth. | Best aesthetics is achieved if the labial surface is preserved. In the mandible, however, access is often much easier from the labial, and aesthetics is less important. | |
| 3. Prepare the cavity outline | (The method is described assuming that access is made through the lingual surface). As soon as the bur enters the cavity, change to a No. ½ or 1 flat fissure bur in the slow-speed handpiece (Fig. 10.3b), and enlarge the cavity from incisal to gingival, shaping the lingual wall so that it becomes almost semi-circular in outline. | Preparing the cavity outline with a slow-speed handpiece is recommended because the cavity is usually small and the pulp may be easily exposed by an inadvertent movement of a high-speed instrument. Creating a semi-circular outline permits adequate access for removal of caries and for subsequent insertion of restorative material. | |
| | Do not extend the cavity outline more than is necessary to remove caries and to provide access for lining and restorative materials. | To place the incisal and labial walls in cleansable areas, and the gingival floor in the less caries-susceptible sub-gingival area, would require considerable enlargement of a small cavity; this is not justified. | |

(*continued overleaf*)

| Procedure | Method | Rationale | Notes |
|---|---|---|---|
| | Define the incisal, labial and gingival margins using a small chisel or marginal trimmer (Fig. 10.3c), gaining access to these margins through the cavity. | Hand instruments are preferred to burs for defining the interstitial margins of the cavity because access with appropriate burs would be difficult and would risk damage to the adjacent tooth. | |
| 4. Remove any remaining caries | Use an excavator or a round bur in a slow-speed handpiece to remove caries from the floor and/or walls of the cavity (Fig. 10.3d). If a bur is chosen, run it at slow speed and with light pressure. | | |
| 5. Wash, dry, and assess the cavity preparation. | Wash the cavity with water and dry with compressed air. Using a probe, confirm that all caries has been removed and that there is sufficient retention for a restoration. If retention is considered inadequate (particularly in the larger cavity), use a No. ½ or 1 round bur to produce a groove in the dentine of the gingival floor (Fig. 10.3e) and a pit in the incisal corner (Fig. 10.3f). Alternatively, and especially in a large cavity with a weak lingual wall, prepare a retentive 'lock' in the lingual surface, using a small flat fissure bur (Fig. 10.3g); this lock should be about 2 mm deep, i.e. just into dentine. Check the enamel margins and smooth if necessary with a chisel or marginal trimmer. | In small cavities, a slight general undercut of the walls is sufficient; this may be more pronounced on the gingival and incisal aspects.<br><br><br>It is important to remove unsupported enamel prisms. | Care must be taken when making an incisal pit because the incisal edge of the tooth may be weakened. |
| 6. Line the cavity | Apply a small amount of hard-setting calcium hydroxide cement, carried on the end of a fine instrument, to the pulpal wall of the cavity. When the cement is set, remove any excess from retentive grooves or pits, or from cavity margins, using a small excavator. | The aim is to cover the pulpal wall but not to obliterate retention in the cavity. | |
| 7. Etch the enamel at the margin of the cavity | Apply 30–50% phosphoric acid to the enamel with a cotton pledget, foam pad or small brush. After 1 minute, wash with water and dry thoroughly. | Etching ensures that the composite resin bonds to the enamel to produce a good marginal seal. | The adjacent tooth should be protected from acid by a matrix strip. |
| 8. Fit a matrix | Use a cellulose acetate or other suitable matrix strip. Check its fit around the cavity, noting especially its fit at the cervical margin. If possible, wedge it firmly at the cervical margin (Fig. 10.3h), placing the wedge from the labial or lingual side; otherwise hold the strip in place with a finger. | It is often impossible to fit the strip tightly to all margins of the cavity, but fitting to the cervical margin is especially important because it is there that any excess filling material will be most difficult to trim when it is hardened. | Cellulose acetate matrix strips are most commonly used, but specially-coated soft metal strips are also available. One type of soft metal matrix has adhesive ends which help to maintain it in position around the tooth; when the matrix is positioned, a thin covering film is peeled off and the adhesive end is pressed onto adjacent teeth (Fig. 10.3i). |

| Procedure | Method | Rationale | Notes |
|---|---|---|---|
| 9. Fill the cavity | Mix the composite resin material according to the manufacturer's instructions (if using an autopolymerising material). Estimate the amount required to half fill the cavity, carry it to the tooth on a suitable plastic instrument, and work it into the cavity undercuts. | | A thin layer of unfilled resin may be applied to the etched enamel before placing the restorative material, but this is not essential. |
| | Alternatively, use a special syringe to insert composite into the cavity. If using an autopolymerising resin, fill the cavity within 1 minute. If using a light-sensitive resin, working time is unlimited. | | Several special syringes are commercially available. |
| | Fold one end of the matrix strip around the lingual surface of the tooth and place an index finger firmly on it, in the lingual concavity. With the other hand, pull the other end of the strip across the labial aspect of the crown and pull it tightly, making sure that it is correctly placed at the cervical margin. | | |
| | Hold the strip in this way, without movement, for the length of time recommended by the manufacturer for polymerisation to take place. | Moving the strip might disturb the composite resin before it has polymerised, and result in poor adaptation to the cavity margins. | Most composite resin materials polymerise in about 2 minutes, but those catalysed by ultra-violet or visible light polymerise more quickly. |
| 10. Finish the restoration | Remove the matrix strip and trim excess beyond the cavity margins with a sharp excavator. | | |
| | If possible, limit any further trimming to the margins of the restoration, using fine diamond or tungsten carbide instruments for accessible margins, and an abrasive composite finishing strip for the cervical margin. | The smoothest surface obtainable on a composite material is that which polymerises against a smooth matrix strip. | If the bulk of the restoration needs some trimming, zirconium silicate discs are available which leave a smooth surface. Composite polishing paste may also be used. |

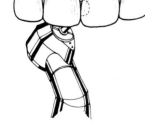

**Fig. 10.3a**

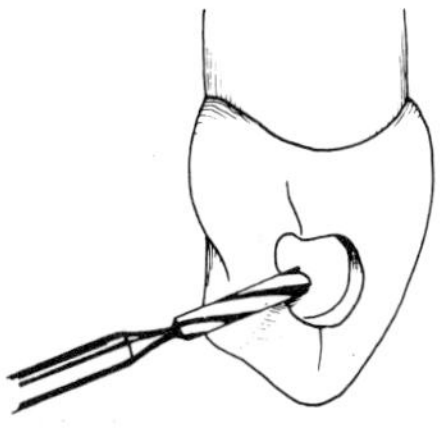

**Fig. 10.3b**

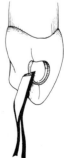

**Fig. 10.3c**

*(illustrations continued overleaf)*

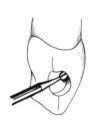

Fig. 10.3d

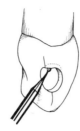

Fig. 10.3e

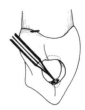

Fig. 10.3f

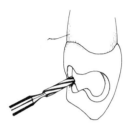

Fig. 10.3g

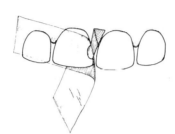

Fig. 10.3h

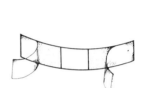

Fig. 10.3i

## Technique: Class IV composite resin restoration

| Procedure | Method | Rationale | Notes |
|---|---|---|---|
| 1. Prepare and line the cavity | The Class IV cavity preparation is similar to the Class III, but that part of the incisal edge that is undermined by caries is cut back. Line the cavity with calcium hydroxide. | | |
| 2. Select and trim a crown form | Select a crown form and cut it to fit over the cavity, overlapping the cavity margin by about 4 mm labially, incisally and palatally (Fig. 10.4a). | The margin of the crown form outlines the periphery of the planned restoration. | |
| 3. Clean the tooth surface<br>4. Isolate the tooth<br>5. Etch the enamel<br>6. Wash and dry the enamel | See 'composite resin crown restoration' (Ch. 28). Etching is extended about 6 mm from the labial, incisal and palatal cavity margins (Fig. 10.4b). | Etching must be carried beyond the planned periphery of the restoration, to ensure that the margin of the restoration is placed on etched enamel. | |

| Procedure | Method | Rationale | Notes |
|---|---|---|---|
| 7. Place the composite resin | Fill the cavity and the crown form with composite resin, and carefully position the crown form on the tooth (Fig. 10.4c). | | A thin layer of unfilled resin may be applied to the etched enamel before placing the restorative material, but this is not essential. |
| 8. Remove excess composite<br>9. Trim and finish the restoration | See 'composite resin crown restoration.' (page 202) | | |

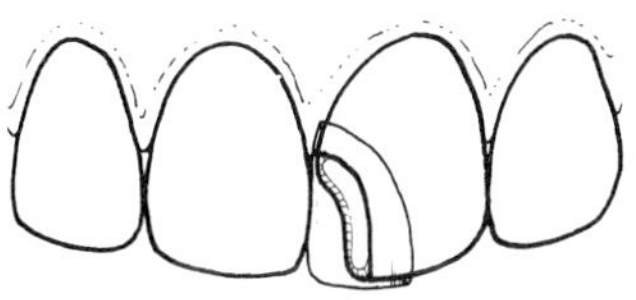

Fig. 10.4a 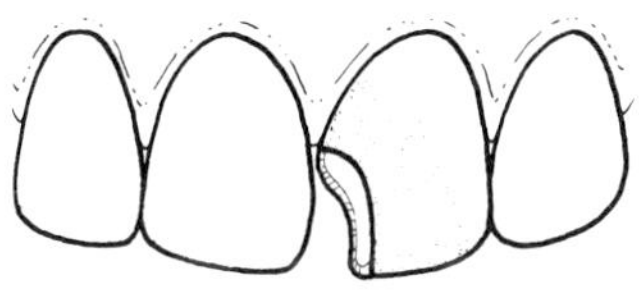      Fig. 10.4b 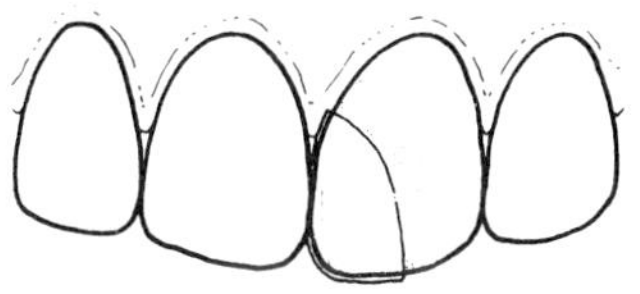      Fig. 10.4c

## STAINLESS STEEL CROWNS FOR FIRST PERMANENT MOLARS

The use of stainless steel crowns for primary molars has been described in Chapter 8. These crowns are also available in sizes suitable for first permanent molars and are particularly useful for restoring very carious or hypoplastic teeth, either semi-permanently before replacement with gold crowns when the child is older, or only temporarily for a year or two before extracting the teeth at the optimum stage of dental development (Ch. 22).

REFERENCES

Anderson R J 1981 The changes in the dental health of 12-year-old schoolchildren in two Somerset schools. British Dental Journal 150:218–221

Andlaw R J, Burchell C K, Tucker G J 1981 Comparison of dental health of 11-year-old children in 1970 and 1979, and of 14-year-old children in 1973 and 1979: studies in Bristol, England. Caries Research 16:257–264

Berman D S, Slack G L 1972 Dental caries in English school children: a longitudinal study. British Dental Journal 133:529–538

Going R E 1984 Sealant effect on incipient caries, enamel maturation, and future caries susceptibility. Journal of Dental Education 48:35–41

Hargreaves J A 1964 The problem of caries in child dental health. British Dental Journal 116:386–390

Houpt M, Eidelman E, Shey Z, Fuks A, Chosack A, Shapira J 1985 Occlusal composite restorations: 4-year results. Journal of the American Dental Association 110:351–353

Raadal M 1978 Follow-up study of sealing and filling with composite resins in the prevention of occlusal caries. Community Dentistry and Oral Epidemiology 6:176–180

Simonsen R J 1980 Preventive resin restorations: three-year results. Journal of the American Dental Association 100:535–539

Simonsen R J 1985 Conservation of tooth structure in restorative dentistry. Quintessence International 16:15–24

Simonsen R J, Stallard R E 1977 Sealant restorations utilising a diluted filled composite resin. Quintessence International, report no. 1514

Todd J E and Dodd T 1985 Children's dental health in the United Kingdom 1983. Her Majesty's Stationery Office, London, p 18

# PART FOUR

# Treatment of abnormalities of the primary and mixed dentitions

# 11

# Normal development of occlusion

The primary dentition
Eruption of first permanent molars
Eruption of permanent incisors
Eruption of premolars and canines

This Part of the book is concerned with the treatment of abnormalities of the primary and mixed dentitions. However, before considering abnormalities, a short account is given in this Chapter of normal development of the occlusion.

Formation of the primary dentition begins after 4 to 5 months of intra-uterine life (Table 11.1). The first teeth usually erupt 6 or 7 months after birth and all primary teeth have usually erupted by 2½ or 3 years of age.

**Table 11.1** Chronology of development of the primary dentition (from Lunt and Law, 1974).

| Teeth | Calcification begins (weeks in utero) | Crown complete (months) | Eruption (months) |
|---|---|---|---|
| Incisors | 13–16 | 1½–3 | 6–9 |
| Canines | 15–18 | 9 | 18–20 |
| First molars | 14–17 | 6 | 12–15 |
| Second molars | 16–23 | 10–11 | 24–36 |

Root development is complete 1–1½ years after tooth eruption.

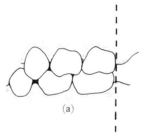

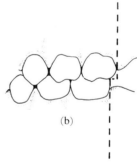

**Fig. 11.1** Primary dentition with (a) 'straight' second molar relationship, and (b) 'mesial step' second molar relationship.

## THE PRIMARY DENTITION

Many opinions have been expressed about the features that characterise a normal primary dentition, but three features are seen frequently enough for them to be considered normal:

1. *'Straight' second molar relationship.* In most dentitions the second primary molars are in cusp-to-cusp occlusion so that the terminal plane of the dentition is straight (Fig. 11.1a). In some dentitions the mandibular second molar is more mesially placed than the maxillary, creating a mesial 'step' (Fig. 11.1b); this can also be considered normal (Baume, 1950; Ravn, 1975). Distal 'steps' also occur (Foster and Hamilton, 1969), and indicate a Class II arch relationship.

2. *Incisor spacing.* Spacing between the primary incisors is normal, and indicates that the permanent teeth will probably have adequate space into which to erupt. Lack of spacing or imbrication of primary incisors are signs that the permanent incisors will probably be crowded when they erupt.

3. *Anthropoid (primate) spaces.* The most common sites for spaces in the primary dentition are in

the canine regions (Foster and Hamilton, 1969). The 'anthropoid spaces' are mesial to the maxillary canines and distal to the mandibular canines.

Considerable variations occur in the overbite and overjet of incisors and it is difficult to define normality (Foster, 1982).

### The primary dentition between age three and six years

Once the primary dentition is completed, the dimensions and form of the arches change very little until permanent teeth begin to erupt; any increases in width and length that have been reported are small (Baume, 1950; Clinch 1951; Foster, Grundy and Lavelle, 1972). Interdental spaces in spaced dentitions do not increase in width, nor do spaces develop in unspaced dentitions. However, two changes may be seen during this period: attrition of teeth (especially of anterior teeth), and reduction of overbite and overjet, so that the incisors may occlude 'edge to edge'.

## ERUPTION OF FIRST PERMANENT MOLARS

The normal or Class I occlusal relationship of first permanent molars is shown when the tip of the mesio-buccal cusp of the maxillary molar occludes in the buccal groove of the mandibular molar. Baume (1950) suggested three ways by which this relationship may be achieved:

1. In primary dentitions which terminate in marked mesial 'steps', the first permanent

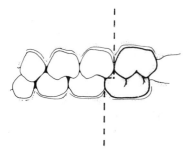

**Fig. 11.2** Eruption of first permanent molars directly into Class I relationship.

molars erupt directly into Class I occlusion (Fig. 11.2).

2. In spaced primary dentitions with straight terminal planes, eruption of first permanent molars pushes the mandibular primary molars forward into the anthropoid spaces so that mesial-step terminal planes are created. The mandibular first permanent molars are then able to erupt into Class I occlusion (Fig. 11.3).

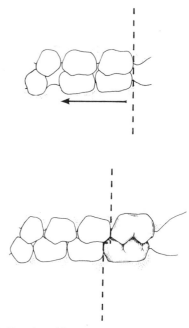

**Fig. 11.3** Eruption of first permanent molars into Class I relationship after mesial movement of mandibular primary molars into the anthropoid spaces.

3. In 'closed' primary dentitions (i.e. those having no interdental spaces), mesial movement of the mandibular primary molars cannot occur. The permanent molars therefore erupt cusp-to-cusp, and normal occlusion is only achieved when the second primary molars are replaced by the smaller second premolars (Fig. 11.4a and b). The permanent molars move forward into the spaces that become available, and since these are greater in the mandible than in the maxilla (because mandibular second primary molars are particularly large teeth), the mandibular permanent molars are able to move forward more than the maxillary molars, and establish Class I relationships.

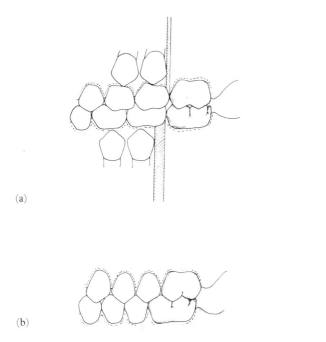

(a)

(b)

**Fig. 11.4** (a) Eruption of first permanent molars into cusp-to-cusp relationship and (b) establishment of Class I relationship after exfoliation of primary molars.

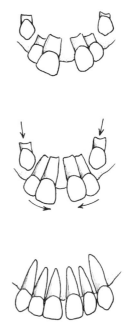

**Fig. 11.5** Eruption of permanent incisors.

## ERUPTION OF PERMANENT INCISORS

Spacing between primary incisors is an important factor in allowing the relatively large permanent incisors to be accomodated in the arch. Further space is provided by labial proclination of permanent incisors, which increases the arch perimeter, and by alveolar bone growth, which increases the intercanine width of the arch. This growth is usually complete when the lateral incisors reach full eruption, so that crowding of incisors at that stage of development does not improve: indeed it may worsen in later years due to pressure from crowded posterior teeth.

Eruption of each tooth pair is usually symmetrical: delay of a few months in the eruption of a tooth after the contralateral tooth has erupted usually indicates an abnormality.

Maxillary incisors often erupt with some distal inclination of their crowns, an appearance sometimes referred to as 'the ugly duckling stage'; usually they straighten gradually with the eruption of lateral incisors and canines (Fig. 11.5).

## ERUPTION OF PREMOLARS AND CANINES

The sum of the mesio-distal dimensions of the primary canine and molars in each quadrant of the dentition always exceeds that of the successional canine and premolars (Fig. 11.6); the excess is accounted for chiefly by the difference in size between the second primary molar and the premolar that replaces it. The excess space, sometimes referred to as the 'leeway space', is important in some dentitions for allowing final adjustment of first molar occlusion. Also, it ensures (if the primary teeth are not prematurely removed) that there will be adequate space for the eruption of permanent canines and premolars.

The occlusion does not remain static but undergoes some changes during adolescence. These changes may include a decrease in arch length and in intercanine width, and an increase in incisor irregularity. However, it is not possible to predict the changes that will occur in an individual patient (Sinclair and Little, 1983).

The chronology of development of the permanent dentition is presented in Table 11.2.

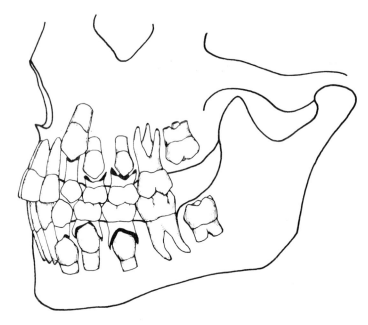

**Fig. 11.6** Eruption of permanent canines and premolars. The sum of the mesio-distal dimensions of the primary teeth is greater than that of their successors.

**Table 11.2** Chronology of development of the permanent dentition (from Schour and Massler, 1940)

| Teeth | Calcification begins | Crown complete (years) | Eruption (years) |
|---|---|---|---|
| First molars | Birth | 2½–3 | 5½–6 |
| Mandibular central incisor | 3–4 months | 4–5 | 6–7 |
| Mandibular lateral incisor | 3–4 months | 4–5 | 7–8 |
| Maxillary central incisor | 3–4 months | 4–5 | 7–8 |
| Maxillary lateral incisor | 10–12 months | 4–5 | 8–9 |
| Mandibular canine | 4–5 months | 6–7 | 9–10 |
| Maxillary first premolar | 1½–1¾ years | 5–6 | 10–11 |
| Mandibular first premolar | 1¾–2 years | 5–6 | 10–12 |
| Maxillary canine | 4–5 months | 6–7 | 11–12 |
| Maxillary second premolar | 2–2¼ years | 6–7 | 10–12 |
| Mandibular second premolar | 2¼–2½ years | 6–7 | 11–12 |
| Second molars | 2½–3 years | 7–8 | 12–13 |
| Third molars | 7–10 years | 12–16 | 16–21 |

Root development is complete about 3 years after tooth eruption.

REFERENCES

Baume L J 1950 Physiological tooth migration and its significance to the development of occlusion. Journal of Dental Research 29:133–132, 331–337, 338–348, 440–447
Clinch L M 1951 An analysis of serial models between three and eight years of age. Dental Record 71:61–72
Foster T D 1982 A textbook of orthodontics, 2nd edn. Oxford, Blackwell, p 47–48
Foster T D, Hamilton M C 1969 Occlusion in the primary dentition. British Dental Journal 126:76–79
Foster T D, Grundy M C, Lavelle C L B 1972 Changes in occlusion in the primary dentition between 2½ and 5½ years of age. Transaction of the European Orthodontic Society 1972:75–84
Lunt R C, Law D B 1974 A review of the chronology of calcification of deciduous teeth. Journal of the American Dental Association 89:599–606
Ravn J J 1975 Occlusion in the primary dentition in three year old children. Scandinavian Journal of Dental Research 83:123–130
Schour I, Massler M 1940 Studies in tooth development: The growth pattern of human teeth. Journal of the American Dental Association 27:1918–1931
Sinclair PM, Little RM 1983 Maturation of untreated normal occlusions. American Journal of Orthodontics 83:114–123

RECOMMENDED READING

Van der Linden PGM 1983 Development of the dentition. Quintessence, Chicago

# 12

# Abnormalities of tooth eruption

Natal teeth
'Teething'
Eruption cyst
Submerged primary molars
Ectopic eruption of first permanent molars
Delayed eruption of permanent teeth

## NATAL TEETH

Occasionally one or more teeth are erupted at birth and are described as natal teeth. They are usually members of the normal series, not supernumerary elements, and are found most commonly in the mandibular incisor region. The enamel is usually hypoplastic and, since there is no root formation at the time of birth, the teeth are only loosely attached.

### Treatment

Since a natal tooth is part of the normal dentition, it should be retained unless it causes the mother discomfort (if the baby is breast fed), or if it is so loose that it might become dislodged and inhaled. Root growth takes place normally after birth and the attachment of the tooth gradually improves.

## 'TEETHING'

Eruption of the primary dentition usually begins in the fifth or sixth month of a child's life. The first appearance of normal teeth is eagerly awaited by the parents since it represents an important early milestone in development. In most cases eruption of teeth causes no distress to the child or parents but sometimes the process causes local irritation, which is usually minor but which may be severe enough to interfere with the child's sleep. The small primary incisors usually erupt without difficulty; 'teething' problems are more commonly associated with eruption of the relatively large molars.

The signs of teething may be manifested both locally (Seward, 1971) and systemically (Seward, 1972a):

Local.     Redness or swelling of the gingiva over the erupting tooth.
           Patches of erythema on the cheeks.
Systemic.  General irritability, and crying.
           Loss of appetite.
           Sleeplessness.
           Increased salivation and drooling.
           Reduced appetite.
           Increased thirst.
           Circumoral rash.

### Treatment

*Local*

*1. Teething toys.* A baby uses hands and mouth to explore unfamiliar objects. A variety of teething rings, rattles and keys are available in mothercraft shops. They are designed to satisfy the natural tendency of the child to bite and suck. The baby may obtain relief from soreness by the pressure of biting, and teething toys have a useful function. Parents should be advised to purchase only well made, smooth toys; poorly made, rough toys can increase irritation in the mouth, and some cheap products have been shown to have high lead contents.

*2. Teething foods.* Hard rusk or biscuit preparations are used in the same way as teething toys. Teething foods consist mainly of flour and fat. It is important that they should contain no sugar or sweetening, since this might contribute to the development of a 'sweet tooth'.

*3. Topical medicaments.* Various types of ointments and jellies are available for topical appli-

**Table 12.1** Active ingredients in preparations used for the control of teething problems.

| Name | Local analgesic | Antiseptic | Analgesic/anti-inflammatory agent |
|---|---|---|---|
| Bonjela | none | 0.01% cetalkonium chloride<br>4.6% glycerin<br>39% alcohol | 8.7% choline salicylate<br>0.05% menthol |
| Dentinox | 0.3% lignocaine hydrochloride | 0.1% cetylpyridinium<br>chloride<br>0.3% polyethoxdodecane<br>3% alcohol | 0.06% menthol<br>0.08% myrrh tincture |
| Moore's Teething Jelly (Teejel Gel) | none | 0.01% cetalkonium chloride | 8.7% choline salicylate |
| Steedman's Teething Jelly | none | 0.02% cetylpyridinium<br>chloride<br>0.0025% ethyl nicotinate | none |

cation to the gingiva. Common ingredients include salicylates, which combine local counter-irritant and anti-inflammatory properties with systemic analgesic and antipyretic effects; antiseptics, which control infection at the site of tooth eruption; and local analgesics, which provide rapid but short-lived pain relief. Some topical preparations for the control of teething problems are listed in Table 12.1.

*Systemic*

Two main types of drugs are used to treat teething problems: analgesics (to relieve pain) and hypnotics (to aid sleep).

*1. Analgesics.* Paracetamol Elixir Paediatric B.P.C. 5 ml contains 120 mg of paracetamol. A sugar-free preparation is now available.
Dosage: Up to 1 year — 5 ml at bedtime.
1–5 years — 10 ml at bedtime.

*2. Hypnotics and sedatives.* There is understandable reluctance to prescribe these drugs for very young children. However, a succession of sleepless nights imposes a severe strain on parents and other members of the family, and a short course of a hypnotic drug will help to restore normal rhythms of sleep. It may be necessary to use hypnotics in combination with local and systemic analgesics.

Chloral Elixir Paediatric B.P.C. 5 ml contains 200 mg of chloral hydrate.

Dosage: Up to 1 year — 2.5 ml twice daily.
1–5 years — 2.5 to 5 ml three times daily.
Dichloralphenazone Elixir B.P.C. (Welldorm Elixir). 5 ml contains 225 mg of dichloralphenazone.
Dosage: Up to 1 year — 2.5 to 5 ml at bedtime.
1–5 years — 5 to 10 ml at bedtime.

The treatment of teething has been reviewed by Seward (1972b). Guidance for the selection of treatment is given below:

| *Complaint* | *Treatment* |
|---|---|
| Irritation at site of tooth eruption. | Topical application. |
| Daytime irritability and fretfulness. | Topical application and systemic analgesic. |
| Disturbed sleep. | Topical application, systemic analgesic and hypnotic. |

## ERUPTION CYST

An eruption cyst may develop in relation to an erupting primary tooth. The normal follicular space around the crown is dilated by accumulation of tissue fluid or blood, forming a type of dentigerous cyst (Shafer, Hine and Levy, 1974; Shear, 1983). Eruption cysts occur most commonly over the large occlusal surfaces of primary molars. At first there is a bluish area over the erupting tooth, and later there may be redness and swelling of the mucosa. Enlargement of the cyst causes it to be bitten upon by opposing teeth, and this increases the child's discomfort.

## Treatment

Many eruption cysts are transient and the trouble is resolved by rupture of the cyst and eruption of the tooth. Sometimes the problem becomes more serious, causing prolonged crying and loss of sleep. If conservative treatment, as given for teething problems, is ineffective, it may be necessary to incise the cyst.

Simple incision of the cyst with a scalpel under topical or local analgesia may be effective. However, a single incision may heal rapidly and allow recurrence of the cyst; because of this possibility, the more thorough technique advocated by Seward (1972b) may be preferred. A longitudinal incision is made along the side of the swelling and a blade of a pair of 'mosquito' forceps is inserted into the cystic space over the crown of the tooth. The roof of the cyst is then held taut whilst an elliptical portion is removed by means of a second incision.

## SUBMERGED PRIMARY MOLARS

A submerged tooth is one that has failed to maintain its position relative to adjacent teeth in the developing dentition, and is therefore below the occlusal level. Surveys conducted in various countries have reported prevalence figures ranging from 1.3 per cent to 8.9 per cent in children up to 12 years of age (Andlaw, 1977; Kurol, 1981).

Mandibular primary molars are affected more commonly than maxillary molars. In most studies the tooth most commonly affected was the first primary molar, but in others it was the second molar. The second molar tends to become grossly submerged, perhaps below gingival level, more frequently than does the first molar.

The mechanism of submergence is not properly understood, but appears to be related to ankylosis (Kurol and Magnusson, 1984), possibly brought about by excessive bone deposition during the alternating resorption and repair phases that characterise normal root resorption of primary teeth; further occlusal movement of the tooth is retarded or arrested, and it therefore falls below the occlusal level of neighbouring teeth.

Although submergence is usually associated with primary molars, permanent molars are occasionally affected (Oliver, Richmond and Hunter, 1986).

## Treatment

A submerged primary molar need not always be extracted: many submerged primary teeth (especially first molars) exfoliate normally and do not interfere with the eruption of premolars (Brearley and McKibben, 1973). However, some form of treatment becomes necessary if there are radiological signs of interference with premolar eruption, or if there is a possibility of adjacent teeth tilting over the submerged tooth, or if there is a danger that the tooth may become submerged below gingival level.

The type of treatment required depends on the degree of infra-occlusion (Andlaw, 1974).

1. Minimal infra-occlusion (marginal ridge of submerged tooth occlusal to adjacent contact areas);
Observe to determine whether the condition worsens. Study models are an essential aid to observation. Take radiographs every 6 to 12 months to determine if premolar eruption is being affected.
2. Moderate infra-occlusion (marginal ridge of submerged tooth just cervical to adjacent contact areas):
A short period of clinical and radiological observation, as outlined above, may again be appropriate, but in the case of moderate infra-occlusion it is more likely that one or more indications for treatment will be present. There are two alternatives:
a. Extract the submerged tooth. It is probable, but not inevitable, that because of ankylosis the tooth will be more difficult to extract than a normal tooth. A surgical approach may be necessary, and appropriate pre-

operative arrangements for this should be made.

It is wrong to remove any primary tooth without considering the effects that the extraction may have on the development of the dentition; the need to balance or compensate the extraction, or to fit a space maintainer, should be considered (Ch. 17).

b. Retain the submerged tooth. If there are no indications of interference with premolar eruption, the submerged tooth may be retained. However, it may be necessary to restore normal contacts with adjacent teeth; this may be achieved by fitting a stainless steel crown (Ch. 8), or by building up the occlusal surface with composite resin (Gorelick, 1977).

3. Severe infra-occlusion (marginal ridge at gingival level):
Extract the submerged molar unless a radiograph shows that resorption of the tooth is almost complete and that eruption of the successional premolar is imminent. Consideration should again be given to the need to balance the extraction or maintain the space.

Submerged permanent molars must be extracted.

## ECTOPIC ERUPTION OF FIRST PERMANENT MOLARS

Ectopic eruption of a first permanent molar results in premature, atypical, resorption of the second primary molar and impaction of the permanent tooth against the crown or root of the primary molar. Usually, further eruption of the permanent tooth is prevented, but occasionally the impaction is temporary (Young, 1957). Almost always it is a maxillary molar that is affected.

The aetiology of the condition is uncertain, but associated factors are mesial inclination and larger-than-average size of the first permanent molars (Bjerklin and Kurol, 1983), and a high tooth-tissue ratio, that is, large teeth in a short maxilla (Pulver, 1968).

## Treatment

Initially, treatment should be instituted to disimpact the first molar; if this is unsuccessful it may be necessary to extract the second primary molar.

If the tooth is impacted against the crown of the primary molar (Fig. 12.1a) it may be possible to disimpact it using soft brass ligature wire (0.5–0.7 mm diameter), as follows:

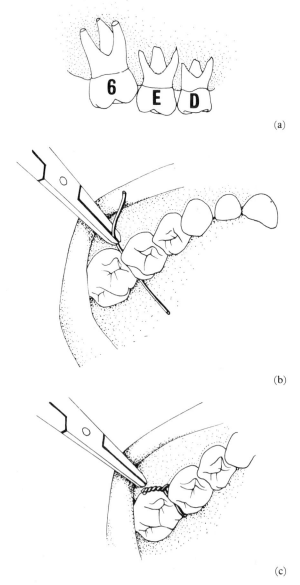

(a)

(b)

(c)

**Fig. 12.1** One of the methods of treating ectopic eruption of a first permanent molar.

1. Anaesthetise the gingiva buccal and palatal to the tooth.
2. Holding the wire in Spencer Wells forceps, pass it under the contact point from buccal to palatal (Fig. 12.1b).
3. Twist the ends together over the contact point; do not overtighten or the wire will snap.
4. Cut off ends, leaving about 5 mm twisted together.
5. Tuck in neatly to avoid traumatising the cheeks or gingiva (Fig. .12.1c).
6. Review every two weeks and retighten.

Although this method is sometimes successful, more reliable results are obtained by using an orthodontic appliance. Various designs of appliance have been described, but the main features are a band on the second primary molar and a spring engaging on the first permanent molar, usually on its occlusal surface (Braden, 1964; Groper, 1985). Cervical traction applied to the first molar with headgear, after extracting the second primary molar, has also been used (Kurol and Bjerklin, 1984).

If this treatment is not practicable the second primary molar must be extracted, and consideration should be given to compensating the extraction or to fitting a space maintainer.

## DELAYED ERUPTION OF PERMANENT TEETH

The data on tooth development given in Table 11.2 conceal the fact that there are considerable normal variations between children. Although a delay in tooth eruption may be associated with a specific condition (e.g. Down's Syndrome), most cases of apparent delay are in fact within the normal range. Parents should be reassured, and occlusal development reviewed. However, as contralateral teeth usually erupt together, a delay of more than a month or two in the eruption of one of the teeth gives cause for concern.

Localised eruption delay is more common in the permanent dentition than in the primary dentition; some of the causes are listed below:

Incisors:  Delayed resorption of a primary incisor following trauma and death of the pulp.
Dilaceration (Ch. 14).
Supernumerary teeth (Ch. 15).
Very early loss of primary tooth, followed by formation of bone in the tooth socket.

Canines:  Abnormal eruption path of maxillary canines.

Premolars:  Impaction against other teeth due to abnormal angulation or crowding.
Retarded resorption of a primary molar.
Submerged primary molar (p. 128).

Molars:  Impaction against other teeth; especially affecting third molars.

Other conditions, such as a dentigerous cyst, may affect any tooth.

## REFERENCES

Andlaw R J 1974 Submerged deciduous molars: a review with special reference to the rationale of treatment. Journal of the International Association of Dentistry for Children 5:59–66

Andlaw R J 1977 Submerged deciduous molars: a prevalence survey in Somerset. Journal of the International Association of Dentistry for Children 8:42–45

Bjerklin K, Kurol J 1983 Ectopic eruption of the maxillary first permanent molar: etiologic factors. American Journal of Orthodontics 84:147–155

Brearley L J, McKibben D H 1973 Ankylosis of primary teeth. Journal of Dentistry for Children 40:54–63

Braden R E 1964 Ectopic eruption of maxillary permanent first molars. Dental Clinics of North America (July) 441–448

Gorelick L 1977 Direct bonding in the management of an ankylosed second deciduous molar. Journal of the American Dental Association 95:307–309

Groper J N 1985 A simplified treatment for correcting an ectopically erupting maxillary first permanent molar. Journal of Dentistry for Children 52:374–376

Kurol J 1981 Infraocclusion of primary molars: an epidemiologic and familial study. Community Dentistry Oral Epidemiology 9:94–102

Kurol J, Bjerklin K 1984 Treatment of children with ectopic eruption of the children with ectopic eruption of the maxillary first permanent molar by cervical traction. American Journal of Orthodontics 86:483–492

Kurol J, Magnusson B C 1984 Infraocclusion of primary molars: a histological study. Scandinavian Journal of Dental Research 92:564–576

Oliver R G, Richmond S, Hunter 1986 Submerged permanent molars: four case reports. British Dental Journal 160:128–130

Pulver F 1968 Ectopic eruption of first permanent molars. Journal of Dentistry for Children 35:138–147

Seward M H 1971 Local disturbances attributable to eruption of the human primary dentition. British Dental Journal 130:72–72

Seward M H 1972a General disturbances attributable to eruption of the human primary dentition. Journal of Dentistry for Children 39:178–183

Seward M H 1972b Treatment of teething in infants. British Dental Journal 132:33–36

Shafer W G, Hine M K, Levy B M 1974 A textbook of oral pathology. Saunders, Philadelphia, p 239

Shear M 1983 Cysts of the oral region, 2nd edn. Wright, Bristol, Ch 6

Young D 1957 Ectopic eruption of the first permanent molars. Journal of Dentistry for Children 24:153–162

RECOMMENDED READING

Davis J M, Law D B, Lewis T M 1981 An atlas of pedodontics, 2nd edn. Saunders, Philadelphia, ch 3

Rapp R, Winter G B 1979 A colour atlas of clinical conditions in paedodontics. Wolfe, London

# Abnormalities of tooth structure

Dental tissues are formed in two stages: the organic matrix is deposited first, and then mineralisation takes place. Disturbance of either of these stages may cause abnormalities of tooth structure, which are particularly important when enamel is involved. A disturbance of matrix deposition produces hypoplasia, characterised by enamel that is irregular in thickness or deficient in structure; defects may range from small pits or grooves in the enamel surface to gross deficiency. Disturbance in the second stage of development causes hypomineralisation; although the enamel is of normal thickness, part of it, at least, is poorly mineralised.

## ENAMEL HYPOPLASIA AND HYPOMINERALISATION

### Local

Developing permanent teeth may be damaged by trauma or infection associated with their predecessors.

Intrusion or severe displacement of a primary incisor as a result of trauma may affect the developing permanent incisor. The younger the child at the time of injury the greater the chance that the enamel of the permanent tooth will be hypoplastic. If the injury occurs after 4 years of age, hypomineralisation rather than hypoplasia is more common, often showing as white or brown patches on the labial surface.

The trauma associated with extraction of a primary molar may damage the developing premolar, expecially if the child is under 4 or 5 years of age when premolar development is at an early stage.

Similarly, the type of damage that may be caused by infection of a primary tooth depends on the stage of development of the permanent successor.

### Systemic

Formation of primary teeth begins *in utero* (Table 11.1). Until birth, the dentition is protected against all but the most severe systemic disturbances; therefore, prenatal enamel usually has a regular, homogeneous structure. There are microscopic differences between pre- and postnatal enamel and sometimes the difference is sufficiently marked to be seen clinically as 'neonatal lines' across the crowns of the teeth that were developing at birth. A well-marked neonatal line, or defective postnatal enamel, are related to systemic upsets at birth or during postnatal development.

The many systemic factors that may affect developing teeth have been reviewed by Pindborg (1982); they include genetically-transmitted factors (e.g. those causing amelogenesis imperfecta), inborn errors of metabolism (e.g. phenylketonuria), neonatal disturbances (e.g. premature birth, hypocalcaemia, haemolytic anaemia), endocrinopathies (e.g. hypoparathyroidism), nephropathies (e.g. nephrotic syndrome), gastro-intestinal disease, liver disease and excessive ingestion of fluoride. The common viral infections are often considered to be causes of enamel hypoplasia, but supporting evidence only exists in relation to rubella syndrome.

### Treatment of anterior teeth

Small areas of hypomineralised labial enamel may

not cause concern to the child or parent and therefore not require treatment. On the other hand severely hypoplastic teeth may be not only unsightly but also sensitive because of exposed dentine. Although the porcelain jacket crown may be regarded as the most satisfactory long-term restoration for a severely hypoplastic or discoloured tooth, it is not an appropriate restoration for children: it is generally agreed that the amount of tooth reduction necessary to make a porcelain jacket crown places at risk the relatively large pulp of a child's tooth. The more conservative veneering methods described below have been considered to offer only a temporary solution (Smith and Pulver, 1982; Cooley 1984), but new developments in materials and techniques have raised hopes that they might provide satisfactory long-term alternatives to the porcelain jacket crown.

Before proceeding with any veneering technique, the decision must be made whether to reduce the thickness of labial enamel before placing the veneer.

If enamel thickness is not reduced (the approach often preferred, especially in children) it is inevitable that the labial bulk of the tooth will be increased, which may not be acceptable. On the other hand, the appearance of an instanding or rotated tooth can be improved by the addition of a labial veneer. The decision to reduce the thickness of labial enamel is usually taken when it is considered undesirable to increase the labial bulk of the tooth, and also if the tooth is very discoloured, since additional layers of composite resin may be required to mask severe discolourations (p. 135).

## Composite resin veneer

Composite resin may be used to cover either localised areas of abnormal enamel or the entire labial surface (Black, 1982). Resins that polymerise when exposed to visible light are generally preferred to autopolymerising resins because they allow unlimited working time; shades may be mixed on the tooth surface until a pleasing result is obtained, and excess may be removed from the margins, before initiating polymerisation with the light source. The microfilled resins, which contain very small filler particles, are usually preferred

because they can be polished to a smoother finish than can other types of composite.

## Technique for full labial veneer

(If it is decided not to reduce the thickness of labial enamel, proceed to stage 4)

1. Use a cylindrical or tapered diamond to reduce the thickness of labial enamel by about 0.5 mm. Depressions or grooves 0.5 mm deep may be made first to facilitate this procedure.
2. Finish the preparation 0.5 mm short of the gingival margin (Fig. 13.1a). However, if the cervical part of the tooth crown is hypoplastic or discoloured, finish the preparation subgingivally.
3. Mesially and distally, finish the preparation just labial to the contact points but, if the enamel is hypoplastic or discoloured in those areas, carry the preparation palatal to the contact points.
4. Clean the tooth with a slurry of pumice in water, or with an oil-free prophylaxis paste. Wash the paste away with a water spray and dry the tooth.
5. Isolate the tooth and place a suitable matrix. Use either a conventional straight matrix strip or a shaped strip made specially for the purpose (Contour Strip, Vivadent) (Fig. 13.1b).
6. Etch, wash and dry the labial enamel as previously described (p. 56).
7. Apply a thin layer of unfilled resin ('bonding agent') to the etched and dried enamel with a fine brush or other suitable applicator (Fig. 13.1c). Direct the air syringe gently over the surface to remove excess resin. If the enamel is discoloured, a colour neutraliser or an opaquer may be used at this stage (p. 135).
8. Apply a small amount of filled composite resin of appropriate shade to the central part of the labial surface. Currently available materials vary considerably in their viscosity. The more viscous materials need to be spread with a dental instrument, and may then be smoothed with a small brush; the less viscous materials may be spread easily with the brush. Add further increments of composite resin as

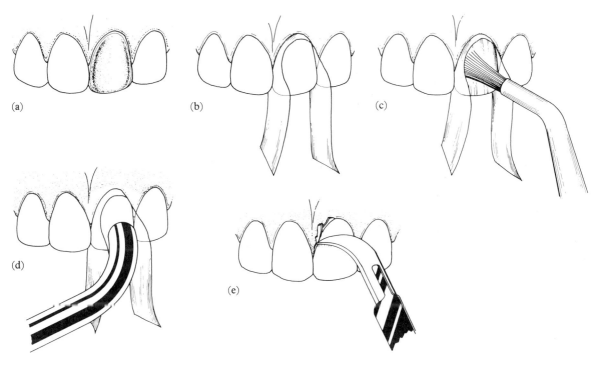

**Fig. 13.1**

required, using different shades if necessary to produce a good colour match with adjacent teeth and to achieve a gradual transition from a relatively dark gingival area to a lighter, more translucent, incisal region.

If using an autopolymering resin, the time available for placing the resin is limited, and it is therefore advisable to use a crown form. Cut off the palatal part of the crown form, and trim the mesial, distal and cervical margins to the planned periphery of the veneer; but leave the incisal margin overlapping the incisal edge of the tooth, to facilitate accurate placement of the crown form on the tooth. If several teeth are to be treated, it might be preferable to prepare the crown forms beforehand on a model (King and Rule, 1980).

9. If using a light-sensitive resin, carefully remove excess from around the margin before applying the light source (Fig. 13.1d).
10. After the resin has polymerised, remove the matrix, explore the margin carefully and smooth with finishing burs and polishing discs. A scalpel is useful to remove excess at the margin (Fig. 13.1e).

The use of composite resin can dramatically improve the appearance of hypomineralised, hypoplastic or discoloured teeth. Unfortunately the surface of composite resin becomes abraded and stained, and therefore the appearance of veneers tends to deteriorate. The more recently introduced microfilled composites stain less than do the larger-particle composites.

### Modification of tooth colour

Composite resin is a translucent material and cannot mask tooth discolouration unless it is used in thick layers, which is usually undesirable. For this reason, colour tints or opaquers are included with products that are marketed specifically as veneering materials.

A colour tint is used to neutralise the colour of the discoloured tooth to the neutral colour of grey. The colour wheel (Fig. 13.2) indicates which

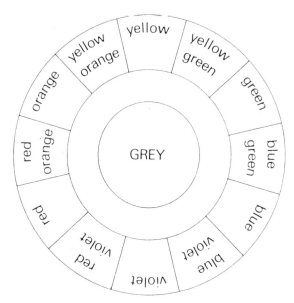

**Fig. 13.2** The colour wheel used in selecting colours for colour modification.

colour must be used to neutralise another. Colours on opposite sides of the wheel neutralise one another; for example, a yellow discolouration is neutralised by the addition of violet.

After the neutral grey colour has been obtained it must be lightened to the desired tooth colour. This can be done by applying one or more thin layers of either a tooth-coloured tint or an opaquer. Opaquers are tooth-coloured and act as reflective screens.

Not all manufacturers provide both colour tints and opaquers, and the recommended methods of using the materials differ. The vehicle for colour tints and opaquers is either the unfilled resin bonding agent, which is applied to etched enamel, or the composite paste that is used to cement the porcelain veneer. It is, of course, essential to follow the manufacturer's instructions carefully, but it is always important to apply layers of colour tint or opaquer very thinly; multiple thin layers may be used if necessary, but thick layers produce a dull, non- translucent appearance.

*Preformed acrylic veneer*

Preformed acrylic veneers (Mastique, L. D. Caulk) are available in a number of sizes for anterior maxillary teeth; they are cemented to etched labial enamel with composite resin. These veneers show little or no colour change up to four years after placement (Roberts, 1983; Rivkin and Warren, 1985).

*Techniques*

It must be decided either to reduce the thickness of enamel (as described for stages 1–3 of the composite resin veneer technique) or to fit the veneer to the normal tooth surface. The techniques are well illustrated by Murray and Bennett, 1985). There are two alternative techniques for fitting acrylic veneers: *direct*, in which the veneer is prepared in the surgery to fit the natural tooth, or *indirect*, in which an impression is taken of the teeth and the veneer is then prepared in the laboratory on a stone model.

*Direct technique*
1. Select a veneer of the correct size and shape.
2. With a stone mounted in a handpiece, carefully grind the fitting surface of the veneer until close adaptation with the labial surface of the tooth is obtained (Fig. 13.3a). The incisal edge of the veneer should be placed just on but not beyond the incisal edge of the tooth.
3. Apply a thin layer of 'primer' to the dry fitting surface of the veneer (Fig. 13.3b) and allow this to dry for 10 minutes; the primer ensures good adhesion of composite resin to the veneer.
4. Clean the labial surface of the tooth with a pumice slurry in water or with an oil-free prophylaxis paste. Wash the paste away with a water spray and dry the tooth.
5. Isolate the tooth and place a suitable matrix: either a conventional straight strip or a shaped strip made specially for veneering techniques (Contour Strip, Vivadent) (Fig. 13.1b).
6. Etch, wash and dry the labial enamel.
7. Apply a thin layer of unfilled resin to the etched and dried enamel with a small brush or other suitable applicator, and polymerise. If the enamel is discoloured, it is necessary to mask the colour (p. 135).
8. Place composite paste of previously selected shade on to the fitting surface of the veneer and press it gently into place on the tooth (Fig. 13.3c).

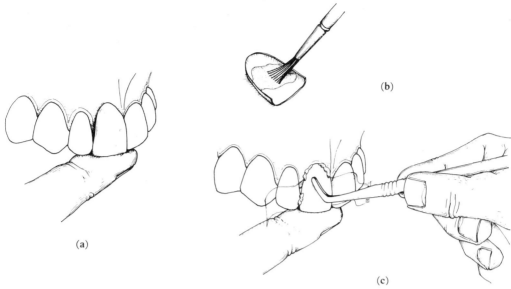

(b)

(a)

(c)

Fig. 13.3

9. Polymerise the resin and trim the margin (see under 'Composite resin veneer' stages 8 and 9).

*Indirect technique.* The indirect technique involves laboratory time but reduces surgery time, especially when several veneers are to be fitted. In addition, veneers can be adapted more closely to the teeth in the laboratory, by warming and applying pressure on them; this is done by fitting the veneers to the model, securing them with wide elastic bands placed around the model, and heating them in hot water (about 75°C) for several minutes.

Acrylic veneers have been found to give satisfactory results in the treatment of hypoplastic and discoloured teeth in children. However, acrylic is not highly resistant to abrasion and can cause gingival irritation if placed subgingivally. When veneers fracture it is invariably the veneer that breaks away from the underlying composite, indicating that the bond between acrylic and composite is weaker than that between composite and enamel, despite the use of primer on the fitting surface of the acrylic veneer.

### Porcelain veneers

Porcelain has several advantages over acrylic as a veneering material: its appearance is superior, it has better resistance to abrasion, it is well tolerated by gingival tissues and, because it can be etched, the bond to the composite resin used for cementing the veneer is greatly increased.

Because the veneers are individually made in the laboratory, they fit more closely than do the performed acrylic veneers, even if the latter are heat-adapted as described above. Therefore a porcelain veneer produces less bulk than an acrylic veneer if placed on a natural tooth surface. Despite this, a conservative enamel preparation is generally preferred (Calamia, 1985).

### Technique

1. The enamel preparation is similar to that described for the composite resin or acrylic veneer, but an incisal edge preparation may also be done. Alternative incisal edge preparations are illustrated in Figure 13.4; the preparations shown in c and d make it easier to locate the veneer accurately on the tooth surface, and also place the porcelain-tooth junction out of sight on the palatal surface of the tooth.
2. Take an impression with a rubber-based impression material. If the incisal edge has been prepared it may also be necessary to take an

impression of the lower arch and a wax registration of the teeth in occlusion.

3. If it is considered necessary to place a temporary restoration, flow a layer of acrylic or composite resin on to the labial enamel (which, of course, should not be etched). This usually remains in place if the patient is careful when toothbrushing.

4. Write precise instructions to the laboratory technician. Indicate the shade of tooth to be matched and make a simple drawing to show the area to be covered by the veneer; this is especially important if the veneer is to be placed on an unprepared tooth surface. If facilities are available for clinical photography, a colour print showing the anterior teeth would be helpful to the technician.

5. (The patient's next visit)

The veneers must be handled carefully not only because they are small and brittle but also because their fitting surfaces have been etched in the laboratory, and contamination of the etched surfaces must be avoided.

Brush a thin layer of silane coupling agent on to the fitting surface of the veneer, allow it to dry for 5 minutes.

6. Clean the tooth surface with a slurry of pumice in water or with an oil-free prophylaxis paste. Wash the pumice away with water, dry the tooth and then place the veneer in position to confirm that it fits properly.

7. Place a layer of try-in paste (composite resin not containing the light-sensitive catalyst) on the fitting surface of the veneer and try it in again. Check the colour match and invite the patient to comment on it.

8. In colour modification is required, proceed as described on page 135.

9. Remove the try-in paste by placing the veneer in acetone and gently dabbing the paste off with a small foam pad.

10. Isolate the tooth and place a matrix (Fig. 13.1b).

11. Etch, wash and dry the labial enamel.

12. Apply a thin layer of bonding agent to the etched enamel surface and to the fitting surface of the veneer, and polymerise.

13. Place a layer of composite paste on the veneer (just enough to cover the previously placed bonding agent). Position the veneer on the tooth and gently press it into place.

14. Maintain the veneer in position while removing excess composite with a probe or other convenient dental instrument.

If the incisal edge of the tooth was reduced, the veneer is firmly located in position but, if not, the veneer may easily be moved out of position while removing excess composite from the margin. To prevent this, use the polymerising light for 5 seconds; this stabilises the veneer while still allowing removal of excess composite.

15. When all excess composite has been removed, polymerise fully with the light.

16. Remove the matrix, check all margins carefully with a probe, and trim and polish as necessary with diamond or tungsten carbide finishing burs, and with abrasive discs.

17. A final polish of trimmed margins may be given with composite polishing paste.

Horn (1983) and Calamia (1985) have reported excellent results with porcelain veneers, but long-term assessment or the durability of the veneers must be awaited.

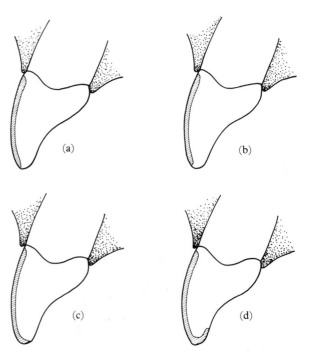

**Fig. 13.4** Alternative incisal edge preparations for a porcelain veneer.

### Castable apatite ceramic veneer

A very recent development is a castable apatite ceramic material that has physical and mechanical properties similar to those of enamel. A technique for making labial veneers (and other restorations) has been described (Hobo and Iwata, 1985), but no reports have yet been published of the clinical use of this material.

### Acrylic crown

If hypoplasia is severe and involves all surfaces of a tooth, a crown is the most appropriate restoration. For a child, a minimal, shoulderless tooth preparation is recommended, to avoid the possibility of damaging the pulp.

### Technique

1. Reduce the incisal edge by about 2 to 3 mm with a cylindrical diamond bur at high speed (Fig. 13.5a).

2. Slice across the mesial and distal surfaces with a fine pointed diamond (some dentists prefer to use a guarded safe-sided diamond disc at slow speed) (Fig. 13.5b). Angle the bur so that the walls of the preparation converge slightly from the cervical margin to the incisal edge. Do not produce a shoulder at the cervical margin.

3. Continuing with the tapered diamond, reduce the labial and palatal surfaces, again angling the bur to avoid producing a shoulder at the cervical margin (Fig. 13.5c). A tapered diamond with a plane tip is useful, the tip being placed in the gingival crevice. Remove only enough labial enamel to eliminate the natural bulbosity of the labial surface and to ensure that the acrylic crown will not be markedly more bulbous than the natural crown. The amount of palatal reduction depends on the occlusion; it need only be minimal if there is an incomplete overbite or an increased overjet (Fig. 13.5d).

4. Smooth the preparation with a finishing dia-

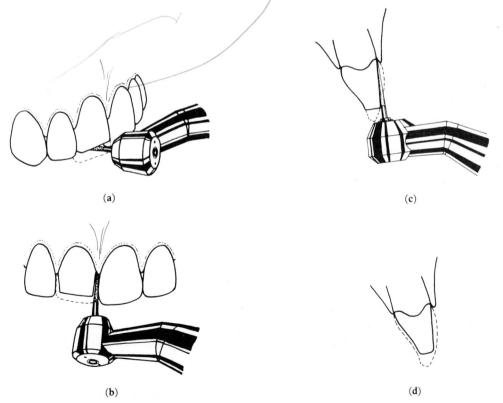

(a)

(b)

(c)

(d)

**Fig. 13.5**

mond, or with abrasive stones or discs; a smooth preparation helps to produce a good impression.

5. Take an impression with a silicone-type impression material in an impression tray, or with impression composition in an accurately trimmed copper ring.

6. Select a colour for the crown, using a shade guide.

7. Make a temporary crown with cold-cure acrylic resin in a cellulose acetate crown form (preformed temporary crowns are not convenient to use when tooth preparation has been minimal). Trim the crown form to fit the cervical margin of the tooth, fill with acrylic and place it on the previously moistened tooth. After about 1½ minutes, when the acrylic has reached its initial set, carefully remove the crown and wait a few minutes for the acrylic to polymerise fully (this may be hastened by placing the crown in warm water). Trim and smooth the margin of the crown and cement to the tooth with quick-setting zinc oxide-eugenol cement.

8. Before cementing the laboratory-made acrylic crown, select the appropriate shade of cement by mixing cement powder with water and placing it in the crown.

### Treatment of posterior teeth

Small areas of hypoplastic enamel in posterior teeth can be restored with amalgam, composite resin or glass ionomer cement. However, crowns are required for more severely affected teeth. Stainless steel crowns are ideal semi-permanent restorations for first permanent molars, but are not made in sizes suitable for premolars. Therefore, cast veneers must be made for premolars.

## AMELOGENESIS IMPERFECTA

Amelogenesis imperfecta is a rare hereditary condition in which enamel structure is defective. A number of genetically distinct types have been described (Witkop, 1965; Winter and Brook, 1975); the most common have autosomal dominant inheritance patterns.

Amelogenesis imperfecta may be broadly sub-divided into types that exhibit hypoplasia or hypomineralisation. The enamel in hypoplasia types may be thin but otherwise of normal appearance, or it may be pitted, grooved or more grossly deficient in structure. The enamel in hypomineralisation types is of normal thickness, and has a smooth surface unless it is chipped and worn away; the areas of hypomineralised enamel vary in size and distribution, and may be opaque white, dull yellow or light brown in colour. In almost all cases, both primary and permanent dentitions are affected. The typical appearances of the different types of amelogenesis imperfecta are illustrated by Rapp and Winter (1979) and by Davis, Law and Lewis (1981).

### Treatment

The principal aims in treatment are to improve appearance, to relieve the pain or discomfort caused by exposed dentine, and to prevent attrition (Winter and Brook, 1975).

It is important to reassure and encourage the child and parents, who may be demoralised by the appearance of the teeth. They should be reassured that treatment is possible and encouraged to take an active interest in the treatment plan. Without their interest and cooperation it is not practicable to embark on the considerable amount of treatment that is necessary to conserve the dentition; the provision of dentures would be the only alternative.

It is not possible to give precise recommendations for treatment because the problems that are presented vary greatly according to the type and severity of the abnormality; however, a guide to treatment is outlined in Table 13.1.

The greatest problem in treatment is presented by severe hypomineralisation, because the soft enamel easily wears away, exposing the dentine; this makes the teeth sensitive to thermal stimuli and allows rapid attrition. In these cases, treatment alternatives are limited: crowning of teeth is usually required.

Table 13.1 suggests that treatment is done only for permanent teeth, starting in the early mixed dentition. However, treatment of primary teeth may be necessary. Stainless steel crowns are ideal restorations for primary molars; conservation of

**Table 13.1** Summary of treatment of amelogenesis imperfecta.

| | *Patient's age* | | |
| --- | --- | --- | --- |
| | 6 | 12 | 18 |
| first permanent molars | amalgam<br>composite resin<br>glass ionomer cement<br>stainless steel crown | —— extraction —————————— | gold<br>veneer<br>crown |
| incisors | composite resin<br>glass ionomer cement<br>composite resin veneer<br>composite resin veneer with preformed acrylic facing<br>porcelain veneer<br>acrylic crown | | porcelain<br>jacket<br>crown |
| canines and premolars | | composite resin<br>glass ionomer cement<br>amalgam<br>full gold veneer | porcelain<br>or<br>porcelain/gold<br>crown |
| | | extraction + denture ———————— | bridge |

these teeth ensures that the first permanent molars erupt in their normal positions. Anterior primary teeth could be conserved by crowning (Ch. 8), but extraction is often justified.

Table 13.1 also indicates that after initial treatment of first permanent molars in the early mixed dentition, a decision must be made either to retain the teeth permanently or to extract them at a time in dental development that will encourage the second molars to occupy their positions. If radiographs show that the unerupted canines and premolars are present, and if it is assessed that there will be insufficient space for their eruption, it may be preferable to extract the first permanent molars when the child is between 8½ and 10 years of age (Ch. 22).

## DENTINOGENESIS IMPERFECTA

Dentinogenesis imperfecta is an hereditary dentinal defect that may occur alone or in association with the skeletal condition of osteogenesis imperfecta (Witkop, 1965; Gage, 1985). The alternative term 'hereditary opalescent dentine' aptly describes the appearance of the teeth, which vary in colour from grey to brownish blue. The crowns of

the teeth are bulbous, being constricted cervically. The enamel, which is usually normal, is poorly supported by the defective dentine and therefore tends to flake away. Attrition of exposed dentine occurs, and the teeth may rapidly be reduced to gingival level. Radiographs often show that the teeth have short, thin roots, and that the pulp chambers and root canals are partly or completely obliterated; there may also be periapical areas of radiolucency. All teeth of both dentitions are affected, but permanent teeth are affected less severely and those teeth that develop later (premolars, and second and third molars) may be normal.

### Treatment

The rationale of treatment is similar to that applied to the treatment of a severe case of amelogenesis imperfecta of the hypomineralisation type; unless teeth (particularly posterior teeth) are crowned they will be worn down by attrition and have to be extracted. Stainless steel crowns are ideal for primary and first permanent molars; in the primary dentition it is sometimes sufficient to crown second molars only. Acrylic crowns may be made for anterior teeth.

A specific problem presented by dentinogenesis

imperfecta is that teeth are often unsuitable for crowning because they are poorly supported by short, thin roots. Therefore, when canines and premolars erupt, an assessment must be made of their suitability for crowning. Much depends on whether the patient is keen to have the considerable amount of treatment that would be required, despite the uncertain prognosis (Mars and Smith, 1981; Mendel, Shawkat and Farman, 1981).

If it is decided not to embark on conservative treatment, the teeth may be retained for as long as possible, but the provision of dentures will eventually be necessary, as it is for the patient who first presents with permanent teeth already worn down by attrition. For a young patient it is preferable to make dentures that fit over the tooth remnants, after rounding and smoothing rough edges. This approach ensures the maintenance of the alveolar ridges, but eventually it may become necessary to extract the teeth and provide normal dentures.

## REFERENCES

Black J B 1982 Esthetic restoration of tetracycline-stained teeth. Journal of the American Dental Association 104:846–852

Calamia J R 1985 Etched porcelain veneers: the current state of the art. Quintessence International 16:5–12

Cooley R O 1984 Status report on enamel bonding of composite, preformed laminate and laboratory fabricated resin veneers. Journal of the American Dental Association 109:782–784

Davis J M, Law D B, Lewis T M 1981 An atlas of pedodontics. Saunders, Philadelphia

Gage J P 1985 Dentinogenesis imperfecta: a new perspective. Australian Dental Journal 30:285–290

Hobo S, Iwata T 1985 A new laminate veneer technique using a castable apatite ceramic material, II: practical procedures. Quintessence International 16:509–517

Horn H 1983 Porcelain laminate veneers bonded to etched enamel. Dental Clinics of North America 27:671–684

King N M, Rule D C 1980 Restoration of hypoplastic teeth — a simplified acid-etch technique. Journal of Dentistry 8:81–84

Mars M, Smith B G N 1981 Dentinogenesis imperfecta — an integrated conservative approach to treatment. British Dental Journal 152:15–18

Mendel R W, Shawkat A H, Farman A G 1981 Management of adolescent dentine — report of a long-term follow up. Journal of the American Dental Association 102:53–55

Murray J J, Bennett T G 1985 A colour atlas of acid etch technique. Wolfe, London

Pindborg J J 1982 Aetiology of developmental enamel defects not related to fluorosis. International Dental Journal 32:123–134

Rapp R, Winter G B 1979 A colour atlas of clinical conditions in paedodontics. Wolfe, London

Rivkin C J, Warren V N 1985 Preformed laminate veneers for children: a clinical study. Journal of Paediatric Dentistry 1:21–26

Roberts G J 1983 Mastique acrylic laminate veneers: clinical evaluation over two years. British Dental Journal 155:85–88

Smith D C, Pulver F 1982 Aesthetic dental veneering materials. International Dental Journal 32:223–239

Winter G B, Brook A H 1975 Enamel hypoplasia and anomolies of the enamel. Dental Clinics of North America (Jan.) 3024

Witkop C J 1965 Genetic disease in the oral cavity. In Tiecke R W (ed) Oral pathology. McGraw Hill, New York, ch 32

# Abnormalities of tooth form

Double teeth
Malformation of the maxillary lateral incisor
Dilaceration

## DOUBLE TEETH

Double teeth may be formed either by fusion of two developing tooth germs or by gemination (partial dichotomy) of one tooth germ. If fusion occurs between two teeth of the normal series, one tooth appears to be missing from the dentition; if, on the other hand, one element is a supernumerary tooth, the normal number of teeth is present in addition to the double tooth. The latter is also the case when the double tooth is formed by gemination of one tooth germ. Therefore, it is sometimes difficult to decide whether an abnormally large tooth is the result of fusion or gemination; use of the term 'double tooth' avoids this difficulty (Brook and Winter, 1970).

Double teeth occur most frequently in the incisor and canine regions, and are more common in the primary dentition than in the permanent dentition. The abnormal nature of a large tooth may be indicated by notching of the incisal edge, or by a longitudinal groove in the crown, or by partial or complete separation of the roots.

### Treatment

No treatment is required for primary double teeth, but in the permanent dentition treatment to improve aesthetics is usually requested by the patient and parent.

If the pulp chanbers and root canals are separate (Fig. 14.1), it is possible to separate the crowns using a fine diamond bur or a guarded diamond disc. To obtain an aesthetic result, it is usually necessary to modify the shapes of the separated parts, which can be done by one of the methods described in Chapter 13. If one part of the double

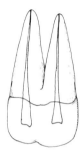

**Fig. 14.1** Double tooth with separate root canals.

tooth is a supernumerary element, its extraction is usually necessary (Smith, 1980; Moore, 1984).

Ideally, separation of a double tooth should be delayed until the late teenage years to allow some recession of pulp horns to occur, thus reducing the risk of pulp exposure. However, the appearance of the double tooth may be so poor that earlier treatment is demanded. Pulp exposure is then more probable, and may be treated by pulpotomy (Gregg, 1985) or pulpectomy (Itkin and Barr, 1975). If treatment is delayed at least until root development is complete (about 11 years), simple root canal treatment may be done if necessary and post crowns considered for one or both parts.

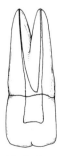

**Fig. 14.2** Double tooth with single root canal.

If there is a single pulp chamber (Fig. 14.2), division of the crown is not feasible. Some improvement of appearance may sometimes be obtained by accentuating the longitudinal groove in the crown, to simulate two separate teeth.

## MALFORMATION OF THE MAXILLARY LATERAL INCISOR

The maxillary lateral incisor is often abnormal in size or shape. The most common abnormalities are 'peg-shaped' crowns and deep palatal invaginations (Fig. 14.3). Peg-shaped lateral incisors have small, conical crowns and resemble conical supernumerary teeth. Palatal pits occur in many lateral incisors, but sometimes the pit is particularly deep and leads to a chamber formed by invagination of the developing tooth germ; this is known as 'dens in dente'. Caries may begin in the depths of a pit or invagination and quickly involve the pulp.

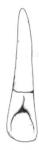

Fig. 14.3 Deep palatal invagination in maxillary lateral incisor.

### Treatment

*Peg-shaped lateral incisor*

If the dental arch is crowded, peg-shaped lateral incisors may be extracted as part of orthodontic treatment.

If extraction is not indicated, composite resin may be used to improve the appearance of the tooth. The acid-etch technique is used, and the method is similar to that used to restore a fractured incisor (Ch. 28). However, a problem arises in adapting a cellulose crown form to the narrow neck of the 'peg' tooth. This may be overcome by making a longitudinal cut in the palatal part of the crown form, overlapping the two sides and sticking with photographic film cement (Fig. 14.4). A

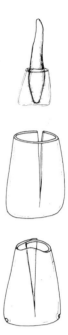

Fig. 14.4 Modifying a crown form to fit a peg-shaped lateral incisor.

crown form is not required if a light-sensitive composite is used; this can be built up in increments.

An alternative treatment is to make a thin porcelain 'thimble' and bond this to acid-etched enamel with composite resin, as described for porcelain veneers on page 138.

*Deep palatal pits*

Ideally, palatal pits should be sealed with composite resin (Ch. 5) as soon as the teeth erupt.

If the teeth have erupted and the pits have not been sealed, careful clinical and radiological examination is required to assess whether they are carious.

## DILACERATION

A dilacerated tooth is one that has a distorted crown or root. Dilaceration affects only permanent teeth, and the maxillary central incisor is the most commonly affected. Severe trauma to primary incisors is a common cause of dilaceration, but some cases are not associated with trauma and simply reflect abnormal development of the tooth (Stewart, 1978).

Severe injury to a maxillary primary incisor (e.g. intrusion or gross displacement) may cause dilaceration of either the crown or the root of the permanent successor, depending on the stage of development of the permanent tooth and its relationship to the root of the primary incisor at the time of injury. Maxillary permanent incisors develop palatal to and very near the root apices of the primary incisors (Fig. 14.5); as they erupt they move over the roots of the primary teeth. Therefore, trauma to the primary incisor in infancy is most likely to displace the permanent tooth crown palatally. Since further development continues normally, the fully developed tooth has its crown bent palatally; it also has hypoplasia of the enamel in the area of the distortion, as evidence of the traumatic incident. After about 1½ years of age, when the roots of the permanent incisors are forming and the teeth are moving over the primary incisor roots, the permanent tooth crown and the partially developed root are more likely to be bent labially; the fully-formed tooth then has a bend in its root, but no enamel hypoplasia.

Dilacerated teeth that are developmental anomalies not associated with trauma are gently curved from crown to root; the crown is bent labially from the crown-root junction and there is no enamel hypoplasia.

A dilacerated tooth usually fails to erupt, but sometimes it erupts into an abnormal position and causes displacement of adjacent teeth.

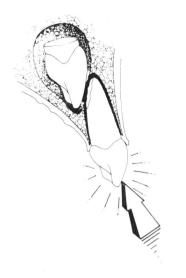

**Fig. 14.5** Relationship of the developing permanent incisor to the root of the primary incisor.

## Treatment

Unerupted dilacerated teeth are usually extracted, but sometimes it is possible to bring a tooth into the arch by a combination of surgery and orthodontics (Howard, 1978; Davies and Lewis, 1984). Erupted teeth in abnormal positions are also usually extracted because it is difficult to move them by orthodontic means. Following extraction, the space must either be maintained with a prosthesis or closed orthodontically, so that tilting of adjacent teeth is minimised.

REFERENCES

Brook A H, Winter G B 1970 Double teeth: a retrospective study of geminated and fused teeth in children. British Dental Journal 129:123–130
Davies P H J, Lewis D H 1984 Dilaceration: a surgical/orthodontic solution. British Dental Journal 156:16–18
Gregg T A 1985 Surgical division and pulpotomy of a double incisor tooth. British Dental Journal 159:254–255
Howard R D 1978 Maxillary anterior displacement and impaction in the mixed dentition. Dental Clinics of North America 22:635–645
Itkin A B, Barr G S 1975 Comprehensive management of the double tooth: report of a case. Journal of the American Dental Association 90:1269–1272
Moore K H 1984 A case report of bilateral double teeth. British Journal of Orthodontics 11:40–41

Smith G A 1980 Double teeth. British Dental Journal 148:163–164
Stewart D J 1978 Dilacerate unerupted maxillary central incisors. British Dental Journal 145:229–233

RECOMMENDED READING

Davis J M, Law D B, Lewis T M 1981 An atlas of pedodontics, 2nd edn. Saunders, Philadelphia, ch 3
Rapp R, Winter G B 1979 A colour atlas of clinical condition in paedodontics. Wolfe, London

# 15

# Abnormalities of tooth number

Congenital absence of teeth
Supernumerary teeth

## CONGENITAL ABSENCE OF TEETH

Congenital absence of all teeth (anodontia) is very rare. However, absence of one or of several teeth is not uncommon; the term 'hypodontia' is now used to define this condition, being preferred to the contradictory term 'partial anodontia'.

Hypodontia in the primary dentition is less common than in the permanent dentition, and when it occurs it is of little clinical significance and usually receives no treatment. However, congenital absence of permanent teeth demands attention. The permanent teeth most commonly congenitally absent are maxillary lateral incisors and mandibular second premolars, but the results of surveys differ about which of these is the more frequently absent. Congenital absence of a tooth may be unilateral or bilateral. Absence of a maxillary lateral incisor is often associated with a small peg-shaped contralateral tooth.

The effects of congenital absence of one or more teeth depend largely on the amount of crowding that would have existed had the dentition been complete. Sometimes the absence of a tooth is sufficient to relieve crowding and permit even alignment of the remaining teeth; in other cases the missing tooth leaves a space.

### Treatment

*Maxillary lateral incisor*

1. In an uncrowded arch: maintain the space (or spaces) by fitting a partial denture, which may be replaced by a bridge in later life.
2. In a crowded arch: approximate the canine and central incisor with an orthodontic appliance.

Improve the appearance by grinding the tip of the canine and, if appropriate, by modifying its shape with etch-retained composite resin to simulate the missing lateral incisor.

*Mandibular second premolar*

1. In an uncrowded arch: Either close the space orthodontically or defer treatment until young adulthood when bridging may be considered. If congenital absence of premolars is diagnosed in the mixed dentition, extraction of second primary molars may be considered, to encourage some closure of premolar spaces by mesial drift of first permanent molars.
2. In a crowded arch: Absence of a premolar, especially if bilateral, is an advantage in an arch that would otherwise be crowded.

## SUPERNUMERARY TEETH

Supernumerary teeth occur most frequently in the premaxilla and are less common in the primary dentition than in the permanent dentition. Primary supernumerary teeth are usually normal or conical in shape. Permanent supernumerary teeth have a greater variety of shapes, and may be classified as follows:

| | |
|---|---|
| Conical | — small, peg-shaped teeth. |
| Tuberculate | — short, barrel-shaped teeth. |
| Supplemental | — teeth resembling a normal incisor, usually a lateral incisor. |
| Odontomes | — variable shapes, unsuitable for inclusion in one of the other groups. |

The majority of supernumerary teeth are either conical or tuberculate; their characteristic features, which differ in many important respects, are summarised in Table 15.1.

**Table 15.1** Features of conical and tuberculate supernumerary teeth (from Foster and Taylor, 1969).

|  | Conical | Tuberculate |
|---|---|---|
| Morphology | Conical, pointed crown | Barrel-shaped crown |
|  | Normal root | Little or no root |
|  | Root development at similar stage to, or ahead of, normal incisors |  |
| Position | Midline of arch, between central incisors | Palatal to permanent incisors |
|  | Occur singly or in pairs | Occur singly or in pairs |
|  | May be inverted | Rarely inverted |
| Eruption | Often erupt with the central incisors | Rarely inverted |
|  | Inverted types do not erupt | Rarely erupt |
| Effect | Median diastema | Usually prevent eruption of incisors |
|  | Usually do not delay eruption of incisors |  |
|  | May cause rotation or other displacement of erupted teeth |  |

## Treatment

Treatment depends on the type and position of the supernumerary tooth, and on the effect it has, or can be expected to have, on adjacent teeth.

1. No treatment. Supernumerary teeth that are not interfering with the eruption of teeth, nor causing displacement of erupted teeth, may be allowed to remain; this is often possible with inverted conical types. Periodic radiographic examination is essential to detect any undesirable changes that may occur.
2. Await eruption and then extract. Most conical supernumeraries that are not inverted may be expected to erupt.
3. Surgical extraction. Most tuberculate and inverted conical types, and odontomes, must be extracted. The timing of treatment is controversial: the advantages and disadvantages of early intervention (before the age of 6 years) and of delayed intervention (between the ages

of 8 and 10 years) have been discussed by Primosch (1981). Early removal of a supernumerary tooth gives the normal developing tooth the best chance of erupting into its normal position; on the other hand, there is a risk of damaging adjacent developing teeth during surgery. Delaying treatment may result in the normal tooth becoming displaced or rotated, and may allow adjacent teeth to drift into the space as they erupt. The later the supernumerary tooth is removed the less eruption potential will the normal tooth have. Each case must be considered individually, but it has been suggested that the most appropriate time to extract midline supernumeraries is when the lateral incisors are just beginning to erupt (Broadway and Gould, 1960).

If there is adequate space in the arch for the unerupted incisor, insert a simple space maintainer. If the space available is inadequate, move adjacent teeth distally with an orthodontic appliance after extracting the primary canines (which are extracted at the same time as the supernumerary tooth); it is important to provide a slight excess of space for the unerupted incisor.

Having removed the supernumerary tooth and provided enough space in the arch, the incisor usually erupts. Sometimes, especially if it has previously been displaced by the supernumerary, the incisor does not erupt, and requires further surgery and orthodontic traction to bring it into the arch (Howard, 1967).

## REFERENCES

Broadway R T, Gould D G 1960 Surgical requirements of the orthodontist. British Dental Journal 108:187–190
Foster T D, Taylor G S 1969 Characteristics of supernumerary teeth in the upper central incisor region. Dental Practitioner 20:8–12
Howard R D 1967 The unerupted incisor. Dental Practitioner 17:332–342
Primosch R E 1981 Anterior supernumerary teeth — assessment and surgical intervention in children. Pediatric Dentistry 3:204–215

## RECOMMENDED READING

Davis J M, Law D B, Lewis T M 1981 An atlas of pedodontics, 2nd edn. Saunders, Philadelphia, ch 3
Rapp R, Winter G B 1979 A colour atlas of clinical conditions in paedodontics. Wolfe, London

# 16

# Intrinsic staining of teeth

Hypomineralised or mottled enamel
Tetracycline staining

Teeth may become discoloured by a variety of intrinsic stains (Baden, 1970; Faunce, 1983). Tetracycline drugs administered during the period of tooth development are a well-known cause and produce discolouration ranging from light yellow-orange to dark grey-brown. White or brown discolouration is associated with hypomineralised enamel, which may be caused by local or systemic disturbances during tooth development. Similar discolouration is associated with mottled enamel caused by excessive ingestion of fluoride, but this is uncommon in the U.K.

There are four possible approaches to treatment: grinding and polishing, bleaching, covering with a veneer, and crowning.

Techniques for veneering and crowning are described in Chapter 13, and for bleaching of non-vital teeth in Chapter 28. The techniques outlined below are for vital teeth.

## HYPOMINERALISED OR MOTTLED ENAMEL

The white or brown discolouration associated with hypomineralisation or with fluorosis is often located in superficial enamel and can therefore be removed by grinding and polishing. Techniques that have been reported involve etching and polishing (Powell and Craig, 1982), etching and bleaching (Boksman and Jordan, 1983), and a combination of etching, bleaching and polishing (Chandra and Chawla, 1975).

**Technique: etching and polishing** (Powell and Craig, 1982)

1. Clean affected surfaces with a pumice-water slurry or with an oil-free prophylaxis paste.

(Powell and Craig used pumice and glycerine, but it may be preferable to avoid the use of glycerine, which is generally contraindicated prior to acid etching of enamel).
2. Etch with 30–37% phosphoric acid for 2 to 3 minutes, wash and dry.
3. Polish with pumice.
4. Repeat steps 2 and 3 several times.
5. Apply topical fluoride gel for 4 minutes to promote remineralisation. (Powell and Craig used 2% sodium fluoride followed by 40% calcium sucrose phosphate).

Powell and Craig reported the successful use of this technique on six patients.

A similar technique using 18% hydrochloric acid has recently been described and beautifully illustrated by Croll and Cavanaugh, 1986.

**Technique: etching and bleaching** (Boksman and Jordan, 1983)

1. Clean affected surfaces with a pumice-water slurry or with an oil-free prophylaxis paste.
2. Isolate the teeth with rubber dam.
3. Etch with 30–37% phosphoric acid for 1 minute, wash and dry.
4. Bleach with a solution of 30% hydrogen peroxide (5 parts) and ether (1 part).
   Take precaution against the caustic properties of hydrogen peroxide: wear rubber gloves, ensure that the rubber dam isolation is effective, and provide the patient with protective spectacles.
   Apply the solution to the teeth on cotton wool pledgets.
5. Place the tip of a suitable heating instrument (see below) on each cotton pledget in turn, and

increase the temperature until the patient reports slight sensitivity. Maintain the highest temperature that the patient can comfortably tolerate for 2 or 3 minutes.

Boksman and Jordan reported that they used the technique successfully on hundreds of patients, but did not give more precise details. The procedure was repeated at weekly intervals; 3 to 6 sessions were required, depending on the severity of the discolouration.

The use of ether is controversial because it is an explosive substance, especially in combination with hydrogen peroxide (Ferguson, 1985). Boksman and Jordan, and others who have used the technique, have not reported any problems, but the fact remains that it is potentially dangerous. Ether is used because it is said to enhance the penetration of bleaching solution into the tooth. Ether should not be stored in a dental surgery; only a small amount of the bleaching solution should be prepared, and it should be discarded after use. Nicholls (1984) concluded that the drawbacks of using ether outweigh its benefits, and recommended using hydrogen peroxide alone.

Heat is commonly used to activate the hydrogen peroxide, and various small heating units have been used successfully. However, light also activates hydrogen peroxide and the use of an infrared or photoflood lamp has been suggested (Nicholls, 1984). More convenient light sources are the ultra-violet or visible light units that are used for polymerising composite resins (Howell, 1980); these may be equally efficient.

### Technique: etching, bleaching and polishing (Chandra and Chawla, 1975)

1. Clean the affected teeth with a pumice-water slurry or with an oil-free prophylaxis paste.
2. Isolate the teeth with rubber dam.
3. Dry the labial surfaces by applying absolute alcohol and using an air syringe for 1 minute.
4. Etch and bleach with a solution made up of 30% hydrogen peroxide (5 parts), 36% hydrochloric acid (5 parts) and ether (1 part).
5. Keep the tooth surface wet with solution while removing superficial enamel with fine cuttle or sandpaper discs fitted to a slow-speed handpiece.

6. Neutralise the solution with 5.25% sodium hypochlorite solution. (This was done by Chandra and Chawla but may not be essential.)
7. Polish the teeth with prophylaxis paste. (Chandra and Chawla used pumice and glycerine, but a fluoride-containing paste might be preferable.)

Chandra and Chawla reported successful results in the treatment of 93 teeth in 22 patients. The majority only required one session of treatment but some required 2 or 3 sessions.

## TETRACYCLINE STAINING

Discoloration caused by tetracycline cannot be polished away because the drug is deposited in both enamel and dentine. Bleaching can be successful in the treatment of light yellow or light grey discolorations, but may not be successful in more severe cases even if repeated several times (Boksman and Jordan, 1983).

### Technique: bleaching

The technique of Boksman and Jordan (1983) is described above.

The technique of Reid and Newman (1977) is similar, but enamel is not etched before bleaching and ether is not included in the bleaching solution. The bleaching procedure, with heating, is continued for 30 minutes. Forty-five patients who received this treatment were examined 5 years later and about a half were still satisfied with the appearance of their teeth (Reid, 1985).

## REFERENCES

Baden E 1970 Environmental pathology of the teeth. In: Gorlin R J, Goldman H M (eds) Thoma's oral pathology, 6th edn. Mosby, St Louis, ch 4

Boksman L, Jordan R E 1983 Conservative treatment of the stained dentition: vital bleaching. Australian Dental Journal 28:67–72

Chandra S, Chawla T N 1975 Clinical evaluation of the sandpaper disk method for removing fluorosis stains from teeth. Journal of the American Dental Association 90:1273–1276

Croll T P, Cavanaugh R R 1986 Enamel color modification by controlled hydrochloric acid-pumice abrasion. Quintessence International 17:81–87 and 157–164

Faunce F 1983 Management of discolored teeth. Dental Clinics of North America 27:657–670

Ferguson M M 1985 (letter) British Dental Journal 159:102

Howell R A 1980 Bleaching discoloured root-filled teeth. British Dental Journal 148:159–162

Nicholls E 1984 Endodontics, 3rd edn. Wright, Bristol, ch 17

Powell K R, Craig G G 1982 A simple technique for the aesthetic improvement of fluorotic-like lesions. Journal of Dentistry for Children 49:112–117

Reid J S, Newman P 1977 A suggested method of bleaching tetracycline-stained vital teeth. British Dental Journal 142:261

Reid J S 1985 Personal communication

# 17

# Premature loss of primary teeth

Factors influencing mesial and distal drift
Assessment of crowding
Treatment planning
Space maintainers

---

Extraction of a primary incisor detracts from the child's appearance but has little or no effect on the development of the permanent dentition. On the other hand, extraction of a primary canine or molar may result in mesial or distal drift of adjacent teeth into the resulting space. Mesial drift of first permanent molars encroaches on space that is required for the eruption of premolars; distal drift of permanent incisors encroaches on the canine spaces. If distal drift occurs on one side only, following unilateral extraction of a primary tooth, the vertical coincidence of maxillary and mandibular centre lines is lost, that is, there is a 'centre line shift'; this is undesirable because it complicates any orthodontic treatment that might be required later.

## FACTORS INFLUENCING MESIAL AND DISTAL DRIFT

The principal factors that influence the rate and extent of mesial and distal drift of teeth are the degree of crowding in the dental arch, the type of primary tooth that is extracted, and the age of the patient.

### Degree of crowding

The rate and extent of drift are directly related to the degree of crowding in the dental arch. In an uncrowded arch there may be little or no movement of teeth, but in a crowded arch adjacent teeth quickly move into spaces provided by the extraction of teeth.

### Tooth extracted

Loss of a primary second molar is especially serious because it allows uninterrupted mesial drift of the first permanent molar; however, centre line shift occurs only in very crowded arches. In contrast, extraction of a primary canine allows permanent incisors to drift distally, but mesial drift of teeth may be minimal. Extraction of a primary first molar allows some mesial and distal drift to occur.

A summary of the relative amounts of mesial and distal drift that may be expected to follow extraction of different primary teeth is given in Table 17.1. Mesial drift of first permanent molars tends to be greater in the maxilla than in the mandible.

**Table 17.1** The relative amounts of mesial and distal drift of teeth that may be expected following extraction of a primary tooth

| Primary tooth extracted | Mesial drift | Distal drift |
|---|---|---|
| second molar | +++ | + |
| first molar | ++ | ++ |
| canine | + | +++ |

### Age of patient

In general, the earlier a primary tooth is extracted the greater the opportunity for drifting of teeth, but over-eruption of opposing teeth may limit movement. If a primary molar is extracted before eruption of the first permanent molar, mesial drift of the latter is inevitable, even in arches that are not crowded. On the other hand, if a primary tooth is extracted shortly before its natural exfoliation, no drift may occur.

## ASSESSMENT OF CROWDING

Because extraction of a primary tooth can have profound effects on the developing permanent dentition, a tooth should never be extracted before first assessing its likely effects and then planning treatment to prevent or alleviate those effects. Since an important factor that determines drifting of teeth is the degree of crowding in the arch, it is essential to assess this before appropriate treatment can be planned.

The degree of crowding in the arch may be assessed by (i) observation of erupting permanent incisors, (ii) examination of radiographs, and (iii) comparison of the space available in the arch for unerupted permanent canines and premolars with the estimated size of the unerupted teeth (Mixed Dentition Analysis).

### Observation of erupting permanent incisors

The erupting incisors may provide early evidence of crowding. Although minimal imbrication may be relieved by growth, which increases the inter-canine arch width up to about 9 years of age, definite overlapping of contact points indicates that the arch is crowded. Signs of severe crowding are rotation or other displacement of the erupting teeth, and resorption of the primary canine root by the lateral incisor.

### Radiographic examination

Signs of arch crowding that may be seen on radiographs include 'stacking' of maxillary molars and

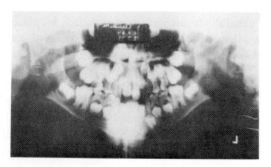

**Fig. 17.1** Radiograph showing 'stacking' of maxillary molars and distal inclination of mandibular molars.

distal inclination of mandibular molars (Fig. 17.1).

### Mixed Dentition Analysis

A quantitative assessment of crowding may be obtained by Mixed Dentition Analysis (M.D.A.). The space available in each dental arch is measured in the mouth or on study models, and the sum of the mesio-distal dimensions of the unerupted teeth is determined in one of the following ways:

1. By using the average mesio-distal dimensions of permanent canines and premolars.
   Mandibular canine and all premolars
                 = 7 mm each (approx.)
   Maxillary canine = 8 mm (approx.)
   Therefore, mandibular canine + two premolars
         = 21 mm
               Maxillary canine + two premolars
               = 22 mm
   This method is useful only as a rough guide because the patient may not have teeth of average size.
2. By measuring the mesio-distal dimensions of the four erupted mandibular permanent incisors, and predicting the combined sizes of the unerupted canines and premolars from the correlation that exists between the sizes of the different groups of teeth.
3. By measuring the unerupted canines and premolars on radiographs.

**Table 17.2** Predicted sum of widths of canines and premolars (75% level of probability) based on the sum of widths of mandibular incisors.*

| Sum of widths of mandibular incisors (mm) | Predicted sum of widths of canines and premolars in each quadrant (mm) | |
| --- | --- | --- |
| | maxilla | mandible |
| 19.5 | 20.6 | 20.1 |
| 20.0 | 20.9 | 20.4 |
| 20.5 | 21.2 | 20.7 |
| 21.0 | 21.5 | 21.0 |
| 21.5 | 21.8 | 21.3 |
| 22.0 | 22.0 | 21.6 |
| 22.5 | 22.3 | 21.9 |
| 23.0 | 22.6 | 22.2 |
| 23.5 | 22.9 | 22.5 |
| 24.0 | 23.1 | 22.8 |
| 24.5 | 23.4 | 23.1 |
| 25.0 | 23.7 | 23.4 |

* For 95% level of probability, add 1.0 mm

**Technique: mixed dentition analysis — method based on measurement of mandibular permanent incisors.**

| Procedure | Method | Rationale | Notes |
|---|---|---|---|
| 1. Measure the mesio-distal widths of each of the four mandibular incisors. | Open a pair of fine-pointed dividers to the greatest mesio-distal width of each incisor in turn (Fig. 17.2a). Mark each width on a straight line (Fig. 17.2b) then measure the combined width (in millimetres) (Fig. 17.2c). | Mesio-distal dimensions of mandibular incisors form the basis for predicting the sizes of unerupted canines and premolars. | If preferred, measurements may be made on study models of the patient's dentition. |
| 2. Determine the predicted sum of widths of canines and premolars. | From a chart (Table 17.2) read the predicted sum of widths of the canine and two premolars in each quadrant, based on the sum of widths of mandibular incisors.* | Correlation between the sizes of the different groups of teeth makes this prediction possible. | Charts are available which give predictions at different levels of probability. |
| | Alternatively, take half the sum of widths of mandibular incisors. If this is x mm then x + 10.5 mm = sum widths mandibular canine and premolars x + 11.0 mm = sum widths maxillary canine and premolars. | | Similar results are obtained by this method, and use of charts is unnecessary (Tanaka and Johnston, 1974). |
| 3. Measure the space available in the arch for the unerupted canines and premolars | With dividers, measure from the distal surface of the lateral incisor to the mesial of the first permanent molar in each quadrant. Make a note of each measurement (in millimetres). If the incisors are imbricated, open the dividers to the combined widths of the central and lateral incisors on one side. Place one point on the centre line and note the position of the other point on the primary canine (or on the gingiva if the canine is absent); measure from this point to the mesial of the first permanent molar (Fig. 17.2d). Repeat for each quadrant. | Measurement of the space available for unerupted canines and premolars must take into account the space required for alignment of crowded incisors. | |
| 4. Estimate the adequacy of space for unerupted canines and premolars. | Compare the measurements made in procedures 2 and 3.† | | |

* The data in Table 17.2 are taken from a much larger chart in which the predicted sum of widths of unerupted canines and premolars are given at different levels of probability ranging from 95% to 5% (Moyers, 1973). The data in Table 17.2 are those given at the 75% level of probability, which means that there is only a 1 in 4 chance that the actual sum of widths of the unerupted teeth exceeds the predicted sum. This is the level of probability generally used in Mixed Dentition Analysis, but if greater certainty is demanded, 1 mm may be added, which will give predicted sum of widths that will be exceeded in only 1 in 20 cases (95% probability level).
† An example of a completed Mixed Dentition Analysis is given in Table 17.3.

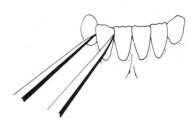

**Fig. 17.2a**

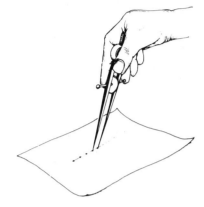

**Fig. 17.2b**

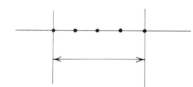

**Fig. 17.2c**

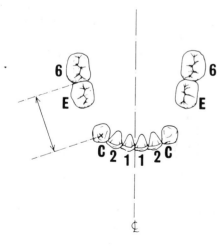

**Fig. 17.2d**

**Table 17.3** Example of Mixed Dentition Analysis

| | Maxilla Right | Left | Mandible Right | Left |
|---|---|---|---|---|
| Sum of widths of mandibular incisors = 22.5 mm | | | | |
| Predicted sum of widths of canine and premolars | 22.3 | 22.3 | 21.9 | 21.9 |
| Space available in quadrant | 22.0 | 22.5 | 20.5 | 19.5 |
| Excess or deficiency of space (mm) | −0.3 | +0.2 | −1.4 | −2.4 |

## Technique: mixed dentition analysis — method based on measurement of unerupted canine and premolars on radiographs

1. Using fine dividers, measure the mesio-distal widths of the unerupted canines and pre-molars, preferably on periapical films (which are less distorted than extra-oral films). Sum the widths of the three teeth in each quadrant.
2. Calculate the magnification due to radiographic distortion by measuring an erupted tooth on each film and the same tooth in the mouth (or on study models); a primary molar or a first permanent molar may be used for this purpose.

Then $\dfrac{\text{clinical measurement}}{\text{radiographic measurement}} = C$

3. Calculate the sum of widths of unerupted teeth in each quadrant, which is: radiographic sum of widths × C.
4. Measure the space available in each quadrant for the unerupted canine and premolars, as described in the previous technique.
5. Subtract the calculated sum of widths of the unerupted teeth in each quadrant from the space available.

Having assessed the degree of dental arch crowding by observation of erupting incisors, from radiographs and by Mixed Dentition Analysis, the dentition may be categorised as one of the following types (Foster, 1982):

Not crowded:   (i) Excess space available for unerupted canines and pre-molars.

               (ii) Just sufficient space for un-erupted canines and pre-molars.

Crowded:  (i) Mild deficiency of space for unerupted canines and premolars.
 (ii) Severe deficiency of space for unerupted canines and premolars.

A summary of the signs of each of these types of dentition is given in Table 17.4.

**Table 17.4** Signs of different types of dentitions

| Type of dentition | Signs |
| --- | --- |
| Not crowded — excess space | Spacing between incisors. Radiograph — long axes of maxillary molars vertical. MDA* — space available in arch exceeds space required for unerupted teeth. |
| Not crowded — just sufficient space | Normal contacts between incisors. Radiograph — long axes of maxillary molars vertical or with slight distal inclination. MDA* — space available in arch equals space required for unerupted teeth. |
| Mild crowding | Slight overlapping of incisors. Radiograph — distal inclination of maxillary molars. MDA* — space available in arch up to 4 mm less than that required for unerupted teeth. |
| Severe crowding | Overlapping, rotation or displacement of incisors. Radiograph — marked distal inclination of maxillary molars, with 'stacking' — distal inclination of mandibular molars. MDA* — space available in arch over 4 mm less than that required for unerupted teeth. |

## TREATMENT PLANNING

Selection of the most appropriate treatment to accompany the extraction of a primary tooth depends greatly on an assessment of the dentition as outlined above. Alternative forms of treatment, which are summarised in Table 17.5, are to balance the extraction or to fit a space maintainer; only when there is excess space in the arch is neither of these forms of treatment necessary.

A *balancing extraction* is the removal of a tooth from the opposite side of the same arch to equalise drift and therefore prevent centre line shift; the tooth extracted is usually, but need not necessarily be, the contralateral tooth. A *compensating extraction*, which is less frequently justified, is the removal of a tooth from the same side of the opposing arch, to equalise drift in the two arches.

A *space maintainer* is an appliance that is fitted to prevent mesial drift of the first permanent molar. Space maintainers are usually not used to prevent centre line shift because this only occurs if the permanent incisors are crowded; in these cases a balancing extraction is generally preferred to provide space for the incisors to spread out. When space maintenance is the selected treatment but is impracticable because of unfavourable parental attitudes or poor patient cooperation, balancing extraction should be performed instead, to equalise drift and retain symmetry in the dental arch.

It should be remembered that the best type of space maintainer is the primary tooth itself. If, after assessing the dentition as a whole, it is decided that maintenance of space is important, every effort should be made to conserve the tooth; only if this is impracticable should an artificial space maintainer be considered.

## SPACE MAINTAINERS

Artificial space maintainers may be fixed or removable. The type of appliance used most commonly to maintain single tooth spaces is the fixed band and loop space maintainer (Fig. 17.3). If the tooth to be banded is very carious, a stainless steel crown is used instead of a band.

Recently, space maintainers made by bonding stainless steel wire to etched enamel with com-

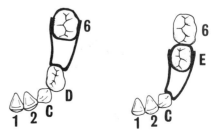

**Fig. 17.3** Fixed space maintainers made with stainless steel bands and wire.

**Table 17.5** Treatment to accompany extraction of a primary tooth from an intact arch.

| Primary tooth to be extracted | Type of dentition | Treatment | Rationale |
|---|---|---|---|
| Canine | Excess space | None | No drifting of teeth is expected. |
| | Just sufficient space | Usually balance, but a period of close observation may be justified | Centre line shift may or may not occur. |
| | Mild crowding | Balance. Compensate also if serial extraction is planned (Ch. 18) | Centre line shift is prevented by balancing the extraction. |
| | Severe crowding | Balance but do not compensate | Serial extraction is not indicated in severely crowded cases because posterior teeth move forward too rapidly. |
| First molar | Excess space | None | No drifting of teeth is expected. |
| | Just sufficient space | Fit space maintainer | A space maintainer ensures that space remains adequate for unerupted canines and premolars. |
| | Mild crowding | Balance | Balancing prevents centre line shift. Space maintenance is not useful because in any case extraction of a permanent tooth from each quadrant will be required later to relieve crowding. |
| | Severe crowding | Fit space maintainer | Space maintenance is justified because further space loss might make it necessary to extract more than one tooth from each quadrant to relieve crowding. |
| Second molar | Excess space | None | No drifting of teeth is expected. |
| | Just sufficient space | Fit space maintainer | (As for first molar above) |
| | Mild crowding | Fit space maintainer | Considerable mesial drift of the first permanent molar can be expected if the space is not maintained. |
| | Severe crowding | Fit space maintainer | Gross mesial drift of the first permanent molar will otherwise occur. |

posite resin have been tested and found to be satisfactory (Artum and Marstrander, 1983).

To maintain bilateral spaces, a lingual arch is used most commonly in the mandible, and a palatal arch or acrylic removable appliance in the maxilla.

Acrylic removable appliances, which are retained with Adams cribs, are more bulky than fixed appliances, but they are well tolerated by children. However, if space maintenance is required for several years, and if active orthodontic treatment is required subsequently, there is a danger that the child's cooperation may become exhausted before treatment begins. Removable appliances are, therefore, most useful for short-term space maintenance.

**Technique: lingual arch space maintainer**

Since most of the procedures in the technique are similar to those used in the band and loop space maintainer, only a few details will be considered here.

1. Fit preformed stainless steel bands to both mandibular first permanent molars. Take an impression, position the bands in the impression and cast a stone model as described previously.

## Technique: band and loop space maintainer

| Procedure | Method | Rationale | Notes |
|---|---|---|---|
| 1. Select and fit a band | Select a preformed stainless steel band to fit the tooth distal to the space — either a second primary molar or a first permanent molar. Try the band on the tooth. The correct sized band should not seat fully with finger pressure but require the use of a band pusher (Fig. 17.4a). The cervical margin of the band should fit just under the gingival margin. With a band pusher, adapt the margins of the band closely to the tooth. | A tight band is necessary for firm retention of the appliance. If the appliance loosens, demineralisation of enamel may occur under the band. If the margin of the band is not subgingival and the patient's oral hygiene is not excellent, cervical caries could occur. | Preformed stainless steel bands are available in a range of sizes. A very secure finger rest is essential when using a band pusher. |
| 2. Take an impression | With the band on the tooth, take an alginate impression of the arch (or of the section of the arch). | | Alternatively, before taking the alginate impression, softened impression compound may be moulded over the occlusal surface of the tooth and over the buccal and lingual surfaces of the band; this provides a more positive surface than alginate on which to place the band in procedure 3. |
| 3. Place the band in the impression | Remove the band from the tooth using band-removing pliers, position it accurately in the impression, and secure it with sticky wax. | The band must be carefully placed and secured in the impression to ensure that it is correctly positioned on the model. | |
| 4. Cast a stone model | Flow the stone into the impression carefully to avoid dislodging the band. Cut off the tooth that is to be extracted. | | Ideally, the space maintainer is made before the tooth is extracted and fitted immediately after the extraction. |
| 5. Adapt a wire loop | Select a preformed wire loop or bend a loop with 0.9 mm or 1.0 mm wire. | The wire loop should be wide enough to allow partial eruption of the premolar, and must not press on the gingiva. | |

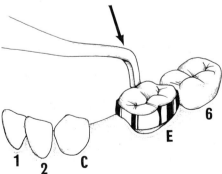

**Fig. 17.4a**

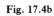

**Fig. 17.4b**

| Procedure | Method | Rationale | Notes |
|---|---|---|---|
| | The ends of the loop should rest tightly against the band buccally and lingually; the arms should run on each side of the alveolar ridge close to, or resting gently on, the gingiva; the anterior part should contact the tooth mesial to the space just under its contact area (Fig. 17.4b). | | |
| 6. Solder the loop to the band | Secure the anterior part of the loop to the model with sticky wax, and cover the wax with plaster. Grind away the stone inside the band on the buccal and lingual sides, that is, inside the parts of the band that are to be soldered to the wire. | Removal of stone inside the band ensures efficient heating of the band, which is essential for soldering. | An alternative method, which makes the grinding out of stone unnecessary, is to flow wax into the band on the buccal and lingual sides immediately after placing the band in the impression (procedure 3), that is, before casting the stone model. |
| | Apply flux to the wire and underlying band, and heat with the soldering flame until the flux dries. Apply silver solder and heat until it flows around the wire. | | The surface of the band and wire must be absolutely clean for satisfactory soldering. |
| 7. Smooth and polish the appliance | Smooth the solder with a stone and a rubber wheel. Remove the band from the model for final polishing and to clean the inside of the band. | Smoothing on the model prevents distortion of the appliance. | |
| 8. Try in | Try the appliance in the mouth and check that it fits correctly. | | The appliance should be fitted as soon as possible after extraction of the tooth. |
| 9. Cement the band | Clean and dry the tooth. Isolate with cotton rolls and saliva ejector. Apply a creamy mix of polycarboxylate cement to the inside of the band; seat first with finger pressure and then with band pusher and band seater. Remove excess cement when it has set. | | |

2. Bend a lingual arch with 0.9 or 1.0 mm stainless steel wire. The ends of the wire should rest against the middle of the lingual surfaces of the bands. The arch should run mesially on each side level with the crests of the interdental papillae, and contact the lingual surfaces of the mandibular incisors just above the interdental papillae (Fig.17.5). If both primary molars on one or both sides are missing, bend the wire down to rest gently on, or just off, the gingiva, on the lingual side of the alveolar ridge. U-loops may be incorporated into the arch; these permit some adjustment of the arch should this be necessary.

3. Check that the arch is passive when placed in position on the model before proceeding to solder.

A lingual arch prevents mesial drift by bracing one first molar against the other. Contact with the mandibular incisors is not essential; indeed, in cases where spontaneous improvement of incisor crowding is desired (for example in serial extraction cases) close contact of the arch against the incisors is undesirable.

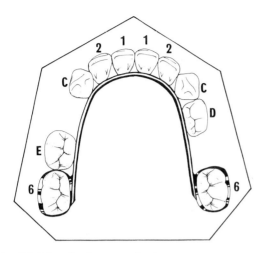

Fig. 17.5 Lingual arch space maintainer.

## Technique: bonded wire space maintainer

The technique outlined below is that described by
Artum and Marstrander (1983). They found
round, multistrand orthodontic wire (0.032 inch
diameter) to be more satisfactory than ordinary
round wire, and they used an autopolymerising
composite resin ('Concise').

1. Bend the wire as shown in Figure 17.6. This
   may be done at the chairside, or in the laboratory on a stone model of the patient's dentition.
2. Follow the procedures previously described for
   acid etching (p. 56): clean the buccal surfaces
   of the teeth to which the wire is to be bonded,
   isolate and dry the teeth, etch the buccal surfaces, wash and dry.
3. Hold the wire in place with a finger and tack
   the mesial end to the mesial abutment tooth
   with a small amount of composite paste thinned
   with unfilled resin:
   paste A 2 parts + resin B 1 part.
   This mixture is fast setting and has the desired
   viscosity.
4. Tack the distal end of the wire in the same
   way.
5. Add a slow setting mixture of composite to
   cover the wire on both teeth:

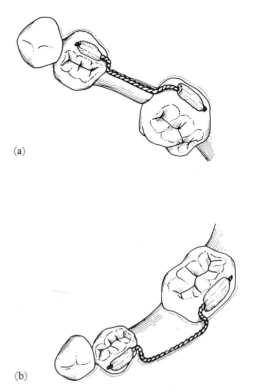

(a)

(b)

Fig. 17.6 Bonded wire space maintainers in (a) maxillary and
(b) mandibular arch.

paste A 1 part + paste B 2 parts + 1 drop
resin B
The drop of resin B reduces the viscosity of the
mixture and makes it easier to apply.
6. Trim and smooth the composite after it has
   polymerised.

REFERENCES

Artum J, Marstrander P B 1983 Clinical efficiency of two
different types of direct bonded space maintainers. Journal
of Dentistry for Children 50:197–204
Foster T D 1982 A textbook of orthodontics. Blackwell,
Oxford, p 136
Moyers R E 1973 A handbook of orthodontics for the student
and the general practitioner. Year Book Medical Publishers,
Chicago, p 369
Tanaka M T, Johnston L E 1974 The prediction of the size of
unerupted canines and premolars in a contemporary
orthodontic population. Journal of the American Dental
Association 88:798–801

# 18

# Crowding of erupting permanent incisors

Serial extraction

The first signs of crowding in the permanent dentition are noted when the permanent incisors begin to erupt; the teeth may be imbricated or, in severe cases, the lateral incisors may resorb the roots of the primary canines or be displaced from the arch.

## SERIAL EXTRACTION

Although most orthodontic treatment is started in children aged between 11 and 13 years, treatment to relieve incisor crowding is sometimes begun in the mixed dentition as part of the technique of Serial Extraction; the technique involves the planned extraction of selected primary and permanent teeth.

## Technique

Classically, the sequence of extractions is as follows (Graber, 1972; Houston, 1982).

*1. Primary canines* — to provide space for the permanent lateral incisors. The canines are extracted when the maxillary permanent lateral incisors are erupting.

*2. First primary molars* — to encourage early eruption of first premolars. The first primary molars are extracted about one year after extraction of the primary canines; the mandibular teeth may require extraction relatively early to ensure that the first premolars erupt before the canines.

*3. First premolars* — to create space for the permanent canines. First premolars are extracted as soon as they erupt.

Before embarking on the serial extraction procedure, a full orthodontic assessment must be made, aided by study models and radiographs. Serial extraction may be considered if the degree of crowding is mild, if the arch relationship is Class 1, and if, radiologically, all unerupted teeth appear in normal positions and normal in structure.

Serial extraction is complicated if crowding is severe, because considerable mesial drift of first permanent molars can be expected to occur following extraction of first primary molars and of first premolars, and this might leave inadequate space for eruption of the canines and second premolars; upper and lower space maintainers would be required in these cases to prevent mesial drift of first molars. Therefore, when there is more than mild crowding, serial extraction treatment must include the use of space maintainers. Alternatively, after extracting the primary canines to encourage spontaneous alignment of incisors, the serial extraction sequence is not persued; instead, the malocclusion is reassessed and treated at a later stage, when premolars have erupted.

## REFERENCES

Graber T M 1972 Orthodontics: principles and practice, 3rd edn.. Saunders, Philadelphia, ch 15
Houston W J B 1982 Orthodontic diagnosis, 3rd edn. Wright, Bristol, p 92

# 19

# Crossbites

## CROSSBITES IN THE PRIMARY DENTITION

Incisor and molar crossbites may occur in the primary dentition; the latter may be unilateral or bilateral. In the U.K., treatment is invariably deferred until the child is older (Leighton, 1966). In the U.S.A., on the other hand, primary dentition crossbites are sometimes treated (Kutin and Hawes, 1969; Lee, 1978).

Some unilateral molar crossbites are due to abnormal premature contacts of primary canines; these may be relieved by grinding the canines.

## FIRST PERMANENT MOLAR CROSSBITE

Crossbites of first permanent molars should not be treated in isolation but as part of an overall orthodontic treatment plan. Treatment is usually delayed until the child is 10 or 11 years of age, when the occlusion is assessed and a plan made to correct the crossbite in the same course of treatment as any other abnormalities that might exist.

## PERMANENT INCISOR CROSSBITE

Incisor crossbite may be associated with a skeletal Class III arch relationship but is more commonly associated with local factors that cause one or more maxillary incisors to be deflected palatally during their eruption (Bodenham and Bodenham, 1969). Some children with mild skeletal Class III jaw relationship posture the mandible forwards to achieve a more comfortable occlusion, and this increases the reversed overjet (Foster, 1982).

### Treatment

Anterior crossbites caused by local factors may be prevented by timely removal of the cause. Thus, extraction of primary canines may allow crowded incisors to erupt in normal alignment, and removal of a primary incisor that is not resorbing normally allows normal eruption of the permanent successor.

When a tooth erupts in crossbite, appliance therapy should be started as soon as a small overbite is established; when the crossbite is corrected, the overbite will retain the tooth in its new position. If there is insufficient space in the arch for the displaced tooth it is, of course, necessary to create space by moving adjacent teeth distally before correcting the crossbite.

### Removable appliances

Anterior crossbites are most commonly treated with removable appliances such as those illustrated in Figure 19.1. Covering of posterior teeth with acrylic is necessary to open the bite sufficiently to allow the teeth to be moved labially.

### Inclined plane

If the number of teeth in the maxillary arch is insufficient to retain a removable appliance, an inclined plane cemented to mandibular incisors may be used. The plane may be made of acrylic or cast metal, and should be inclined at about 45° (Fig. 19.2). This appliance is potentially traumatic and should not be used for more than a few weeks.

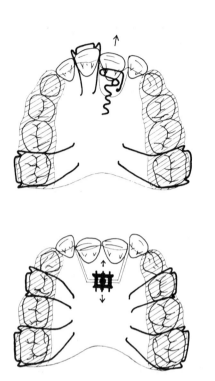

Fig. 19.1 Appliances for the correction of anterior crossbites.

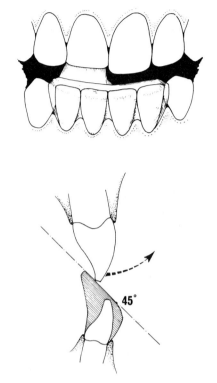

Fig. 19.2 Anterior inclined plane to correct anterior crossbite.

REFERENCES

Bodenham R S, Bodenham J A 1969 The aetiology and
    treatment of anterior crossbites. Dental Practitioner
    20:52–58
Foster T D 1982 A textbook of orthodontics 2nd edn.
    Blackwell, Oxford, p 320–324
Kutin G, Hawes R R 1969 Posterior crossbites in the
    deciduous and mixed dentitions. American Journal of
    Orthodontics 56:491–504
Lee B D 1978 Correction of crossbites. Dental Clinics of North
    America 22:647–668
Leighton B S 1966 The early development of crossbites. Dental
    Practitioner 17:145–152

# 20

# Proclined maxillary permanent incisors

It is an objective of orthodontic treatment to obtain an acceptable result in the minimum possible time; in most cases this is achieved by delaying the start of treatment until all permanent teeth (other than third molars) have erupted (Fletcher, 1958). However, earlier treatment may be considered for some children who have proclined maxillary incisors and increased incisor overjets, to reduce the risk of trauma to the teeth or to eliminate a source of psychological distress. Boys who participate in contact sports are particularly at risk from trauma, especially if the teeth are inadequately covered by the lips. Girls tend to be more concerned about their appearance and more sensitive to the unkind comments of other children.

## Treatment

Early treatment of Class II division I malocclusion has been outlined by Fulstow (1968). The essential stages in treatment are as follows:

1. Confirm radiologically that the permanent canines are in satisfactory positions.
2. Start treatment when the crowns of the permanent canines are distal to the roots of the lateral incisors. Extract the maxillary primary canines if space is required for retraction of incisors.
3. Retract the incisors with a removable appliance.
4. When the incisors are retracted, modify the appliance (or make another appliance) to use for night-time retention for six months.
5. Extract maxillary first premolars as soon as they erupt. Sometimes it is advisable to extract first primary molars to accelerate eruption of first premolars, or to enucleate the latter before their eruption. It is hoped that the permanent canines will erupt into the premolar spaces, but appliance therapy may be required.

Although conventional treatment of Class II Division 1 malocclusion has fewer potential complications and usually is completed more quickly, there are important reasons for considering early treatment in certain cases.

REFERENCES

Fletcher G G T 1958 The age factor in orthodontics. Dental Practitioner 9:31–40
Fulstow E D 1968 The early treatment of Angle's Class II Division I malocclusion. Dental Practitioner 19:137–144

# Persistent digit sucking

Digit sucking occurs so commonly in young children that it must be regarded as normal behaviour. The effects on the dentition vary according to the way in which the thumb or fingers are sucked, but include anterior open bite (usually asymmetrical), proclination of upper incisors, and retroclination of lower incisors.

## Treatment

Parents must be reassured that the dental effects of digit sucking are usually reversible when the habit stops: overbite and overjet return to normal unless prevented by the action of the lips and tongue (Mills, 1982).

The dentist must try to achieve rapport with the child by an understanding and sympathetic approach, so that cessation of the habit becomes a matter of mutual concern. In addition, a simple passive removable appliance may be fitted when the child is about 8 or 9 years of age, mainly to act as a reminder to the child. With or without an appliance, the habit is usually abandoned by about 10 years of age, when children begin to take greater interest in their teeth and in their appearance generally. If the habit persists, insertion of an appliance as part of orthodontic treatment finally breaks the habit.

In the U.S.A., fixed appliances are commonly used which incorporate wire 'cribs' that prevent thumb or fingers from being placed in the mouth (Gellin, 1978); these types of appliances are not in favour in the U.K.

REFERENCES

Gellin M E 1978 Digital sucking and tongue thrusting in children. Dental Clinics of North America 22:603–619
Mills J R E 1982 Principles and practice of orthodontics. Churchill Livingstone, Edinburgh, p 52–54

# First permanent molars of poor prognosis

Assessment of long-term prognosis
Treatment planning

First permanent molars are important teeth in the dentition, and extraction is only considered if their long-term prognosis is poor. Unfortunately, many first molars become carious soon after eruption; by the age of 10 years only 38% of children in the U.K. have not experienced decay in these teeth (Todd and Dodd, 1985). If first permanent molars must be extracted, the undesirable effects on the occlusion may be minimised by balancing and compensating extractions and, if possible, by extracting the teeth at the most appropriate time in dental development, which is usually between the ages of 8½ and 10 years; ideally, the developing second molars then erupt into the first molar spaces and a satisfactory occlusion is established without appliance therapy.

## ASSESSMENT OF LONG-TERM PROGNOSIS

It is an important responsibility of children's dentists to assess the long-term prognosis of first permanent molars in child patients by the age of 8 or 9 years, so that a decision can be made on whether to conserve or extract the teeth. Signs that indicate a poor prognosis include the following:

1. Large amalgam restorations already present.
2. Recurrent caries in teeth already restored.
3. Lingual demineralisation or caries in mandibular molars, and buccal demineralisation or caries in maxillary molars, especially around existing restorations.
4. Abnormal enamel structure (e.g. hypoplasia).
5. Unfavourable attitudes of the child and parent regarding dental care.
6. Poor oral hygiene.
7. Poor patient cooperation.

## TREATMENT PLANNING

When the first permanent molars are assessed to have a poor prognosis, the following factors must be considered before a decision is made to extract the teeth.

### 1. Congenital absence of teeth

Clearly, plans to extract first molars become complicated if other teeth are found to be congenitally absent. However, the absence of third molars has only a marginal effect on the decision. Indeed the germs of the third molars may not have begun to calcify at the age of 8½ to 10 years; therefore the decision to extract first molars must often be made without knowledge of the development of third molars.

### 2. Hypoplasia of premolars

One or more unerupted permanent teeth may be hypoplastic due to infection of the primary predecessors or to trauma during extraction of the primary tooth; second premolars are most commonly affected. It may be possible to detect severe hypoplasia on a radiograph and to decide that the prognosis of the hypoplastic tooth is worse than that of the carious first molar.

### 3. Arch relationship and degree of crowding

In general, the most favourable conditions for

extraction of first molars are a Class 1 arch relationship and mild crowding (i.e. insufficiency of space for eruption of canines and premolars).

## 4. Stage of dental development

Extractions must be timed to maximise bodily mesial movement of the developing second molars, and to minimise mesial tilting. The ideal time to extract mandibular first molars is when root formation of the second molars is just beginning (as shown on a radiograph), which is usually between the ages of 8½ and 10 years; this gives the second molars every opportunity to move forward bodily. Earlier extraction generally is undesirable because mandibular second premolars have a tendency to drift distally, and very early extraction of first molars encourages this tendency. On the other hand, if extractions are delayed till after 10 years of age, the second molars will show less bodily movement and more tilting. Thus, extraction of mandibular first molars at the age of 8½ to 10 years is a compromise between the need to extract early to encourage mesial drift of second molars, and the need to delay to discourage distal drift of second premolars.

In the maxilla, unerupted second molars tend to be distally inclined, especially in a crowded arch, and they readily drift mesially by moving into more upright positions. Therefore, extraction of maxillary molars can often be delayed until about 11 or 12 years of age without affecting the final occlusion.

Under the conditions outlined above, extraction of poor first molars between the ages of 8½ and 10 years is fully justified, and often results in a satisfactory occlusion with acceptable contacts between second premolars and second molars; sometimes, final adjustments with an orthodontic appliance may be required. This outcome is preferable to that resulting from extraction of first molars several years later, following repeated repair and extension of restorations.

If, however, all the conditions outlined above are not satisfied, it would be prudent to consult an orthodontist before proceeding with treatment. For example, if the patient has severe incisor crowding or a Class II malocclusion with increased overjet, it may be preferable to delay (if possible) the extraction of maxillary first molars until the maxillary second molars erupt, and fit an appliance to hold the second molars in position, thus preserving space for retraction of premolars and correction of incisor crowding or overjet (Crabb and Rock, 1971). However, some orthodontists argue against this approach, on the grounds that the patient may be more than 13 years of age before the second molars are erupted sufficiently to be clasped (an age when orthodontic treatment is not always well tolerated) and that retraction of premolars followed by correction of incisor crowding or overjet is lengthy treatment complicated by anchorage problems; they suggest that maxillary first molars should be extracted with the mandibular molars at about 8½ to 10 years and accept that a premolar unit may have to be extracted later to complete treatment (Houston, 1982). This approach ensures that treatment is carried out for a relatively young child and is completed quickly, but the possible loss of premolars in addition to first molars may be considered unacceptable.

## REFERENCES

Crabb J J, Rock W P 1971 Treatment planning in relation to the first permanent molar. British Dental Journal 131:396–401

Houston W J B 1982 Orthodontic diagnosis, 3rd edn. Wright, Bristol, p 19

Todd J E, Dodd T 1985 Children's dental health in the United Kingdom 1983. Her Majesty's Stationery Office, London, p 31

# PART FIVE

# Treatment of common oral soft tissue lesions

# 23

# Periodontal disease

Chronic marginal gingivitis
Gingivitis artefacta
Localised gingival recession
Gingival hyperplasia associated
  with phenytoin therapy

Periodontitis
  Prepubertal periodontitis
  Juvenile periodontitis

## CHRONIC MARGINAL GINGIVITIS

Chronic marginal gingivitis is widespread in children. A survey in 1983 of child dental health in the U.K. (Todd and Dodd, 1985) showed that the condition was present in 18 per cent of 5-year-old children, 40 per cent of 7-year-olds, 54 per cent of 11-year-olds and 49 per cent of 15-year-olds.

Chronic gingivitis is often associated with erupting primary and permanent teeth, and with exfoliating primary teeth, but this resolves spontaneously. Most of the chronic gingivitis in children is associated with the presence of plaque, materia alba and calculus, and therefore is the result of inefficient oral hygiene. Other common local irritants include rough edges of carious cavities and overhanging margins of restorations.

### Treatment

1. Remove local irritating factors by carrying out a prophylaxis, restoring carious cavities, and replacing or smoothing unsatisfactory restorations.
2. Give oral hygiene instruction and dietary advice (Ch. 3).

## GINGIVITIS ARTEFACTA

Gingivitis artefacta is a self-inflicted lesion, most commonly on a gingival margin or papilla; it is usually inflicted with a finger nail. If the child is asked to indicate the site of discomfort, the offending finger points directly to the lesion; this is a useful diagnostic sign. The lesion may be an ulcer or a localised stripping of the gingival margin from the tooth, which may expose the root surface.

This type of behaviour by a child is usually initiated by minor gingival irritation, for example from an inflamed papilla or an exfoliating tooth, but sometimes psychological factors are involved and the injuries are more serious (Stewart and Kernohan, 1972).

### Treatment

1. Examine closely to detect any possible source of local irritation, and treat as necessary.
2. Inform the child that the finger is aggravating the soreness and attempt to gain the child's and the parents' cooperation in breaking the habit. Placing a piece of adhesive bandage on the finger may serve as a useful reminder.
3. Patients with psychological disturbances may needs to be referred for treatment before any improvement in their gingival condition can be achieved.

## LOCALISED GINGIVAL RECESSION

Localised gingival recession in children is seen most frequently on the labial surface of a mandibular incisor; the condition is sometimes referred to as a 'Stillman's cleft'.

Gingival recession is sometimes associated with a labial fraenum that is attached high into the free gingival margin; the latter may be pulled away from the tooth during normal movements of the lips. The high fraenal attachment also makes it difficult for the child to keep the gingival margin clean with a toothbrush. The situation may be further complicated by a very shallow labial sulcus, with little or no attached gingiva over the root of the tooth.

The condition is also often associated with a tooth that is more labially positioned than the other incisors in the arch and therefore has little or no supporting labial bone. Occlusal trauma may also be a factor, and this is sometimes associated with an anterior crossbite.

### Treatment

1. If a high fraenal attachment is the cause, periodontal surgery is required to correct the abnormality and restore a normal gingival contour.
2. If the fraenal attachment is normal but the tooth is positioned labially in the arch or is in traumatic occlusion, orthodontic treatment is required. Either space is created for alignment of the incisors, or the labially-positioned tooth is extracted and the space closed.

## GINGIVAL HYPERPLASIA ASSOCIATED WITH PHENYTOIN THERAPY

Gingival hyperplasia is often seen in children suffering from epilepsy and receiving the drug phenytoin (Epanutin). Not all patients on phenytoin develop gingival hyperplasia, and when it occurs its severity varies considerably. Phenytoin does not directly cause the hyperplastic reaction; the primary cause is dental plaque but the drug appears to induce an exaggerated connective tissue response within the gingival tissues.

### Treatment

1. Give the child and the parents detailed instructions and every possible assistance in establishing and maintaining efficient plaque control.
2. Consult the child's physician. Although phenytoin is a safe and effective drug in the control of epilepsy, it is sometimes possible to change to another drug that does not cause gingival hyperplasia.
3. If the condition is severe, hyperplastic tissue may be removed by surgery, but this will recur

unless plaque control is excellent.
4. Advise the use of chlorhexidine, as mouthwash or toothpaste (Corsodyl Dental Gel). The mouthwash solution may be applied with a toothbrush; handicapped patients may not be capable of mouthrinsing.

## PERIODONTITIS

Periodontal disease in children is usually confined to the gingival tissues. Rarely, however, severe and rapidly progressing periodontitis occurs in children, even in the primary dentition. Alveolar bone is rapidly destroyed, producing deep periodontal pockets.

Two clinical conditions are recognised: prepubertal periodontitis and juvenile periodontitis. These diseases may occur in children who show no other signs of disease, but also may be associated with other diseases, for example Papillon Lefèvre syndrome. The aetiology is not fully understood, but there appears to be impaired response of periodontal tissues to certain bacteria in the gingival crevice (Tsai et al, 1981; Ngan, Tsai and Sweeney, 1985) and abnormal function of monocyte and neutrophil leucocytes (Page et al, 1983).

### Prepubertal periodontitis

Prepubertal periodontitis affects the primary teeth of very young children, and may be localised or generalised (Page et al, 1983). The localised form usually presents by the age of 4 years and affects only a few teeth. Plaque deposits may be minimal and gingival inflammation mild, but deep pockets are detected on probing and seen radiologically, and periodontal bone destruction is rapid. Affected children may also suffer from otitis media and upper respiratory tract infections.

Generalised prepubertal periodontitis begins earlier (at about the time of tooth eruption) and affects all the primary teeth. Both the marginal and attached gingiva is acutely inflamed and, because of this, toothbrushing may be abandoned and the teeth become covered by heavy plaque deposits. Periodontal bone destruction is even more rapid than in the localised form of the disease. The children also suffer from otitis media and from recurrent, often severe upper respiratory infections.

## Treatment

Treatment is difficult because of the rapid progress of the disease and the young age of the patients. However, it is possible to control the localised form of the disease.

1. Perform thorough curettage of affected roots under local or general anaesthesia.
2. Prescribe a course of antibiotics. Penicillin has been used (Page et al, 1983) but other broad-spectrum antibiotics may be preferred. Tetracyclines should not be used for patients of this age, to avoid the risk of causing discolouration of developing teeth.
3. Emphasize to the parents the importance of efficient plaque removal, for which they must be responsible. Demonstrate an efficient technique for brushing and flossing the child's teeth (Ch. 3).
4. Every 2 months, perform a prophylaxis and re-emphasize the importance of meticulous oral hygiene.

The generalised form of the disease cannot be controlled and extraction of teeth will be necessary.

## Juvenile periodontitis

Juvenile periodontitis affects permanent teeth within a few years after their eruption. Localised and generalised forms have been described (Lindhe, 1983). The localised form is more common and typically affects incisors and first molars. The disease most frequently presents in adolescents but may be found in children as young as 10–11 years of age. Plaque deposits may be minimal and the gingiva may appear normal, but the deep periodontal pockets bleed on gentle probing. Severely affected teeth are mobile.

## Treatment

The disease can be controlled but tends to recur (Lindhe, 1983).

1. Reflect a soft tissue flap, curette the diseased tissues and plane the root surfaces.
2. Prescribe tetracycline: 250 mg to be taken four times daily for 2 weeks.
3. Prescribe chlorhexidine mouthwash (0.2% chlorhexidine gluconate solution): to be used several times a day for 2 weeks following surgery.
4. Instruct and motivate the patient to maintain excellent oral hygiene.

Irrigation of the periodontal pockets with antimicrobial solutions during surgery, and later by the patient at home (using an oral irrigation device) has also been recommended (Rams, Keyes and Wright, 1985).

If conservative treatment is unsuccessful, or is not undertaken because the patient is disinterested or uncooperative, extraction and prosthetic replacement of badly affected teeth is the only alternative treatment.

## REFERENCES

Lindhe J 1983 Textbook of clinical periodontology. Munksgaard, Copenhagen, ch 6
Ngan P W H, Tsai C C, Sweeney E 1985 Advanced periodontitis in the primary dentition: case report. Pediatric Dentistry 7:255–258
Page RC, Bowen T, Altman L et al (1983) Prepubertal periodontitis. 1. Definition of a clinical disease entity. Journal of Periodontology 54:257–271
Rams T E, Keyes P H, Wright W E 1985 Treatment of juvenile periodontitis with microbiologically modulated periodontal therapy (Keyes technique). Pediatric Dentistry 7:259–270
Stewart DJ, Kernohan DC (1972) Self-inflicted gingival injuries: gingivitis artefacta, factitial gingivitis. Dental Practitioner 22:418–426

Todd JE, Dodd T 1985 Children's dental health in the United Kingdom 1983. Her Majesty's Stationary Office, London
Tsai CC, McArthur WP, Baehni PC, Evian C, Genco RJ, Taichman NS (1981) Serum neutralizing activity against Actinobacillus actinomycetemcomitans leukotoxin in juvenile periodontitis. Journal of Clinical Periodontology 8:338–348

## RECOMMENDED READING

Armitage G C 1985 Periodontal diseases of children. In: Braham RL, Morris ME (eds) Textbook of pediatric dentistry, 2nd edn. Williams and Wilkins, Baltimore

# 24

# Viral, bacterial and mycotic infections of the mouth

Viral infections
  Acute herpetic gingivostomatitis
  Herpes labialis
  Herpangina
  Hand, foot and mouth disease
  Other viral infections

Bacterial infections
  Acute necrotising ulcerative gingivitis
Mycotic infections
  Candidosis (Candidiasis)

## VIRAL INFECTIONS

### Acute herpetic gingivostomatitis

Acute herpetic gingivostomatitis is caused by the herpes simplex virus; it occurs most frequently in infants between the ages of 1 and 3 years, but adults may also be affected. The patient becomes unwell and refuses to eat. Within about 24 hours, the mouth is very sore, the temperature is raised, and cervical lymph nodes are enlarged and tender. Vesicles about 3 or 4 mm in diameter form on the gingiva and oral mucosa, particularly on the dorsum of the tongue and on the hard and soft palate; the vesicles soon burst and leave shallow, painful ulcers. The gingiva is diffusely inflamed. The lesions heal spontaneously within about 10 days.

*Treatment*

1. Reassure the parent that the disease is self-limiting. Recommend a soft diet of cold rather than hot foods, and a high fluid intake.
2. Although no further treatment is essential, one or more of the following methods may be used:
   a. Systemic anti-viral drugs. Acyclovir (Zovirax): one 200 mg tablet or 5 ml elixir to be taken 5 times a day for 5 days. This drug is used especially for the treatment of herpes simplex infections in immunosuppressed patients.
   b. Topical application to the ulcer.
      (i) Acyclovir cream (Zovirax): Contains 5% acyclovir. The cream should be applied to the lesions as soon as they appear and again every 4 hours for 5 days.
      (ii) Carboxymethylcellulose Gelatin Paste (Orabase): A paste that adheres to mucous membranes and, by covering the ulcers, provides some relief from pain.
      (iii) Choline Salicylate Dental Paste (Bonjela, Teejel): Contains an anti-inflammatory and analgesic substance in a base that adheres to the oral mucosa.

   These preparations must be applied carefully with a cotton applicator several times a day; in practice many parents find this very difficult or impossible.
   c. Mouthwash
      Tetracycline Mouth-bath (Tetracycline Mixture): Contains 125 mg tetracycline hydrochloride in 5 ml. The solution must be rinsed around the mouth for 2 or 3 minutes several times a day; infants and young children are not able to do this.
3. If the child cannot sleep, prescribe a hypnotic drug (Ch. 12).

### Herpes labialis

Following primary herpetic infection, a balance is established in the body between the virus and the immune response. If the balance is upset by a disturbance such as the common cold, a fever or other factors, secondary lesions appear which take the form of small clusters of vesicles around the vermilion borders of the lips. The vesicles enlarge, coalesce, become covered by scabs and heal without scarring within about 10 days.

*Treatment*

Although the lesions heal spontaneously, acyclovir cream has been found helpful if applied as soon as the vesicles start to form. If this is done, the healing period may be halved (Fiddian et al, 1983).

## Herpangina

Herpangina is caused by a Coxsackie group A virus. The disease affects infants and young children and is heralded by fever and sore throat. The child is ill for 3 to 5 days.

Vesicles similar to those of primary herpes infection appear in the throat and on the soft palate, and break down into small ulcers. However, their distribution differs from that in primary herpes: they are mainly confined to the throat, and the gingiva is not affected. Healing occurs rapidly, within 3 or 4 days.

### Treatment

No treatment is necessary, other than reassuring the parent and recommending a soft diet with adequate fluids, but analgesics and antipyretics may be prescribed.

## Hand, foot and mouth disease

Hand, foot and mouth disease is caused by a strain of Coxsackie group A virus, and generally affects children of school age. However, the child may not feel unwell, as there is little, if any, fever; the chief complaint is a rash on the hands and feet. In the mouth there are small ulcers scattered on the oral mucosa, but there are no vesicles; the gingiva is not affected. The rash and oral ulcers disappear within about 1 week.

### Treatment

No treatment is required, but if the oral ulcers are painful they may be treated with Carboxymethylcellulose Gelatin Paste or Choline Salicylate Dental Paste (p. 172).

## Other viral infections

The mouth may be involved in a variety of viral infections, such as chickenpox, glandular fever and mumps. The oral lesions of chickenpox usually accompany the skin lesions and take the form of vesicles which burst to leave small ulcers. Glandular fever is often heralded by a sore throat, and commonly observed oral lesions are superficial erosions. A helpful diagnostic sign in mumps may be inflammation of the papilla at the opening of the parotid duct.

### Treatment

If the mouth lesions are painful, recommend a soft diet, with cold rather than hot food, and the use of Orabase or Bonjela as described above.

# BACTERIAL INFECTIONS

## Acute necrotising ulcerative gingivitis (Vincent's infection)

Acute necrotising ulcerative gingivitis (ANUG) is associated with the organisms Fusobacterium nucleatum and Borellia vincentii. The disease is rare in children under 16 years of age, except in under-developed countries; most cases of acute gingival inflammation in children are caused by the herpes simplex virus. ANUG is most common in young adults, and a number of predisposing factors have been noted, which include mental stress and local irritation from plaque or calculus deposits.

The disease is characterised by rapid destruction of interdental papillae and the formation of grey, punched-out ulcers. The condition may be localised to a single papilla, but in severe cases extensive areas of both the free and attached gingiva may be affected. There may be marked halitosis, which is characteristic of the condition.

### Treatment

1. If it is possible without causing intolerable pain, remove gross calculus and debris from the gingival margins by gentle scaling and by irrigation with hydrogen peroxide solution (20 vols).
2. Prescribe Metronidazole Tablets, one 200 mg tablet to be taken three times a day for 3 days. Metronidazole acts specifically against obligate anaerobes and does not otherwise disturb the normal oral flora.

Although metronidazole is widely used in the U.K., penicillin is equally effective in the treatment of ANUG (Duckworth et al, 1966). Penicillin may be used in the form of a syrup for young or handicapped children who refuse to take a tablet.

Penicillin V Elixir: Contains 250 mg phenoxymethylpenicillin in 5 ml. The dose is 5 ml every 6 hours for 5 days.

Metronidazole is generally preferred because it avoids the danger of developing penicillin-resistant strains of bacteria.

3. After about 1 week, when the acute phase has subsided, carry out more thorough scaling; an ultrasonic scaler provides a rapid and efficient method of doing this.
4. Give detailed oral hygiene instruction. An adequate standard of oral hygiene is necessary to avoid recurrence.

## MYCOTIC INFECTIONS

### Candidosis (Candidiasis)

Candidosis is caused by the fungus Candida albicans, which is commonly present in the mouth as a yeast-like saprophyte. Under certain conditions the fungus grows rapidly and the yeast-like forms are replaced by pathogenic mycelial forms which grow in the epithelium of the oral mucosa and produce characteristic lesions.

Two main types of candidosis are seen in children: acute pseudomembranous candidosis (Thrush) and chronic atrophic candidosis (denture stomatitis).

*Acute pseudomembranous candidosis (Thrush)*

Thrush is not uncommon in the newborn and in weak, undernourished infants, but it may also occur in apparently healthy children. A baby may become infected at birth by direct contact with Candida infection of the mother's vagina, which is not uncommon in pregnant women. Thrush may also result from prolonged use of antibiotics or steroids; Candida albicans is resistant to most of the commonly used antibiotics and may multiply when other microorganisms are suppressed.

The oral lesions are soft, elevated, creamy-white patches that cover small or large areas of the oral mucosa; the patches can be rubbed off, and leave raw, bleeding surfaces.

*Treatment*

1. Prescribe an antifungal drug. The alternatives are:
   a. Miconazole (Daktarin Oral Gel): contains 25 mg miconazole per ml, in a sugar-free gel.
   b. Nystatin (Nystan Pastilles): each pastille contains 100 000 units nystatin. One pastille should be sucked slowly 4 times daily for 7–14 days. The pastilles are more palatable than other nystatin preparations but they contain sugar.
2. Advise the parent to wash the infant's feeding utensils carefully after each meal and to store them in an antiseptic solution (e.g. Milton).

*Chronic atrophic candidosis ('denture stomatitis'):*

This type of candidosis affects the palatal mucosa under a denture or removable orthodontic appliance. The mucosa underlying the appliance becomes inflamed, appearing bright red and spongy. Springs or screws on the appliance may become buried in the inflamed tissue.

Clearly, conditions under the appliance of the affected patient must be favourable for the multiplication of Candida albicans, but local irritation from rough or ill-fitting appliances, or from poor oral hygiene, may also be a factor.

*Treatment*

1. Prescribe an antifungal drug, as for Thrush (above). Advise the child to keep the solution in the mouth for 2 or 3 minutes before swallowing, and also to apply solution to the fitting surface of the appliance; Candida grows on the surface of acrylic dentures as well as on the oral mucosa (Davenport, 1970).
2. Inspect the fitting surface of the appliance and smooth any sharp edges.
3. Give detailed instructions in oral hygiene and

in the care of the appliance. The appliance must be rinsed after meals and, when at home, brushed with a tootbrush.

4. Ideally, the appliance should not be worn until healing has occurred, but this would allow relapse of any orthodontic tooth movement previously achieved. Therefore, instruct the patient to wear the appliance for 2 or 3 weeks at night only (this prevents relapse and allows time for the mucosa to heal) and to keep the appliance in an antiseptic solution.

REFERENCES

Davenport J C 1970 Oral distribution of Candida in denture stomatitis. British Dental Journal 129:151–156
Duckworth R, Waterhouse J P, Britton D E R, Nuki K, Sheiham A, Winter R, Blake G C 1966 Acute ulcerative gingivitis: a double blind clinical controlled trial of metronidazole. British Dental Journal 120:559–602
Fiddian A P, Yeo J M, Stubbings R, Dean D 1983 Successful treatment of herpes labialis with topical acyclovir. British Medical Journal 286:1699–1701

RECOMMENDED READING

Pindborg J J 1980 Atlas of diseases of the oral mucosa, 3rd edn. Munksgaard, Copenhagen
Robinson H B G, Miller A S 1983 Color atlas of oral pathology, 4th edn. Lippincott, Philadelphia

# Miscellaneous soft tissue lesions

## EPULIS

The term 'epulis' is used to describe localised tumours of the gingiva. Three types of epulis occur in children: fibrous epulis, pyogenic granuloma and giant cell epulis. They are the result of local irritation which causes minor injury to the gingiva; this permits infection by oral bacteria, which is followed by chronic inflammation and proliferation of granulation tissue. The epulis remains covered by oral epithelium. Most epulides are found on a gingival margin or papilla in the anterior part of the mouth.

### Fibrous epulis

In the fibrous epulis, which is the most common type, granulation tissue is largely replaced by fibrous tissue. It has a smooth surface, which has the colour of normal oral mucosa.

### Pyogenic granuloma

The pyogenic granuloma contains dilated blood vessels and its colour ranges from dark red or purple to pale red. A pyogenic granuloma may, in time, change its character to that of a fibrous epulis.

### Giant cell epulis

This type of epulis contains large multinucleated osteoclasts ('giant cells') in proliferating granulation tissue. The epulis is soft, maroon or purple in colour, and bleeds easily. It remains localised in the gingiva but occasionally causes superficial resorption of the underlying bone.

### Treatment

1. Excise the epulis and a small area of normal tissue at its base. After removing a giant cell epulis, scrape the underlying bone with a curette. Send the tissue for histological examination to confirm the diagnosis.
2. Examine the area closely to detect any possible sources of gingival irritation that may have initiated the lesion.

## ENDOSTEAL GIANT CELL GRANULOMA

The endosteal giant cell granuloma is similar histologically to a giant cell epulis but originates within the bone and is seen on the gingiva only if it erodes through the bone; it then appears as a purplish nodule on the gingiva. It is more common in the mandible than in the maxilla and is diagnosed radiologically.

### Treatment

The granuloma must be surgically removed.

## PAPILLOMA

A papilloma is a small epithelial tumour consisting of a core of connective tissue covered by stratified squamous epithelium. The surface has a rough, warty appearance. A papilloma may be up to 1 cm in diameter, is pedunculated, and appears most frequently on the soft palate near the uvula, on the gingiva and on the tongue. It may be either soft and red, or firm and white, depending on the degree of keratinisation of the epithelium.

## Treatment

Excise the papilloma as described for an epulis.

## GEOGRAPHIC TONGUE (erythema migrans)

Geographic tongue is a common benign lesion that affects the dorsum of the tongue. The lesions are usually erythematous and have a white or yellow border, and they occur in patches that vary in size, shape and distribution.

## Treatment

No treatment is required, other than reassuring the patient and parent that the condition is harmless.

## APHTHOUS ULCERS ('CANKER SORES')

Aphthous ulcers occur commonly in adults and in children, but rarely in infants. The ulcers are usually shallow and about 2 to 4 mm in diameter, but they may be as large as 1 cm. The number of ulcers may be limited to one or two, or there may be large numbers scattered over the buccal and labial mucosa and floor of the mouth. The ulcers heal in about a week but tend to recur; the frequency of recurrence varies greatly, from only once or twice a year to more than once a month. The ulcers are painful but there is no associated systemic disturbance.

The aetiology of aphthous ulceration is unknown but it has been associated with an alpha-haemolytic streptococcus (S. sanguis) and with various immunological abnormalities (Rennie et al, 1985). Predisposing factors include psychological stress, allergies; trauma and, occasionally, deficiencies in haematinics (e.g. iron, folate or vitamin $B_{12}$) which may be caused by disorders such as coeliac disease.

## Treatment

If the ulcers are not very painful and systemic factors have been excluded, no treatment is required other than reassurance that the condition is self-limiting. However, in more severe cases some form of treatment should be given. Many methods have been tried, which reflects the uncertain aetiology of the condition.

1. Topical application to the ulcers:
   a. Carboxymethylcellulose Gelatin Paste (Orabase):
      The paste adheres to the oral mucosa; covering the ulcers makes them less painful.
   b. Choline Salicylate Dental Paste (Bonjela, Teejel):
      An anti-inflammatory and analgesic agent in a base that adheres to the mucosa.
   c. Triamcinolone Dental Paste B.P.C. (Adcortyl in Orabase):
      A corticosteroid in carboxymethylcellulose gelatin paste.
   These preparations must be applied several times a day by a parent, using a cotton applicator. This is only feasible if the child is reasonably cooperative, if there are not too many ulcers present and if the ulcers are near the front of the mouth.
2. Lozenges to dissolve in the mouth.
   Hydrocortisone Lozenges B.P.C. (Corlan Pellets): Contain 2.5 mg hydrocortisone, to be used two to four times a day, starting as soon as the patient senses that ulcers are developing.
3. Mouthwashes, to be kept in the mouth for 2 or 3 minutes.
   a. Tetracycline Mixture B.P.C.: Contains 125 mg tetracycline hydrochloride in 5 ml, to be used three times a day.
   b. Chlorhexidine gluconate solution (Corsodyl mouthwash): Contains 0.2 per cent w/v chlorhexidine gluconate, to be used three or four times a day.

## MUCOCELE

There are two types of mucocele: the mucous extravasation cyst, and the mucous retention cyst. They occur most commonly on the lower lip.

Extravasation cysts are much more common than retention cysts and they occur as a result of trauma to a small duct of a minor salivary gland, for example by biting the lip. Saliva escapes into the tissues and appears as a bluish blister up to

1 cm in diameter. They are not true cysts because they do not have epithelial linings.

## Treatment

Excise the mucocele together with the underlying mucous gland tissue.

REFERENCES

Rennie J S, Reade P C, Hay KD, Scully C 1985 Recurrent aphthous stomatitis. British Dental Journal 159:361–367

# PART SIX

# Treatment of traumatic injuries

# 26

# Prevention of trauma to teeth

Mouthprotectors
Early treatment of proclined maxillary incisors

Trauma to children's teeth occurs quite commonly. Permanent incisors showed signs of having been traumatised in 10 per cent of 8-year-old children and in 23 per cent of 12-year-old children examined in England and Wales in 1983 (Todd and Dodd, 1985). At all ages, the prevalence was higher in boys than in girls; for example, among 12-year-old children, 29 per cent of boys and only 16 per cent of girls showed evidence of trauma. Predisposing factors are Class II Division I malocclusion, increased incisor overjet and inadequate lip coverage of maxillary incisors (Hallett, 1953; O'Mullane, 1973; Todd and Dodd, 1985).

## MOUTHPROTECTORS

Mouthprotectors are used most commonly by young adults who participate in contact sports. Because less than 10 per cent of injuries to the anterior teeth of children under 15 years of age are associated with contact sports (O'Mullane, 1973; Winter and Kernohan, 1966), there is little justification for recommending mouthprotectors for all these children. However, mouthprotectors can be strongly recommended for certain children who are particularly at risk during contact sports; for example, those with increased incisor overjet and incompetent lips. In addition, because some sports (e.g. rugby football) become progressively rougher during the teenage years, the use of mouthprotectors by these children should be encouraged; their value in protecting children playing American football has been shown (American Dental Association, 1973).

Three types of mouthprotector are available (Stevens, 1972; Turner, 1977):

*1. The stock protector.* Made of latex rubber and commonly used by boxers, this type of protector is not recommended for children because it is poorly retained in the mouth, being held in position only by the opposing teeth; a near-fatal accident has been reported in which a protector of this type occluded the airway of an injured rugby player.

*2. The protector made in the mouth.* These are of two types:
   a. A firm outer 'shell' shaped in the form of a dental arch which is filled with acrylic resin and placed in the mouth; the resin sets in the mouth but remains resilient at mouth temperatures (Coe Dental Guard).
   b. A 'blank' of polyvinyl acetate-polyethylene material, 3 mm thick, which is softened by inserting into hot water (75°C), placed in the mouth, and moulded with the tongue and fingers (Coe Rediguard).

Both these types of protector are satisfactory if they are accurately fitted in the mouth. To ensure this, professional supervision is required.

*3. The protector made on a model.* This type of protector is the most satisfactory because it is made on an accurate model of the patient's maxillary teeth; however, since it is made professionally, it is the most expensive. Various materials are available, but polyvinyl acetatepolyethylene is most commonly used, in sheets 3–6 mm thick.

## Technique: mouthprotector

| Procedure | Method | Rationale | Notes |
|---|---|---|---|
| 1. Take an alginate impression | Take an alginate impression of the maxillary teeth and cast a plaster/stone model. | The mouthprotector will be made on the model. | |
| 2. Outline the periphery of the mouth-protector | Draw a pencil line on the model (Fig. 26.1a)<br>(i) *buccally and labially* — about 3 mm from the muco-buccal fold, avoiding the fraena;<br>(ii) *palatally* — about 10 mm from the molar gingival margins and behind the rugae;<br>(iii) *distally* — about 3 mm behind the most distal tooth in the arch.<br>OPTIONAL — Scribe a shallow groove along the pencil line. | The pencil line defines the outline to which the vinyl material will later be cut. This amount of coverage provides adequate support and sufficient retention.<br><br>The groove will show as a ridge on the vinyl and be an aid when trimming. | |
| 3. Mould the vinyl material to the model | Place a sheet of polyvinyl acetate-polyethylene material on the model. Ideally, use a mechanical apparatus which heats the vinyl and uses either vacuum, pressure, or both, to adapt the sheet over the model.<br>If the apparatus is not available, heat the vinyl either in hot water (75°C) or with a bunsen flame, and mould it by hand. | The mechanical apparatus moulds the vinyl quickly and efficiently. | |
| 4. Trim the vinyl | After allowing the vinyl to cool, remove it from the model and trim with scissors to the previously marked outline (Fig. 26.1b). | | |
| 5. Smooth the cut margin | Smooth the cut margin by passing it lightly over a flame.<br>Replace the mouthprotector on the model and ensure that it has not become distorted during trimming and smoothing. | Rough edges would cause discomfort to the patient by traumatising the soft tissues. | |
| 6. Try in the mouth and adjust if necessary | Try the mouthprotector in the mouth and further trim the margin if necessary to ensure the patient's comfort.<br>If the occlusion of the opposing teeth on the mouthprotector is uneven, place it again on the model and soften the area(s) of premature contact by heating with a flame. Replace it in the mouth (after checking that it is not too hot) and ask the patient to close firmly. | | |

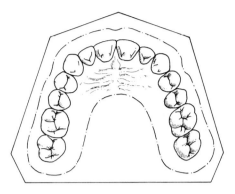

**Fig. 26.1a**

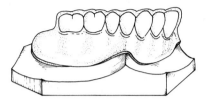

**Fig. 26.1b**

## EARLY TREATMENT OF PROCLINED MAXILLARY INCISORS

A child with a gross Class II Division I malocclusion is particularly at risk from trauma to anterior teeth. If, in addition, the child participates in contact sports or has already suffered trauma, there is a strong case for early correction of the malocclusion. This treatment is discussed in Chapter 20.

### REFERENCES

American Dental Association (1973) Mouth protectors: 11 years later. Report of bureau of dental health education, council on dental materials and devices. Journal of the American Dental Association 86:1365–1367

Hallett G E M 1953 Problems of common interest to the paedodontist and orthodontist with special reference to traumatised incisor cases. Transactions of the European Orthodontic Society 266–270

O'Mullane D M 1973 Some factors predisposing to injuries of permanent incisors in school children. British Dental Journal 134:328–332

Stevens O O 1981 Prevention of dental and oral injuries. In: Andreasen J O (ed) Traumatic injuries of the teeth, 2nd edn. Munksgaard, Copenhagen, ch 12

Todd J E, Dodd T 1985 Children's dental health in the United Kingdom 1983. Her Majesty's Stationery Office, London, ch 13

Turner C H 1977 Mouth protectors. British Dental Journal 143:82–86

Winter G B, Kernohan D C 1966 The importance of mouthguards. British Dental Journal 120:564–565

# 27

# Assessment and immediate treatment of traumatised anterior permanent teeth

## ASSESSMENT

When a child is brought to the dentist following an injury, the first essential is to assess the child and the nature of the injury; only when the relevant information is gained can the appropriate treatment be planned. A suggested outline for history-taking and examination is given below:

### History and examination

| Information sought | Rationale |
|---|---|
| **History** | |
| *Dental* | |
| How did the injury occur? | Indirect trauma, e.g. a blow on the chin, is more likely to cause jaw |
| Direct or indirect trauma to the teeth? | fracture than is a direct blow on a tooth. |
| Where did the injury occur? | If the wound is contaminated with soil, a tetanus toxoid injection may be indicated (see below). |
| When did the injury occur? | If the crown is fractured (especially through the pulp), the longer the interval between injury and treatment the poorer the prognosis. |
| Is a tooth fractured? If so, where is the fractured piece? | If the fractured piece cannot be accounted for, a chest radiograph should be obtained to exclude the possibility of its inhalation. |
| Is the child in pain? If so, from a tooth or elsewhere? | Pain suggests the site of injury; however, many fractured teeth are not painful immediately after injury, and pain is an unreliable indication of the degree of injury. |
| Was the child concussed, or has he suffered from headache, vomiting or amnesia since the injury? | The possibility of brain damage must be excluded. If any suggestive symptoms are reported, the patient should be referred to a hospital or to his doctor for further investigation. |
| Has the child received dental care in the past? | Regular attenders are more likely to be interested and co-operative in receiving treatment to save injured teeth. |
| *Medical* | |
| Is the child in good general health? Congenital heart defect or history of rheumatic fever? | If the child has a congenital heart defect, endodontic treatment may be justified only if the tooth is vital, and should be carried out under antibiotic cover to avoid the risk of causing a bacteraemia and bacterial endocarditis. |
| | If the tooth has a necrotic pulp, infected tissue would remain in lateral canals even after endodontic treatment, and be a possible source of bacteraemia in the future. |
| | However, all congenital heart defects do not carry the same risks of bacterial endocarditis. Therefore, the child's paediatrician should be consulted before a decision about endodontic treatment is made. |
| Bleeding disorders? | Bleeding disorders are relevant if soft tissues are lacerated, or if teeth are to be extracted. |
| Allergies? | If antibiotics are to be given, penicillin should be avoided if there is a history of allergy. |
| Tetanus immunisation status | If the wound is contaminated with soil and the child has not had a 'booster' injection within the last 5 years, he should be referred to a hospital or to his doctor for a tetanus toxoid injection. |

| Information sought | Rationale |
| --- | --- |
| **Examination** | |
| *Extra-oral* | |
| During history-taking, observe the following: | |
| (i) Facial swelling, bruising or lacerations? | Lacerations of the face may require suturing. |
| (ii) Limitation of mandibular movement, or mandibular deviation on opening or closing the mouth? | These are signs that the jaw may be fractured. |
| (iii) Are wounds clean or contaminated? | Antibiotics and/or tetanus toxoid may be required if wounds are contaminated. |
| Carefully palpate the face and jaws and note any painful areas. | |
| *Intra-oral* | |
| If a tooth is fractured, note whether the fracture is through enamel only, or whether it also involves dentine or pulp. | Treatment will differ according to the extent of fracture. |
| Note any tooth displacement. | Displaced teeth will need to be repositioned, and mobile teeth may require splinting. |
| Palpate teeth and alveolus to detect any mobility. | |
| If soft tissues are lacerated, examine carefully to detect any embedded tooth fragments. | Lacerations of the lips or tongue require suturing, but those of the oral mucosa heal quickly and usually do not need suturing. |
| *Radiographic* | |
| Take periapical radiographs of traumatised teeth; take two radiographs from different angles. | Periapical views show any root fractures and the stage of root development. Two radiographs are preferable because a root fracture may not be detectable from only one angle. |
| If the lips are lacerated, take radiographs to determine whether tooth fragments are embedded: | |
|     lower lip — occlusal view | |
|     upper lip — lateral view with occlusal film | |
| If there is a suspicion of jaw fracture, other radiographs will be required, e.g. | |
|     lateral oblique | |
|     panoramic | |
|     lateral skull | |
|     anterior-posterior skull | |

Pulp vitality tests are often misleading at this stage because the teeth may be concussed. However, a positive response to pulp testing indicates a good long-term prognosis for pulp vitality (Rock et al, 1974). During history-taking and examination, signs that might suggest child abuse should not be overlooked (Ch. 30).

## TREATMENT OF CROWN FRACTURES

### PULP PROTECTION

A traumatised tooth that is not fractured, or fractured through enamel only, requires no immediate treatment other than smoothing of rough edges, unless the tooth is loose in which case splinting may be necessary (see below). As in all cases of trauma, pulp vitality should be reviewed for at least 2 years; first, after about 1 month, and then at 3- to 6-month intervals. However, a tooth that is fractured through the dentine requires immediate treatment. The pulp must be protected against the irritation it would suffer from thermal stimuli passing through the exposed dentine, and from bacteria that might invade the pulp through the dentinal tubules. It is also important to stabilise the position of the tooth by restoring crown shape.

The pulp is protected by covering exposed dentine with a suitable insulating material, usually calcium hydroxide; but this material must in turn be protected if it is to remain in place and fulfil its function. Various materials and methods that may be used for this purpose are described below.

### Composite resin

Composite resin is the material used most frequently to cover and protect the calcium hydroxide dressing placed over fractured dentine. As an emergency procedure, either unfilled or filled resin is layered over the dressing and is retained on acid-etched labial and palatal enamel; but if time allows the fractured crown may also be restored (Ch. 28).

## Technique: composite resin cover

| Procedure | Method | Rationale | Notes |
|---|---|---|---|
| 1. Polish the labial and palatal enamel surfaces. | Use a slurry of pumice and water or an oil-free prophylaxis paste to polish labial and palatal surfaces of the fractured tooth. Wash off the pumice with a water spray. | Polishing removes plaque and pellicle that might interfere with subsequent acid etching. Pumice is preferred to commercial prophylactic pastes because the latter may contain fluoride and/or oily constituents that reduce the effectiveness of acid etching. | |
| 2. Isolate the tooth | Isolate the tooth by placing a cotton roll in the labial sulcus, and use a saliva ejector. | For the treatment to be successful it is essential that the tooth is kept isolated from saliva. | Although ideal isolation is obtained by placing a rubber dam, this is often not practicable in the emergency treatment of a fractured tooth. |
| 3. Etch labial and palatal enamel | After drying the tooth, apply a proprietary acid etchant in gel form with a small cotton pledget or fine brush. Apply the gel to labial and palatal enamel, extending about 4 mm from the fractured edge along the full mesio-distal width of the tooth. | Using a gel avoids the risk of acid flowing on to the fractured surface.<br><br>Etching about 4 mm from the fractured edge provides sufficient area for bonding of the composite resin. | |
| | Do not apply acid to the fractured incisal surface. | Although the fractured dentine has been protected with calcium hydroxide, it is prudent to avoid the possibility of acid seeping beneath it. | |
| | It is not necessary to etch the mesial or distal surfaces. | Approximal surfaces need not be etched because crown restoration is not the aim of this treatment. | If time is available and it is decided to restore the crown at the same session, mesial and distal surface enamel must also be etched. |
| | Keep the labial and palatal enamel wet with acid for 1 minute. | A 1-minute application has been found to produce the optimal etching pattern that ensures a strong bond with composite resin. | |
| 4. Wash and dry the enamel surface. | With an assistant holding the tip of a high-volume aspirator suction tube close to the tooth, wash the acid off with a stream of water directed at each surface for 15 seconds. Do not allow the patient to rinse. | Simultaneous washing and aspiration prevents acid from entering the mouth and giving the patient an unpleasant taste. Inadequate washing, or contamination of the etched surface by saliva, reduces the subsequent bond strength of resin to enamel. | |
| | Holding the lip away from the tooth, remove the wet cotton roll from the sulcus and replace with a dry one.<br>Dry the etched surface thoroughly by directing oil-free compressed air to each surface for 30 seconds. | Inadequate drying, or contamination by oil, also reduces the subsequent bond strength. | |

| Procedure | Method | Rationale | Notes |
|---|---|---|---|
| 5. Apply unfilled resin ('bonding agent') | Apply unfilled resin to the etched enamel and over the calcium hydroxide dressing previously placed over the incisal surface. | Unfilled resin readily permeates the etched enamel and forms a strong bond. | Although it seems logical to apply unfilled resin before the filled resin restorative material, it is not certain that this increases the bond strength. |
|  | Keep resin *within* the etched area. | Resin applied beyond the etched area would not bond to the enamel and, if not removed later, might create a 'pocket' in which plaque would accumulate. | Etched enamel remaining uncovered by resin quickly remineralises and is not more susceptible to caries. |
| 6. Apply filled resin (i.e. composite paste) | When the unfilled resin has polymerised, add a layer of composite paste, adapting it to the unfilled resin with any convenient instrument (Fig. 27.1). Allow the material to polymerise and smooth if necessary with a fine stone or abrasive disc. | Composite paste is stronger than the unfilled resin and therefore provides a more reliable protection for the tooth. The paste bonds directly with the resin. | Unfilled resin alone may provide adequate protection. Whether using unfilled resin alone or layers of unfilled and filled resins, this method of retaining the pulp dressing without restoring the crown is convenient as an emergency measure. |

Arrange to see the patient within 3 or 4 weeks to test pulp vitality and to restore the crown (Ch. 28). Crown restoration is important not only for aesthetic reasons but also to prevent (a) movement of adjacent teeth into the space, (b) over-eruption of the opposing tooth, and (c) labial drift of the fractured tooth (if the incisal edge is no longer under the control of the lower lip).

ALTERNATIVE METHODS
1. Instead of the 2-stage procedure described in 6 and 7 above, involving first unfilled resin and then paste, a 1-stage procedure could be employed by using a thin mix of paste. This may be made by mixing equal parts of catalyst resin and universal paste.
2. A 1-stage procedure may also be used if one of the following types of materials is available:-
    i) a filled resin fissure sealant
    ii) a low viscosity filled resin restorative material.
3. If time is available at the emergency visit, the crown may be restored as described in Chapter 28

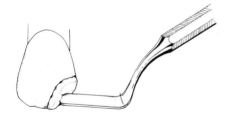

**Fig. 27.1**

Although careful precautions are taken in this technique to avoid endangering the pulp during the etching procedure, some dentists prefer to confine this method to cases where the area of exposed dentine is small.

## Stainless steel crown

Composite resin cannot be used when the extent of fracture is such that there is insufficient enamel available to retain the composite. In these cases, stainless steel crowns, which have long been used in the emergency treatment of fractured incisors, are very useful. They require no tooth preparation (unless the tooth has tight contacts with adjacent teeth), they are fairly easy to fit and they are strong. Their only disadvantage is that their appearance is poor, but this is rarely a problem with a child patient if it is explained that pulp protection is the essential treatment at this stage and that an aesthetic crown will be made later.

### Copper ring

A copper ring normally used for taking impressions may be used to retain a protective dressing on a fractured tooth. A ring of the correct size is cut and fitted as illustrated in Figure 27.2; like the stainless steel crown, it is fairly easy to fit and it is strong, but its appearance is very poor.

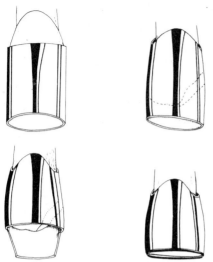

**Fig. 27.2** Method of using a copper ring to protect a fractured incisor.

## Orthodontic band

A preformed othodontic band may be cemented to the tooth, using the cementing material to cover the calcium hydroxide material over the fractured dentine.

## Acrylic, epimine or composite resin crown

A reasonably aesthetic crown may be made with a crown form filled with acrylic, epimine or composite resin. However, this method is only suitable if there is spacing between the fractured and adjacent teeth because, to provide adequate thickness of resin, a crown form must be selected that is larger than the natural teeth; the alternative of cutting the tooth is not considered an appropriate form of immediate treatment.

## Technique: stainless steel crown

| Procedure | Method | Rationale | Notes |
|---|---|---|---|
| 1. Select a crown | Measure the mesio-distal width of the fractured tooth at the gingival margin using dividers or a Vernier gauge. Select a crown of the same size, or slightly larger. Check the fit by placing it on the tooth. | If a crown of the exact size is not available, a slightly larger size should be used; later the edge can be crimped with contouring pliers to produce a tight fit. | If dividers or gauge are not available, the crown may be selected by trial and error. |
| 2. Trim the crown | Place the beaks of the dividers at the incisal edge and gingival margin of the tooth, in the centre of the labial aspect (Fig. 27.3a). Transfer this measurement to the stainless steel crown and mark the position of the gingival edge with a dental instrument or bur. Similarly, mark the position of the gingival margin on the mesial, distal and palatal aspects. With a pair of strong crown scissors, join the marks; this will approximate the gingival contour. (OPTIONAL) Cut a notch from the palatal aspect of the crown; this allows pulp testing without removal of the crown. | | The notch is also helpful when removing the crown. |
| 3. Try the crown on the tooth | After smoothing the cut edge of the steel crown with a stone, try it on the tooth. If necessary, reduce the crown further by cutting or stoning the edge. | A rough edge would traumatise the gingiva when trying the crown in place. The margin of the crown should be placed just within the gingival crevice. | |
| 4. Contour the margin of the crown | Use a Johnson No. 114 plier to contour the margin of the crown so that it is a tight fit (Fig. 27.3b). | Contouring is necessary to produce a good fit at the gingival margin; this is essential to ensure good retention and to avoid gingival irritation. | |

| Procedure | Method | Rationale | Notes |
|---|---|---|---|
| (OPTIONAL)<br>Cut away the labial face of the steel crown | Note the area of labial tooth surface that is to be left uncovered and, with a diamond bur in a high-speed handpiece, make a hole in a part of the crown that would cover this area. Enlarge the hole as required to produce a 'window', as in Fig. 27.3c or d. | Removing the labial face of the crown improves aesthetics and permits subsequent vitality testing without removing the crown. | |
| 5. Smooth the margin of the crown | Smooth all cut margins of the crown with a stone and finally with a rubber wheel. | | |
| 6. Cement the crown | Cover the dentine on the fractured surface with calcium hydroxide (if this has not previously been done). Cement the crown with quick-setting zinc oxide-eugenol.<br><br>If the entire labial surface of the steel crown has been cut away (as in Fig. 27.3d), add composite resin to replace the fractured portion of crown. | A very adhesive cement (e.g. polycarboxylate) would make it difficult to remove the crown for pulp testing. | If a palatal notch or labial 'window' has been made, the crown may be cemented with polycarboxylate cement. |

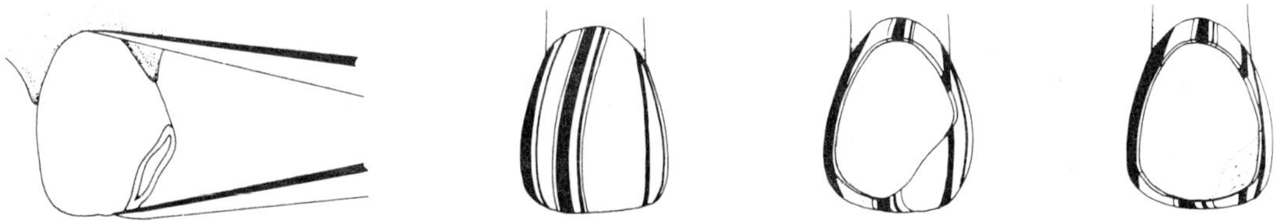

**Fig. 27.3a**    **Fig. 27.3b**    **Fig. 27.3c**    **Fig. 27.3d**

A crown form is trimmed to the gingival margin of the tooth and filled with the selected shade of resin. After moistening the tooth (or covering it with a thin layer of petroleum jelly), the filled crown form is placed over it. After 1 to 2 minutes, before the resin has completely polymerised, it is removed from the tooth and allowed to fully polymerise. After trimming and polishing the margin, the crown is cemented to the tooth with quick-setting zinc oxide–eugenol cement.

### PULP CAPPING

When a tooth is fractured through the dentine, it is necessary merely to protect the pulp. However, when the fracture involves the pulp, some form of pulp treatment becomes necessary. Sometimes the pulp is not actually exposed but can be seen as a reddish shadow beneath a thin layer of dentine; such cases should be treated as if the pulp were exposed, because infection will inevitably have reached the pulp before treatment can be started.

If the pulp exposure is pin-point in size and the child presents within a few hours of injury, pulp capping with calcium hydroxide may be justified (Andreasen, 1981). However, pulp capping has been found to be less successful than pulpotomy (Fuks et al, 1982), presumably because the pulp becomes contaminated before treatment is carried out. It may be argued that pulp capping is justified only for teeth with completed root development because, should the pulp die, root canal treatment is an uncomplicated procedure. In contrast, if the pulp dies in a tooth with immature root development, the problems in treatment are much greater (Ch. 28); for this reason pulpotomy is the treatment of choice in these cases.

Even when pulpotomy is the planned treatment, pulp capping may sometimes be done as an emergency measure. Time may not be available to complete a pulpotomy at the emergency visit and, moreover, the child may be upset and uncooperative as a result of his injuries. However, the child should be seen again as soon as possible (ideally within 24 hours) for the pulpotomy to be done.

Before pulp capping, the exposed pulp and surrounding dentine should be cleaned gently with a cotton pledget moistened in sterile saline or sterile water, and then dried with a cotton pledget; water or compressed air from a 'triplespray' should not be used as these would irritate the pulp and cause pain. A hard-setting type of calcium hydroxide usually is used, and it must be protected by one of the methods described above.

## PULPOTOMY

Pulpotomy involves removal of coronal pulp; the objectives are to remove infected pulp tissue and to preserve healthy radicular pulp so that root development can continue. If the radicular pulp dies, the root apex will remain open, and this would present a problem in endodontic treatment. Therefore, pulpotomy is especially indicated for immature teeth in which root development is incomplete.

## Technique: vital pulpotomy

| Procedure | Method | Rationale | Notes |
|---|---|---|---|
| 1. Prepare equipment and materials | Use a sterile pre-packed tray containing all the instruments and materials required. | | |
| 2. Prepare the patient and the site of operation | Administer local analgesia. Place rubber dam (unless there is good reason for not doing so). | The maintenance of a sterile field is so important for the success of this treatment that every precaution should be taken to ensure it. | If it is not possible to use rubber dam, isolate the tooth using cotton wool rolls and saliva ejector. |
| 3. Gain access to the pulp chamber | Use a diamond or tungsten carbide bur at high speed to outline the access cavity in the palatal surface of the tooth. Prepare this cavity in dentine but do not extend into the pulp (Fig. 27.4a). Make the cavity large enough to permit good access to the pulp chamber and to the pulp horns (Fig. 27.4b). Dry the area, and then wipe the tooth, adjacent teeth and rubber dam with a cotton pledget soaked in hibitane solution (1:1000) or other disinfectant. Using a sterile round bur (size 4–6) deepen the access cavity until pulp is exposed. Either with the same bur or with a similar-sized fissure bur, remove the entire roof of the pulp chamber (Fig. 27.4c). | The pulp chamber will later be opened with a sterile bur.   All instrumentation from this stage must be under strictly sterile conditions. | It is very important to provide good access to the pulp chamber. Since the final restoration is usually a post crown, it is unnecessary to conserve coronal tissue. |
| 4. Amputate the coronal pulp | With a round bur revolving slowly, or with a sharp excavator, amputate the pulp at the floor of the pulp chamber. | | The use of a bur or excavator to amputate the pulp is equally satisfactory; each method has its adherents. |

| Procedure | Method | Rationale | Notes |
|---|---|---|---|
| | Remove amputated coronal pulp, including pulp horns, with an excavator (Fig. 27.4d), and wash the pulp chamber with sterile saline or sterile water using a disposable syringe. Dry and control haemorrhage with sterile cotton wool pledgets, avoiding pressure. | | |
| 5. Apply calcium hydroxide | When haemorrhage has ceased, place calcium hydroxide paste or powder in the floor of the pulp chamber (Fig. 27.4e). Paste is best applied fairly thickly on the end of a small instrument; powder is insufflated through a 'Jiffy' tube. Do not exert pressure on the radicular pulp. | Pressure on the pulp could cause after-pain and provoke an inflammatory response in the pulp. | Many calcium hydroxide pastes are available. Only non-setting preparations have been extensively tested in this technique and should therefore be used rather than a hard-setting type. |
| 6. Seal the cavity | Seal the cavity with a thick mix of quick-setting zinc oxide-eugenol (Fig. 27.4f). Avoid pressure by smearing the cement over the opening of the cavity; do not pack it in. | An effective seal from the oral fluids is essential to the success of the treatment. | Alternatively, a cement base may be placed and the cavity sealed with glass ionomer cement. |

Arrange to see the patient within a few weeks to test pulp vitality and to restore the crown (Ch. 28). Part of the pulp chamber may be used to contribute to the retention of a composite resin restoration.

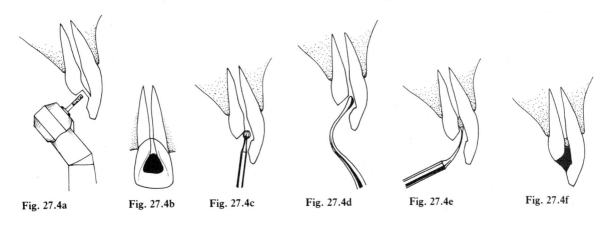

Fig. 27.4a          Fig. 27.4b          Fig. 27.4c          Fig. 27.4d          Fig. 27.4e          Fig. 27.4f

Assessed radiologically, root development of maxillary incisors appears complete by the age of about 10 or 11 years, but it has been shown that further closure of the apex occurs up to 14 or 15 years of age (Friend, 1966).

Although pulpotomy should be performed as soon as possible after injury, the immediate treatment sometimes may be pulp capping, for reasons given above.

PARTIAL PULPOTOMY

The traditional view that pulpotomy (i.e. removal of all coronal pulp) is the correct treatment for teeth with exposed vital pulps has been challenged by Cvek (1978), who has obtained successful results with a partial pulpotomy technique.

Instead of making access to the pulp chamber through the palatal surface of the tooth, partial pulpectomy is carried out through the pulp ex-

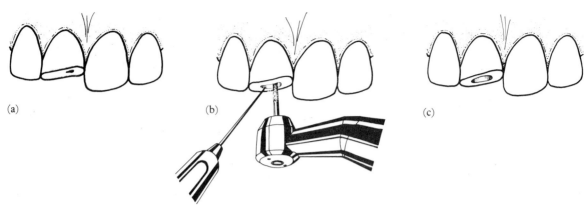

(a)          (b)          (c)

**Fig. 27.5**

posure site (Fig. 27.5a). A sterile cylindrical or cone-shaped diamond instrument is used at high speed, while cooling and washing with sterile water or saline delivered from a syringe (Fig. 27.5b). This technique is claimed to cause minimal irritation to the underlying pulp, which is removed to a depth of about 2 mm. After controlling bleeding with sterile cotton wool pledgets, a layer of calcium hydroxide is placed over the pulp and a quick-setting zinc oxide-eugenol cement is inserted without pressure, to seal the cavity (Fig. 27.5c).

This technique is more conservative than the standard pulpotomy technique not only in the amount of pulp removed but also in the amount of tooth substance destroyed. Cvek (1978) found that the size of the pulp exposure and the time elapsed before treatment were not critical for the success of treatment. The technique must be accepted as an attractive alternative to the standard pulpotomy, although it is not yet supported by the same weight of experimental evidence.

PULPECTOMY

Pulpectomy (removal of coronal and radicular pulp) is the usual treatment when a tooth with a fully developed root becomes fractured through the pulp. However, if the pulp exposure is pinpoint in size and the patient presents within a few hours of injury, pulp capping may be adequate treatment. Pulpectomy must be followed by root canal treatment and root filling.

Pulpectomy need not be done as part of im-

mediate treatment; the exposed pulp may be capped with calcium hydroxide (retained by one of the methods described above), and arrangements made for further observation or treatment as necessary.

The techniques of pulpectomy and root canal treatment will not be described here; the reader is referred to textbooks of endodontics.

TREATMENT OF ROOT FRACTURES

The treatment of a tooth that has sustained a root fracture depends on whether it has been loosened as a result of the fracture. When a fracture occurs in the apical third of a root (Fig. 27.6a) the tooth is not loosened; when it occurs in the middle third of a root (Fig. 27.6b) the tooth is usually loosened; when it occurs in the cervical third (Fig. 27.6c) the tooth is always loosened.

Teeth with apical third root fractures require no treatment, but the immediate treatment of teeth with middle third root fractures, and of some with cervical third fractures, involves splinting of the teeth; this is discussed in the next section. The prognosis for most root-fractured teeth is good (Zachrisson and Jacobsen, 1975). However, when a fracture is close to the gingival crevice (Fig. 27.6d) the prognosis is poor and splinting is not recommended; in these cases a decision must be made either to extract the coronal portion and retain the apical portion for construction of a post crown (Fig. 27.6 e and f), or to extract the two fragments and make a prosthetic replacement.

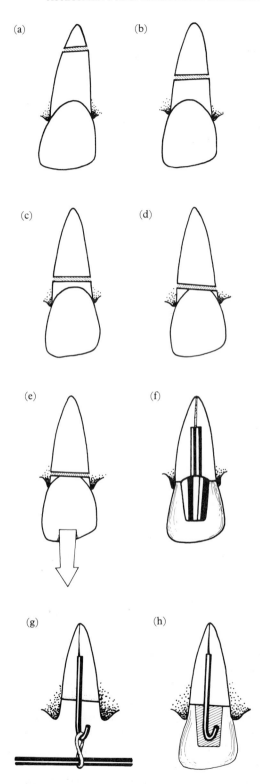

**Fig. 27.6**

When the decision is made to extract the coronal portion only, immediate treatment must also include removal of the pulp and the placement of a temporary dressing in the remaining root portion. However, this treatment (extraction and pulpectomy) may be postponed, and the coronal fragment temporarily splinted in position; this course of action might be indicated if the child is upset and uncooperative as a result of the traumatic experience.

After a coronal fragment is extracted, it may be found that the face of the remaining root lies too far subgingival to permit adequate access for its preparation and for taking an impression. This problem may be resolved by either surgical or orthodontic means; the latter approach is preferred. A piece of steel wire, bent into a hook at one end, may be cemented into the root canal (after pulp extirpation), and traction applied by an orthodontic elastic band attached to a labial arch wire (Fig. 27.6g). Alternatively, a composite resin core or even a crown may be made over the wire hook and an orthodontic bracket bonded to its labial surface (Fig. 27.6h). When the root has been extended sufficiently, root canal treatment is completed and a post crown made.

## SPLINTING

Trauma may loosen a tooth either by breaking the periodontal attachment to the alveolar bone or by fracturing the root. Splinting may be required to stabilise a loosened tooth until healing of the periodontal ligament occurs or until repair of the root fracture takes place.

### Periodontal healing

Splinting is not an essential pre-requisite for periodontal healing; indeed, prolonged splinting delays healing and encourages root resorption. However, it is often desirable to splint the tooth to protect it from further trauma during the healing period. The decision on whether to make a splint depends principally on the degree of tooth mobility; grossly mobile teeth should be splinted, but less mobile teeth may be left unsplinted if the child is sensible enough to follow instructions and to take obvious precautions.

The splinting period is kept as short as possible. Even for the severest cases, for example a replanted tooth, the splint can be removed after about a week; but it would not be unreasonable to prolong this to 2 to 3 weeks, or to 3 to 4 weeks if alveolar bone is fractured (Andreasen, 1981).

### Repair of root fractures

A longer splinting period, 2 to 3 months, is recommended in the treatment of root fractures (Andreasen, 1981), when the aim is to promote repair of the fractured root.

Ideally a hard tissue repair occurs and the fragments become firmly united, but a connective tissue repair may be satisfactory. Sometimes, however, little or no repair takes place, the fracture site becomes filled with inflamed granulation tissue, and the tooth remains loose.

Teeth with apical third root fractures do not require splinting because such fractures do not cause loosening; the teeth have adequate periodontal support and it is not necessary to promote repair of the root.

Splinting is required for teeth with middle third and cervical third root fractures (except those described above) because these types of fracture do cause loosening of the teeth. Periodontal support is inadequate to maintain normal function and additional support is required by repair of the fractured root.

REPOSITIONING OF DISPLACED TEETH

Teeth that have been displaced must be repositioned before they are splinted. Teeth that have been displaced labially or palatally, or that have been extruded, may be repositioned by digital pressure. If there has been delay in presenting for treatment and the teeth have become firm in abnormal positions, they must be repositioned by orthodontic treatment.

Teeth that have been intruded do not need to be splinted because they are supported by alveolar bone, but they present special problems because rapid pulp death and external root resorption occur frequently. These complications have been found to occur especially when intruded teeth are surgically repositioned by the use of forceps; for this reason more gentle extrusion by orthodontic means is the recommended treatment (Andreasen 1981; Spalding et al, 1985). To do this, an orthodontic bracket is bonded with composite resin to the labial surface of the tooth. If the tooth is completely intruded it must be pulled down gently with forceps just far enough to allow a bracket to be attached.

Although intruded teeth with incompletely formed roots sometimes re-erupt spontaneously, early orthodontic treatment is recommended for these as well as for mature teeth (which do not re-erupt). Pulp death may occur and root resorption may begin within 2 to 3 weeks and it is important that the teeth are extruded sufficiently to allow access to the pulp chamber for endodontic treatment. Orthodontic treatment may be delayed only when an immature tooth has suffered a minor degree of intrusion and access to the pulp chamber has not been compromised; the tooth may be given the opportunity to re-erupt spontaneously.

Endodontic treatment should be carried out as soon as possible for teeth with completely formed roots because pulp death is inevitable. After pulpectomy, the root canal should be filled with calcium hydroxide paste (p. 211) which inhibits external root resorption. However, this treatment can be delayed for immature teeth because it is possible that the pulp will survive; close observation is essential, and radiographs should be taken every 2 to 3 months to check for the earliest signs of external root resorption.

METHODS OF MAKING SPLINTS

Splints may be made either by the direct method, in which the splint is constructed in the patient's mouth, or by the indirect method, in which the splint is made in the laboratory.

### Direct method

The most obvious advantage of the direct method is that laboratory services are not required, thus avoiding delay and expense.

The most commonly used splints are made with acrylic, epimine or composite resin. These ma-

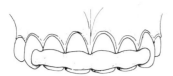

**Fig. 27.7** Resin splint

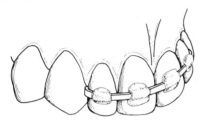

**Fig. 27.8** Arch wire and resin splint

terials can either be applied across the labial surfaces of the teeth (Fig. 27.7) or used to bond an arch wire to the teeth (Fig. 27.8).

The tooth to be splinted must be supported while the splint is being made, and this is usually done with a finger placed over its incisal edge. An alternative method utilises impression compound (Croll and Johnson, 1982). A piece of softened compound is placed on the incisal edges of the mandibular incisors (assuming the traumatised tooth is a maxillary incisor), the patient is asked to close his teeth together and the compound is moulded over the palatal surfaces and incisal edges of the maxillary incisors (but kept away from the labial surfaces). The traumatised tooth is supported in this way while the splint is made.

*Acrylic or epimine resin splint*

Although retention can be obtained by flowing resin between the teeth and on to the palatal surfaces (Freedman and Hooley, 1968), it is more usual to provide retention by etching the labial enamel. However, it is important to ensure that the splint can be easily removed at the end of the splinting period, and for this reason acrylic or epimine resin are preferred to composite resin. The latter bonds very strongly to etched enamel and is difficult to remove; even after careful polishing of the enamel surface it is difficult to ensure that all composite is removed and that the enamel is restored to its original state. On the other hand,

acrylic and epimine resins are easily removed yet are retained satisfactorily on etched enamel for the short splinting periods that are required.

*Technique: acrylic or epimine resin splint*

1. The teeth to be splinted should include at least one tooth mesial and distal to the loose tooth. Clean the labial surfaces of the teeth with a pumice–water slurry or an oil-free prophylaxis paste. The traumatised tooth must be cleaned very gently while supporting it firmly as described above; if, despite these precautions, the tooth is painful, cleaning may be limited to gentle rubbing with a moist cotton wool roll.
2. Isolate and dry the teeth.
3. Etch the incisal third of the labial surfaces of the teeth for one minute with 30–50% phosphoric acid. A gel form of etchant is preferable if control of gingival bleeding is incomplete because gel is less easily displaced from the tooth surface than a solution.
4. Wash and dry the etched surfaces.
5. Mix the resin according to the manufacturer's instructions and flow it across the teeth, over the etched areas.
6. When the resin begins to harden, remove excess and, when it is set, smooth any rough edges.

*Arch wire bonded with acrylic or epimine resin*

Although composite resin has been used successfully to bond an arch wire to enamel for splinting purposes (Toplis, 1980), acrylic or epimine resin may be preferred because they are more easily removed from the teeth at the end of the splinting period. In a study comparing an acrylic resin (Trim), an epimine resin (Scutan) and a composite resin (Durafill) it was found that the acrylic resin formed the weakest bond to etched enamel but that this was sufficient to retain a wire splint for at least 10 days; since this material was also the easiest to remove from the teeth it was concluded that this is the material of choice for splint construction (Awang, Hill and Davies, 1985).

*Technique: wire and resin splint*

1. Use either round or rectangular wire (about 0.020″ diameter or about 0.018″ × 0.025″ mm).

If suitable orthodontic wire is not readily available, a paper clip may be used.

2. Bend the wire to fit the incisal third of the labial surfaces of the teeth to be splinted; it should fit closely, but not necessarily very accurately. It is helpful to bend a short tag to fit around the distal surface of a tooth that will be at one end of the splint; this helps to re-locate the wire in exactly the same position after making adjustments to its shape.

3. Clean the labial surfaces of the teeth to be splinted, isolate and dry the teeth, and etch the labial enamel.

4. Place a small amount of resin on the etched areas, position the wire over the teeth and add more resin until the parts of the wire lying over the labial surfaces are covered.

The two types of splint described above fulfil most of the requirements of an ideal splint: they are easy to make and are retained reliably; they do not impinge on the gingiva; they allow access for pulp testing, and for endodontic treatment should this be required; and they are easy to remove. The only possible disadvantage is that the progress of periodontal re-attachment cannot be assessed without first removing the splint; although the general guidelines regarding splinting periods are usually satisfactory, some teeth may be splinted longer than necessary and others not long enough. Removable splints have an advantage in this respect.

*Other splints*

Other types of splint have been used successfully, but have little to commend them when they are compared with those described above. Preformed stainless steel bands with labial brackets have been used, cemented to the teeth and joined with a strip of acrylic resin labially. Interdental 'figure-of-eight' wiring has been used, or an arch wire ligated to the teeth with ligature wire. No doubt these methods are satisfactory in expert hands but they cannot be recommended for general use.

## Indirect method

The indirect method can be used at any time in preference to the direct method, but it is particu-larly useful when it would be difficult or impossible to make a satisfactory splint by the direct method. For example, a 7 or 8-year-old child with traumatised maxillary central incisors may not have lateral incisors sufficiently erupted to provide support, or deciduous teeth suitable for the purpose. One of the splints described below would offer a solution to this problem.

Alginate is a suitable impression material, but precautions must be taken to avoid displacing, or even extracting, the mobile tooth. Moderately mobile teeth need only be covered with petroleum jelly (Vaseline), but grossly mobile teeth, for example a replanted tooth, should either be supported with a suitably bent piece of wire or dental instrument (Fig. 27.9), or covered with thin casting wax or metal foil (Fig. 27.10); the wax or foil is adapted closely to the labial and palatal surfaces of the teeth but not pressed between the teeth, so that it comes away in the impression.

Unless facilities are available for making the splint immediately, there is inevitably some delay,

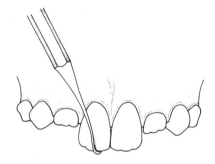

**Fig. 27.9** Stabilising a very mobile tooth with a bent dental instrument while taking an impression.

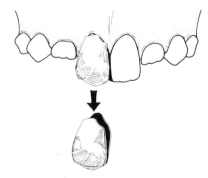

**Fig. 27.10** The use of thin metal foil to facilitate taking an impression of a very mobile tooth.

perhaps of up to a few days, before it can be fitted. Therefore a temporary splint is required to stabilise the tooth during this period. Suitable temporary splints may be made with soft metal and zinc oxide–eugenol cement, or with adhesive bandage material.

*Soft metal/cement temporary splint*

A convenient source of soft metal, available in most dental surgeries, is a 'galley' pot; other sources are milk bottle tops and the foil inside X-ray film packets.

1. Cut the metal to size, long enough to extend over two or three teeth mesial and distal to the loose tooth, and wide enough to extend over the incisal edges and 3–4 mm over the labial and palatal gingiva.
2. Place the metal over the teeth and bend it down over the labial and palatal surfaces. Note where it is unnecessarily over-extended, remove it from the mouth and modify its shape accordingly.
3. Replace the metal over the teeth and, with gentle finger pressure, adapt it as closely as possible to the teeth labially and palatally (Fig. 27.11).
4. Cement the metal to the teeth with quick-setting zinc oxide–eugenol cement; since the splint will be removed within a few days it is unwise to use a more adhesive cement.

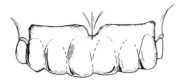

**Fig. 27.11** Soft metal/cement temporary splint

*Adhesive bandage temporary splint*

A proprietary material is available (Stomahesive, Squibb), composed of pectin, gelatin, carboxymethylcellulose and polyisobutylene, which is sandwiched between a smooth polyethylene film on one side and a removable backing paper on the other. It adheres to moist hard or soft tissues, and gradually disintegrates in the mouth; within 24 to 72 hours it completely disappears or is reduced to

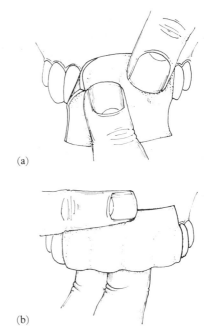

(a)

(b)

**Fig. 27.12** Adhesive bandage temporary splint

small remnants which are easily removed (Rule, 1969).

1. Before removing the backing paper, cut a piece similar in shape to that described above for the soft metal splint.
2. Adapt one half of the bandage to the labial surfaces (Fig. 27.12a) and then bend it over the incisal edges of the teeth on to the palatal surfaces (Fig. 27.12b). Modify its shape as necessary.
3. Remove the backing paper and place the bandage on moist teeth and gingiva; the material is hydrophilic and therefore adheres to moist surfaces. Use finger pressure to adapt it as closely as possible, and then use a flat dental instrument to push it interdentally, avoiding pressure to the traumatised tooth.

The patient should be recalled within a few days for replacement of the temporary splint with a sturdier, more reliable splint. One of the following types of splint is recommended.

*Removable acrylic splint*

This type of splint is retained by Adams cribs and is removable by the patient.

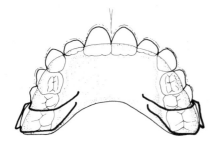

**Fig. 27.13** Removable splint, showing occlusal coverage.

In designing the splint, two decisions must be made: whether to extend acrylic over the occlusal surfaces of posterior teeth, and which teeth to crib. It is usually necessary to cover occlusal surfaces of posterior teeth (Fig. 27.13); if this is not done the only occlusal contact would be between mandibular incisors and palatal acrylic . The slight opening of the bite produced by occlusal coverage is easily tolerated by child patients. However, if the patient has an incomplete overbite there might be sufficient clearance for palatal acrylic, making it unnecessary to cover posterior teeth.

Cribs on first permanent molars give adequate retention in most cases. However, there may be a tendency for the anterior part of the splint to drop and therefore it is advisable to place cribs or clasps on other teeth if possible. First premolars are obvious choices, but in a younger child a first primary molar or a non-traumatised incisor may be used. Splints in the lower arch (which are much less frequently required) are adequately retained by cribs on first permanent molars.

The patient is instructed to remove the splint for cleaning after meals and before retiring to bed.

Although it has been asserted that these removable splints are suitable only for stabilising slightly mobile teeth (Hargreaves, Craig and Needleman, 1981), they have been found to be effective in treating very loose teeth, including replanted teeth (Saunders, 1972); in these cases, the child is instructed to keep the splint in place continuously for the first 3 days.

*Removable thermoplastic vinyl splint*

Various thermoplastic materials are available which may be used for making splints. A suitable material is polyvinyl-acetate-polyethylene, which is also used for making mouth-protectors (Skyberg, 1978). The splint is made in the same way as a mouth-protector; the technique is described in Chapter 26. The splint is removable and the patient is given the same instructions as those outlined for the removable acrylic splint.

The fact that removable splints can be removed by the patient may be considered to be a disadvantage. However, the experience of those who use removable splints is that patients do not remove them because they feel more comfortable and secure wearing them. If the patient's sense of responsibility is in doubt a removable splint should not be used. The main disadvantages of using a removable splint are the laboratory time required for its construction and the need to make

## Technique: replantation

| Procedure | Method | Rationale | Notes |
|---|---|---|---|
| 1. Prepare the patient | Inform the patient and parent of the need to splint the tooth for 1–2 weeks, of the probable need for root canal treatment, and of the uncertain prognosis. | Unless the tooth is replanted under ideal conditions, root resorption and eventual loss of the tooth is inevitable. If the patient is not keen to receive the necessary treatment, immediate prosthetic replacement may be preferable. | If the patient has incisor crowding and/or an increased overjet, orthodontic treatment involving closure of the space may be preferable to replantation. |
| 2. Prepare the tooth | When the patient brings the avulsed tooth to the surgery, place it immediately in a dish containing sterile saline or water. Hold the tooth by its crown and gently wash or dab away any mud or dirt (Fig. 27.14a). Do not remove or damage adherent periodontal tissues. | Preservation of undamaged periodontal tissues greatly improves the prognosis of replantation. | |

| Procedure | Method | Rationale | Notes |
|---|---|---|---|
| | OPTIONAL — If the tooth has a fully developed root, open the pulp chamber through the palatal surface of the crown, remove the entire pulp with a barbed broach, ream the canal to the root apex, wash the canal with sterile saline or water, dry the canal with paper points, and fill the canal with cement (e.g. zinc oxide-eugenol) using a rotary filler in a slow-speed handpiece. | The pulp of a tooth with a fully-developed root will almost certainly die following replantation, so that immediate root canal treatment can be justified. The pulp of an immature tooth may remain vital in ideal circumstances. | The available evidence suggests that it is preferable to replant the tooth immediately and to defer root canal treatment for a few weeks until the tooth is firm again after splinting. |
| | Cut off 2–3 mm of the root apex with a bur or disc. During this entire procedure hold the tooth by the crown and not by the root. | The apical region of the root canal usually contains many accessory canals (the apical 'delta') which might provide a focus for infection later. | |
| 3. Prepare the tooth socket | Anaesthetise the area. Inspect the socket and surrounding tissues and clean if necessary with sterile saline or water. Do not disturb the blood clot in the socket. | | If a firm blood clot has already formed, it is necessary to break it up gently with a sterile instrument, or aspirate it from the socket. |
| 4. Replant the tooth | Replace the tooth carefully in its socket (Fig. 27.14b), without using force. | | |
| 5. Make a splint | Splint the tooth by one of the methods described on pages | | |
| 6. Prescribe antibiotic | Prescribe a course of oral penicillin. | The tissues will certainly have become infected. | If the patient is allergic to penicillin, or has received penicillin during the previous 3 months, erythromycin should be prescribed. |
| 7. Check tetanus immunisati- on status | Arrange for tetanus toxoid injection if necessary (Ch. 27). | | |

FOLLOW-UP

*After 1–2 weeks*: remove the splint carefully. The tooth will not yet be firm, but a longer splinting period encourages root resorption.

*3–4 weeks after replantation:*
  (i) take a radiograph of the tooth
  (ii) carry out endodontic treatment if the tooth has a completely formed root; an immature tooth with a wide open root apex may be kept under observation for a longer period (p 209)
  (iii) test the vitality of adjacent teeth that might also have been traumatised. A replanted immature tooth, if it remains vital, may be expected to give a vital response to pulp testing only after about 6 months
  (iv) if the patient wishes to participate in contact sports, make a mouthprotector (Ch. 26).

*At about 3–4 week intervals:*
  (i) take further radiographs of replanted immature teeth that have not been root filled, carry out root canal treatment and fill the canal with calcium hydroxide (p. 211) at the first sign of root resorption
  (ii) test pulp vitality of replanted immature teeth and of adjacent teeth.

*At about 3-month intervals*: take radiographs of replanted mature teeth that have been root filled with calcium hydroxide; replace the root dressing if necessary.

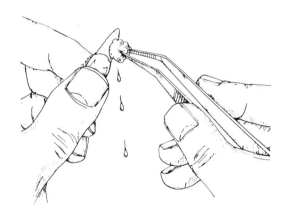
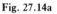

**Fig. 27.14a**

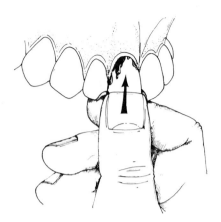

**Fig. 27.14b**

a temporary splint. On the other hand, an advantage of using a removable splint is the case with which the progress of periodontal re-attachment can be assessed, which ensures that the splint is discarded at the optimal time.

*Other splints made by the indirect method*

Thin thermoplastic materials (e.g. cellulose acetate) have been used. They can be pressure- or vacuum-moulded to the model, cut to fit accurately around the gingival margins of all the teeth on the model, and cemented to the teeth. Acrylic resin has been used to make a similar type of full-coverage splint which is cemented to the teeth; this type of splint can be restricted to anterior teeth if the patient has a large overjet or an incomplete overbite. However, fixed splints of this type cannot be recommended; they cause gingival irritation and do not give access to the teeth for pulp testing or for endodontic treatment.

## REPLANTATION (REIMPLANTATION)

Replantation is the replacement in its socket of a tooth that has been avulsed. The tooth usually becomes firm within a few weeks, but its long-term prognosis is dependent on many factors. The prognosis is most favourable if the tooth is replanted within half an hour of avulsion and if, before replantation, the periodontal tissues at-

tached to the root are kept moist and not disturbed.

Under ideal conditions, normal healing occurs and the tooth remains healthy. Unfortunately, the majority of replanted teeth show progressive root resorption: either inflammatory resorption, or replacement resorption and ankylosis (Andreasen 1981). The rate of progress of resorption varies greatly; the tooth may be lost within a few months or it may survive for several years.

After replanting the tooth, it must be stabilised by splinting, but only for 1 to 2 weeks; a longer splinting period encourages root resorption (Andreasen, 1981). Root canal treatment almost certainly will be required if the replanted tooth had a fully developed root, but may not be necessary if the root apex was open. Root resorption sometimes may be arrested by root canal treatment and filling with calcium hydroxide.

If a parent telephones to report avulsion of a tooth, the following instructions may be given:

1. Hold the tooth by its crown (not by its root). If the root appears dirty, clean it very gently with a handkerchief moistened with saliva. Do not touch the root any more than is absolutely necessary.
2. Replace the tooth in its socket. (It is necessary to ensure that the parent can differentiate between the labial and palatal surfaces of the tooth).

3. Report to the surgery as soon as possible, maintaining the tooth in position by biting on a handkerchief.

If the parents are unwilling or unable to carry out these instructions, they should be advised to place the tooth in milk (Blomlof and Otteskog, 1980) or, if this is not available, in a clean handkerchief moistened with saliva. The child's or the parent's mouth would provide excellent conditions for transporting the tooth, but difficulty might be expected in persuading them to place an avulsed tooth in their mouths. Unfortunately, water is not a suitable medium for the periodontal tissues.

REFERENCES

Andreasen J O 1981 Traumatic injuries of the teeth, 2nd edn. Munksgaard, Copenhagen
Awang H, Hill F J, Davies E H 1985 An investigation of three polymeric materials for acid-etch splint construction. Journal of Paediatric Dentistry 1:55–60
Blomlof L, Otteskog P 1980 Viability of human periodontal ligament cells after storage in milk or saliva. Scandinavian Journal of Dental Research 88:436–440
Croll T P, Johnson R 1982 Stabilisation of a traumatised tooth for application of a splint. Journal of Dentistry for Children 49:357–358
Cvek M 1978 A clinical report on partial pulpotomy and capping with calcium hydroxide in permanent incisors with complicated crown fractures. Journal of Endodontics 4:232–237
Freedman G L, Hooley J R 1968 Immobilisation of anterior alveolar injuries with cold-curing acrylic resins. Journal of the American Dental Association 76:785 786
Friend L A 1966 The root treatment of teeth with open apices. Proceedings of the Royal Society of Medicine 59:1035–1036
Fuks A B, Bielak S, Chosak A 1982 Clinical and radiographic assessment of direct pulp capping and pulpotomy in young permanent teeth. Pediatric Dentistry 4:240–244
Hargreaves J A, Craig J W, Needleman H L 1981 The management of traumatised teeth in children, 2nd edn. Churchill Livingstone, Edinburgh, p 50
Massler M 1974 Tooth replantation. Dental Clinics of North America 18:445–452
Rock W P, Gordon P H, Friend L A, Grundy M C 1974 The relationship between trauma and pulp death in incisor teeth. British Dental Journal 136:236–239
Rule D C 1969 The temporary stabilisation of mobile teeth: a use for adhesive bandage. British Dental Journal 126:228–229
Saunders I D F 1972 Removable appliances in the stabilisation of traumatised anterior teeth: a preliminary report. Proceedings of the British Paedodontic Society 2:19–22
Skyberg R L 1978 Stabilisation of avulsed teeth in children with the flexible mouthguard splint. Journal of the American Dental Association 96:797–800
Spalding P M, Fields H W, Torney D, Cobb H B, Johnson J 1985 The changing role of endodontics and orthodontics in the management of traumatically intruded permanent incisors. Pediatric Dentistry 7:104–110
Toplis J W 1980 An aesthetic anterior splint. British Dental Journal 149:263–264
Zachrisson B J, Jacobsen I 1975 Long-term prognosis of 66 permanent anterior teeth with root fracture. Scandinavian Journal of Dental Research 83:345–354

RECOMMENDED READING

Andreasen J O 1981 Traumatic injuries of the teeth, 2nd edn. Munksgaard, Copenhagen
Hargreaves J A, Craig J W, Needleman H L 1981 The Management of traumatised anterior teeth of children, 2nd edn. Churchill Livingstone, Edinburgh

# 28

# Intermediate and final treatment of traumatised anterior permanent teeth

Restoration of the crown
  Teeth with fractures not involving the pulp
  Teeth with fractures involving the pulp
Pulp vitality tests

Pulpectomy
  Mature teeth
  Root-fractured teeth
  Immature teeth

Partial pulpectomy
Retrograde root canal filling
Bleaching of discoloured
  pulpless teeth

## RESTORATION OF THE CROWN

### Teeth with fractures not involving the pulp

A fractured tooth may be restored with composite resin as part of immediate treatment (Ch. 27), in which case the restoration is retained semi-permanently until such time that it is no longer satisfactory, usually for aesthetic reasons. If, on the other hand, immediate treatment involved only the placing of a protective layer of composite resin, the crown should be restored within a few weeks to prevent either drifting of the tooth labially (if the fracture shortened the length of the crown and released it from control of the lower lip) or tilting of adjacent teeth over it (if there is incisor crowding). If a stainless steel crown or copper ring was used in immediate treatment, a more aesthetic replacement is usually welcomed by the child and parents.

The material most commonly used to restore a fractured incisor is composite resin. This type of restoration has been evaluated in numerous studies (Jordan et al, 1977; Watkins and Andlaw, 1977).

Satisfactory results have been obtained, but the main problem has been the gradual discolouration of the composite resin; these restorations are therefore only acceptable at present as semi-permanent restorations. In attempts to overcome the problem of discolouration, manufacturers have produced resins containing fillers of different types and particle size; the most satisfactory for the restoration of fractured incisors appear at present to be the 'hybrid' types, which contain a mixture of 'macro' and 'micro'-sized particles.

Because of the limitations of composite resin, the porcelain jacket crown is still considered to be the ultimate restoration for a fractured incisor. However, this should be delayed until the patient is at least 18 years of age, by which time the pulp horns have receded and the tooth reduction that is required can be done safely. A possible alternative to the procelain jacket crown is the recently introduced porcelain veneer, which is bonded to etched enamel with composite resin (p. 137); since tooth reduction for this restoration is very conservative it can be done for children.

### Technique: composite resin crown restoration

| Procedure | Method | Rationale | Notes |
| --- | --- | --- | --- |
| 1. Clean the tooth surface | Use a slurry of pumice in water or an oil-free prophylaxis paste to clean all surfaces of the crown. Ensure that dentine on the fractured surface is covered with calcium hydroxide. | | |
| | If composite was used previously to provide pulp protection (Ch. 27), stone and then pumice to produce a 'fresh' composite surface. | New composite will bond to old composite if the latter has a clean, uncontaminated surface. | |

| Procedure | Method | Rationale | Notes |
|---|---|---|---|
| 2. Prepare a crown form | Select a cellulose acetate crown form matching the tooth size and shape. | | An alternative technique, not using a crown form, is to apply the composite directly to the tooth. Unless the fracture is very small, this technique is only feasible if a light-sensitive composite is used; the material is applied in increments, polymerising each before adding the next. |
| | Cut the crown form so that its margin lies about 4 mm from the fractured edge of the tooth (Fig. 28.1a). If labial enamel thickness was reduced, the margin of the crown form should lie over the periphery of the tooth preparation. With a probe, punch a small hole through the crown form at the incisal corner. | The crown form is cut so that its margin lies at the desired periphery of the restoration. About 4 mm from the fractured edge provides sufficient area for adequate bonding.<br><br>Small holes incisally allow any air incorporated into the composite during mixing or when filling the crown form to escape when the crown form is placed on the tooth, thus preventing the formation of voids in the restoration. | When the fracture is oblique, less than 4 mm will be available mesially or distally. This deficiency must be compensated for by allowing more coverage elsewhere. |
| 3. Isolate the tooth | Isolate the tooth, ideally with rubber dam but otherwise with cotton wool rolls and a saliva ejector. | For successful bonding of composite resin to enamel to occur, it is essential that the tooth is kept isolated from saliva. | |
| 4. Etch the enamel | As described on page 56, but extend the area of etching *beyond* the planned periphery of the composite restoration, i.e. at least 5 mm from the fractured edge if possible (Fig. 28.1b). | | |
| 5. Wash and dry the enamel surface | See page 56. | | |
| 6. Apply unfilled resin | See page 56. | | |
| 7. Apply filled resin (i.e. composite 'paste') in the crown form | Fill the crown form with composite paste of the appropriate colour, place it on the tooth and vibrate it gently by hand into its previously determined position (Fig. 28.1c). | Vibrating the crown form into position encourages any entrapped air to escape through the holes made in the incisal corners. | |
| 8. Remove excess composite | It using a light-sensitive material, support the crown form in position with a finger and, with a probe or other hand instrument, remove excess material that extruded from the crown form. Polymerise the composite by applying an appropriate light source to labial and palatal surfaces in turn.<br><br>If using an autopolymerising resin, less time is available for removing excess; the material polymerises within a few minutes. | | |

| Procedure | Method | Rationale | Notes |
|---|---|---|---|
| 9. Trim and finish the restoration | When the composite has polymerised, remove the crown form by splitting it palatally with a probe or excavator and lifting it off. | | |
| | If possible, limit finishing procedures to the margin of the restoration, but if the whole restoration is too bulky it must be reduced. Use diamond or tungsten carbide finishing burs in a high-speed handpiece, or abrasive discs in a slow-speed handpiece. For final polishing, use a tungsten carbide finishing bur, or the finest abrasive disc, or composite polishing paste. | No known method of polishing a composite restoration leaves its surface as smooth as that which polymerises against a crown form or matrix strip. | However closely the crown form fitted initially, it inevitably becomes distorted to some extent when it is filled with composite and pressed into position on the tooth. It is therefore always necessary to trim the margin of the restoration. |

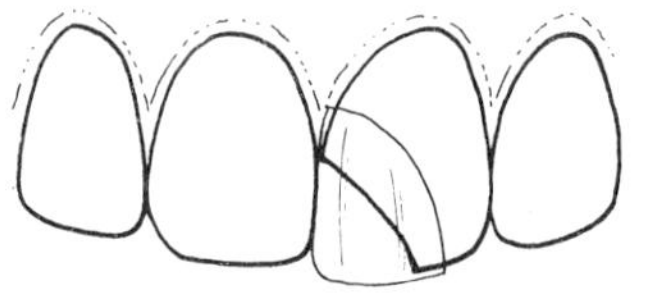

Fig. 28.1a 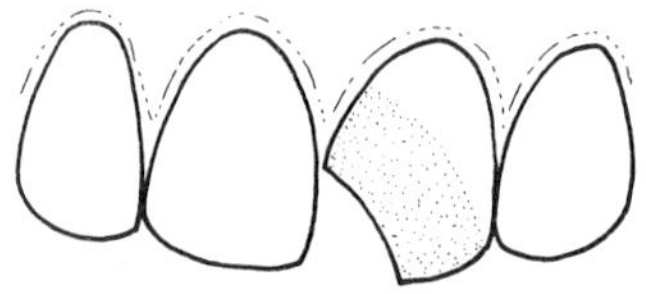                Fig. 28.1b 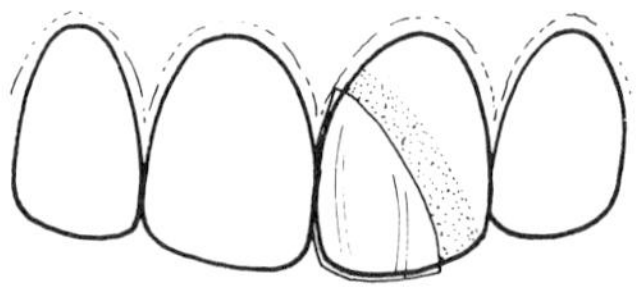                Fig. 28.1c

Despite its limitations, composite resin provides the most satisfactory means of restoring a child's fractured incisor, at least semi-permanently. Before proceeding, the decision must be made either to apply the composite to the existing labial surface or to first reduce the thickness of labial enamel; these alternatives were discussed in relation to veneering techniques on page 136.

If it is decided not to reduce enamel thickness, the only mechanical preparation recommended is to bevel the enamel at the labial edge of the fracture line (Fig. 13.4), to increase the thickness of composite at this point.

If enamel reduction is decided upon, about 0.5 mm of labial enamel is removed with a diamond bur at high speed, extending 4–5 mm from the fractured edge.

## Teeth with fractures involving the pulp

Retention of the composite crown restoration described above is dependent on its bond to etched enamel. When fractures involve the pulp, less natural crown remains, and the available enamel may be inadequate to retain the relatively large restoration that is required. If at least half of the crown remains and the tooth has received endodontic treatment, satisfactory retention can be obtained by utilising part of the pulp chamber; a retentive cavity is prepared palatally into which composite resin is packed at the time of making the restoration.

If less than half of the crown remains, restoration with a post crown may be the most obvious solution, but this is not feasible for an immature tooth with a wide open root apex. In such a case, further measures are required to retain a crown for a few years until further closure of the root apex occurs. Pins and a dentine adhesive may be used to aid retention. Self-shearing pins are available which are inserted into dentine with a slow-speed handpiece and shear off at the depth of a previously prepared hole (Fig. 28.2). Dentine adhesives are used instead of the unfilled resin.

If less than half of the crown remains but the tooth has a fully developed root, there are no

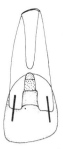

**Fig. 28.2** Use of pins and pulp chamber retention for a composite resin crown.

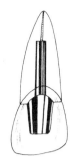

**Fig. 28.3** Post and core and porcelain jacket crown.

special difficulties in restoring the tooth with a conventional post crown (Fig. 28.3). However, for an active child prone to accidents or involved in contact sports, it may be preferable to use a short cast or preformed post (Fig. 28.4), to reduce the risk of root fracture should further trauma occur. In either case, it is prudent to provide a mouth protector for a patient who engages in contact sports.

A summary of intermediate and final treatments for crown restoration is given in Table 28.1.

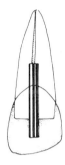

**Fig. 28.4** Short post and composite resin crown.

**Table 28.1** Summary of intermediate and final treatments for crown restoration

| Type of fracture | Root development | Immediate treatment previously performed | INTERMEDIATE TREATMENT | FINAL TREATMENT (after age 18) |
|---|---|---|---|---|
| Class II (through dentine) | open apex closed apex | pulp protection | composite resin restoration (acid etch technique) | porcelain jacket crown (or composite resin restoration) |
| Class III (through pulp) | | | | |
| at least ½ crown remaining | open apex closed apex | pulpotomy pulpotomy or pulpectomy and root filling | composite resin restoration (acid etch technique + extra retention in pulp chamber) | root canal treatment, reduction of crown to gingival margin and preparation for post and core (cast or preformed), porcelain crown |
| less than ½ crown remaining | open apex | pulpotomy | composite resin restoration (acid etch technique + extra retention in pulp chamber, from pins and from dentine adhesive) | root canal treatment and post crown, as above. |
| less than ½ crown remaining | closed apex | pulpectomy and root filling | i) short post, core projecting through fractured crown, composite resin restoration | removal of short post, reduction of crown to gingival margin, preparation of conventional post and core, porcelain crown |
| | | | ii) reduction of crown to gingival margin and preparation for post and core, porcelain crown | if the margin of the crown is supra-gingival and therefore not aesthetic — cutting of porcelain crown from post, re-establishment of margin, making of new porcelain crown |

## PULP VITALITY TESTS

Root canal therapy does not usually form part of the immediate treatment of fractured teeth, except when a tooth with a fully developed root is fractured through the pulp. However, the pulp of any traumatised tooth may die, either quickly (within a few weeks) or slowly (during the next year or two). Therefore, regular assessment of pulp vitality is essential for at least 2 years after trauma, and root canal therapy is required if the pulp becomes non-vital.

Tests of pulp vitality are, in fact, tests of the sensitivity of pulpal nerves to thermal or electrical stimuli. Although pulp sensitivity is associated with pulp vitality, this is not invariably the case. Thus, a normal response to stimulation usually indicates that the pulp is healthy, and a reduced or a negative response usually indicates that the pulp is partially or totally necrotic. However, it is possible for trauma to injure pulpal nerves and not the blood vessels. In such a case the pulp would be healthy in having a normal blood supply, but would not respond to stimuli (Bhaskar and Rappaport, 1973). This could occur following the immediate replantation of an avulsed tooth; the pulp may remain healthy but the nerve supply may not be re-established for several months.

Conversely, sensitivity to stimulation does not necessarily indicate that the pulp is vital. If the stimulus is transmitted through the tooth to periodontal rather than to pulpal nerves, a false positive response would be given. It has been estimated that a healthy pulp responds to an electrical stimulus of 150 $\mu$A from a monopolar pulp tester, and that stimuli greater than 200 $\mu$A may excite periodontal nerves (Matthews and Searle, 1974).

Thus, pulp testing cannot provide definitive information about pulp vitality; it should be regarded only as an aid in diagnosis (Chambers, 1982), to be considered in conjunction with clinical signs (for example tooth colour, and the presence of a sinus), symptoms, sensitivity to percussion and radiographic evidence.

Thermal or electrical tests may be used to assess pulp vitality. Thermal tests are of two kinds: the application of heat (usually heated gutta percha) or of cold (usually frozen ethyl chloride on a cotton pledget). Electrical tests are made with instruments that are usually of the monopolar type, one electrode contacting the crown of the tooth to be tested, and the indifferent electrode contacting some other part of the body (for example, the hand). During the test the current is gradually increased, and the dial reading at which the patient indicates that the tooth is sensitive is noted.

Electrical tests provide the following important advantages over thermal tests:

## Technique: electric pulp testing

| Procedure | Method | Rationale | Notes |
|---|---|---|---|
| 1. Prepare the patient and the equipment | Explain the purpose of the test in simple terms, e.g. 'to check if the tooth is well' (avoid 'to check if the tooth is dead'). Tell the child that his help is needed to carry out the test. | Cooperation is essential if meaningful information is to be obtained from the test; good patient management is therefore imperative. Encouraging active participation rather than expecting passive acceptance is good practice. | |
| | Explain that (i) the tester will be placed on his tooth, (demonstrate this on a finger nail); (ii) he will feel nothing at first but that, as the test progresses, he *may* feel a 'little tingle' or 'twinge' in the tooth; (iii) if he should feel this, he should 'signal' by raising his arm. | Explaining the type of sensation to be expected prevents the child being surprised and upset by it. | |

| Procedure | Method | Rationale | Notes |
|---|---|---|---|
| 2. Perform the test | If the vitality of a particular tooth is in doubt, test that tooth first. | If a sound tooth is tested first and, despite careful preparation, the child dislikes the sensation, he may later give false positive responses when a non-vital tooth is tested. If the first tooth tested is non-vital, the child will not respond and important information will have been obtained. | Occasionally a response may be obtained when testing a non-vital tooth, probably through stimulation of the periodontal nerves. |
| | Place the electrode tip on the middle of the labial surface, away from the gingival margin (Fig. 28.5). | Contacting the gingival margin would provoke a false positive response. | Different instruments provide different types of electrical contact at the electrode tip e.g. moist cotton wool, toothpaste, conductive rubber. |
| | (If the instrument being used employs a moist cotton electrical contact, prepare the cotton wool small enough to avoid contact with the gingiva and, before using, remove excess water by touching it on a cotton wool roll). | Excess water might run down the tooth surface and cause a gingival response. | |
| | Increase the current *slowly*. If and when the child signals by raising his arm, immediately remove the electrode from the tooth and note the reading on the dial. | Increasing the current quickly might result in the point of first stimulation being exceeded, causing the child unnecessary discomfort. | |
| | Repeat the test on the same tooth. If a similar reading is obtained, the result can be accepted with confidence. If a very different reading is obtained, the reliability of the child's responses must be doubted. Repeat the procedure but place the electrode near, but not in contact with, the tooth. If the child again signals, his responses are clearly meaningless. Explain to the child once again the nature of the sensation to be expected, and encourage him to wait for it. | | The ability to check the patient's responses in this way is an advantage of electrical tests over thermal tests. Response may also be checked by use of the tester with the current switched off. |
| | Having established that the child is responding reliably, proceed to test neighbouring teeth. | In cases of trauma, several teeth may have been injured, even though they are not fractured and appear undamaged. | It has been shown that teeth traumatised but not fractured are more liable to become non-vital than teeth fractured through enamel or dentine (Rock *et al.*, 1974). |
| | If no response is elicited from the first tooth tested, repeat the test two or three times to confirm. Then proceed to test neighbouring teeth. | If no response is elicited from one tooth but a positive response from neighbouring teeth, strong evidence will have been obtained that the first has a necrotic pulp. | |

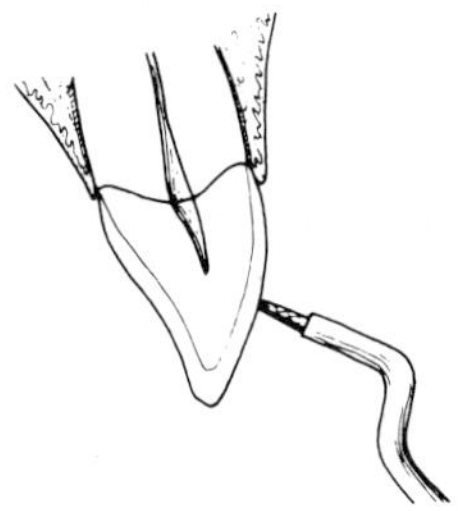

**Fig. 28.5**

1. It is easy to check the reliability of the response. If the patient responds at widely different points on successive tests, the reliability of the response is in doubt. Thermal tests do not allow such a check to be made.
2. Changes in the sensitivity of a tooth may be assessed by comparison with neighbouring teeth. If two or more teeth respond at similar points in one test and then, some time later, one tooth responds at a different point, that tooth would come under some suspicion thereafter. Comparisons of the relative sensitivity of different teeth are not possible with thermal tests.

## PULPECTOMY

All traumatised teeth should be reviewed at regular intervals for at least 2 years, noting signs and symptoms, testing sensitivity to percussion, testing pulp vitality and taking radiographs. Pulpectomy is required if the pulp dies or if root resorption is diagnosed radiologically.

### Mature teeth

Traumatised teeth that are not loosened or, if loosened, suffer little or no displacement, may be kept under observation as outlined above. In these cases, the risk of root resorption is minimal and the reason for endodontic treatment is almost always pulp death. Conventional pulpectomy and root canal filling techniques can be used.

In contrast, endodontic treatment should be carried out within 2 to 3 weeks for teeth that are intruded or avulsed; not only is it almost certain that pulp death will occur but it is probable that this will happen, and that external root resorption will begin, within this short period of time. After removing the pulp, and cleaning and washing the root canal, the canal should be filled with calcium hydroxide, which has been shown to inhibit root resorption; the technique is described on page 211. A radiograph should be taken every 3 to 6 months; if it is noted that the calcium hydroxide is becoming resorbed at the root apex or that root resorption is progressing, it should be washed out and replaced. This treatment may be repeated as

many times as necessary, and the completion of endodontic treatment by obturation of the canal should be delayed until external root resorption appears to have been controlled. Internal root resorption is less common, but should also be treated with calcium hydroxide, which should be replaced every few weeks in an attempt to control the resorptive process.

### Root-fractured teeth

Inflammation and necrosis of a root-fractured tooth is often confined to the coronal fragment, pulp in the apical fragment remaining vital. For this reason, endodontic treatment may be restricted to the coronal fragment, and the apical fragment can be left *in situ* and removed later only if periapical inflammation persists. The recommended treatment again involves the use of calcium hydroxide as a root canal dressing for several months before obturating the canal.

Pulp death in a root-fractured tooth is associated with failure of the repair process at the fracture site. If the fracture occurred in the middle or cervical third of the root the coronal fragment will be loose because periodontal support is insufficient to stabilise the tooth. If the tooth is to be saved, either root canal treatment of both fragments must be carried out and a metal post used to splint both fragments together, or the apical fragment must be removed and a metal implant used to retain the tooth.

### Immature teeth

Calcium hydroxide is used in the endodontic treatment of traumatised mature teeth to prevent or arrest root resorption, after which endodontic treatment is uncomplicated. The treatment of non-vital immature teeth presents an additional problem: the shape of the root canal. The walls of the root apex may be divergent ('blunderbuss'-shape), parallel-sided or convergent (Fig. 28.6), depending on the extent of root development. When the walls are divergent it is impossible to achieve a good apical seal with a conventional root filling; when the walls are parallel-sided or convergent, it is not impossible but still difficult. In these cases calcium hydroxide is used not only to

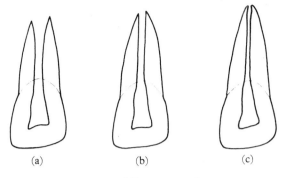

**Fig 28.6** The root apex at different stages of root development: (a) divergent walls, (b) parallel-sided walls, (c) convergent walls.

control root resorption if necessary but also to induce closure of the root apex (Cvek, Hollander and Nord, 1976). Calcium hydroxide stimulates the deposition of a calcific barrier across the root apex or, in some cases, continued root development (Heithersay, 1970). Whether a calcific barrier is formed or root development continues, the treatment with calcium hydroxide makes it easier later to achieve the fundamental objective of root canal therapy: the complete obturation and sealing of the root apex.

The pulp of a replanted immature tooth may survive if the tooth has a wide open root apex (e.g. in a 7 to 9-year-old child), especially if, after avulsion, the tooth was kept under ideal conditions and replanted within about 2 hours. The tooth should be radiographed about 3 weeks after replantation and at 3- to 4-week intervals afterwards. Thermal or electric pulp testing is not useful during this early stage, and the need for endodontic treatment is determined from clinical signs and symptoms or from the radiological diagnosis of external root resorption. Pulpectomy and root filling with calcium hydroxide should be carried out at the first sign of root resorption. In immature teeth that remain vital after replantation, a response to pulp testing may be elicited after about 6 months.

Intruded immature teeth that are being extruded orthodontically or allowed to re-erupt (p. 193) should likewise be treated by pulpectomy and root filling with calcium hydroxide at the first radiological sign of root resorption.

The timing of final root canal filling is decided on the basis of clinical and radiographic assessment of apical barrier formation or of continued root development. Usually, final treatment is carried out about 1 year after the initial treatment with calcium hydroxide.

If the root canal converges towards the apex, filling is uncomplicated and may be achieved with a large gutta percha point, or by condensation of several gutta percha points. However, if the canal is parallel-sided or divergent, it is more difficult to fill adequately. A calcific deposit at the root apex helps, but this cannot be expected to be a complete and impervious barrier. These wide canals may be filled by lateral or vertical condensation of many gutta percha points.

## Technique: pulpectomy of an immature tooth

| Procedure | Method | Rationale | Notes |
|---|---|---|---|
| 1. Prepare instruments and materials | Ideally, use a pre-packed sterile tray containing all the necessary instruments and materials. | | |
| 2. Prepare the site of operation | Place rubber dam (unless there is good reason for not doing so). | Rubber dam ensures good isolation from saliva and eliminates the risk of the patient, particularly if supine, swallowing or inhaling a reamer or other instrument if it should accidentally be dropped into the mouth. | If rubber dam is not used, isolation must be obtained with cotton wool rolls and saliva ejector, and the patient protected by using a 'parachute harness' attached to reamers and files or, at the very least, by placing a piece of gauze behind the anterior teeth. |

| Procedure | Method | Rationale | Notes |
|---|---|---|---|
| 3. Gain access to the pulp chamber | Use a diamond or tungsten carbide bur at high speed to outline the access cavity in the palatal surface of the tooth (Fig. 28.7a). Prepare this cavity in dentine but do not extend into the pulp. Make the cavity large enough to permit good access to the pulp chamber, and extend it over the region of the pulp horns (Fig. 28.7b). Dry the area, and then wipe the tooth, adjacent teeth and rubber dam with a cotton pledget soaked in hibitane solution (1:1000) or other antiseptic. Using a sterile round bur (size 4–6) deepen the access cavity until pulp is exposed. Either with the same bur or with a similar-sized fissure bur, remove the entire roof of the pulp chamber (Fig. 28.7c). | Good access is essential for successful root canal therapy. All instrumentation from this stage must be under sterile conditions; although the necrotic pulp is infected, introduction of further infection should be avoided. | |
| 4. Eliminate the cervical construction of the root canal | With a flame-shaped or tapered fissure bur in a slow-speed handpiece, open out the constricted area to the diameter of the canal immediately apical to it (Fig. 28.7d). | Removal of the cervical constriction is necessary to ensure access to all of the radicular pulp. | |
| 5. Determine the length of the root canal | Place a reamer to the estimated length of the canal (judged from a pre-operative radiograph); support it in position with soft wax or warm gutta-percha, and obtain a periapical radiograph. | | If vital tissue is encountered before reaching the root apex, a partial pulpectomy may be performed (page 212). |
| 6. Extirpate the necrotic pulp | Use barbed broaches and/or reamers to extirpate the necrotic pulp tissue (Fig. 28.7e). Before inserting a broach or reamer into the canal, mark it in some way so that the distance from the mark to its tip is 1–2 mm less than the estimated length of the tooth. Insert each instrument until the mark is level with the incisal edge of the tooth. | The periapical tissues must not be traumatised. | Various methods may be used to mark the working length of root canal instruments. |
| 7. File the walls of the root canal | Use files to cleanse the walls of the root canal, again to 1–2 mm of the root apex (Fig. 28.7f). Work carefully and methodically around the canal. | The use of files is essential because the largest reamer may not engage the walls of the root canal of an immature tooth, and because the root canal is not circular. | Meticulous mechanical cleansing of the root canal is crucial to the success of treatment. |
| 8. Wash the canal | Use a syringe containing sterile water or saline (Fig. 28.7g). Place the needle of the syringe at least half way up the canal; while syringing, hold the nozzle of a high-volume aspirator close to the palatal cavity in the tooth. | Simultaneous syringing and aspirating removes necrotic tissue from the canal. | The canal should be syringed several times during the filing procedure. |
| 9. Dry the canal | Use absorbent paper points to dry the canal (Fig. 28.7h). | | Large diameter paper points are available which are useful when drying wide root canals. |

| Procedure | Method | Rationale | Notes |
|---|---|---|---|
| 10. Fill the canal with calcium hydroxide paste | Use a rotary filling instrument in a slow-speed handpiece (Fig. 28.7i). Mark it as above so that its tip will reach to 1 mm short of the root apex. | | Some clinicians disinfect the canal by dressing with antiseptic solution or polyantibiotic paste on several occasions before filling the canal with calcium hydroxide, but satisfactory results are obtained when the canal is filled with calcium hydroxide at the first visit (Cvek *et al.*, 1976). |
| | Prepare a stiff mix of calcium hydroxide powder and sterile water, or use a proprietary material. Pick up some paste along the length of the rotary filler; do not pick up too much.<br>With the handpiece stationary, insert the filler into the canal and place it in light contact with the canal wall. Run the handpiece at slow speed in the forward direction while withdrawing the filler slowly from the canal; aim to deposit paste in the canal, not to spin it up.<br>Repeat the procedure as often as is necessary to fill the canal completely. | If a large bulk of paste is picked up, it is difficult to carry it beyond the entrance of the root canal. Inserting the filler with the handpiece stationary avoids the risk of it jamming and fracturing.<br><br>If paste is spun up the canal it may pass into the periapical tissues. | A non-setting type of calcium hydroxide paste should be used so that it can easily be washed out of the canal when required.<br><br>Some types of rotary fillers have a flexible connection between spiral and shank; this design greatly reduces the risk of fracture.<br><br>Although calcium hydroxide introduced periapically becomes absorbed, the aim in this technique is to keep it within the root canal. |
| 11. Seal the cavity | See 'vital pulpotomy' (Ch. 27). | | |
| FOLLOW-UP | Check after 1 month, and then at 3- or 6- month intervals.<br>Radiograph 6-monthly to check for evidence of calcific barrier formation or of continued root development.<br>After 6 months, the calcium hydroxide may be washed out with sterile water or saline, and the presence of an apical barrier tested gently with a reamer or a gutta percha point. The canal may either be refilled with calcium hydroxide or filled with a permanent root filling material. | | |

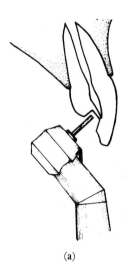
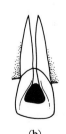
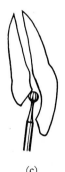
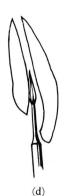
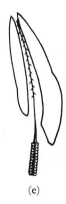

(a)          (b)          (c)          (d)          (e)

Fig. 28.7

(continued overleaf)

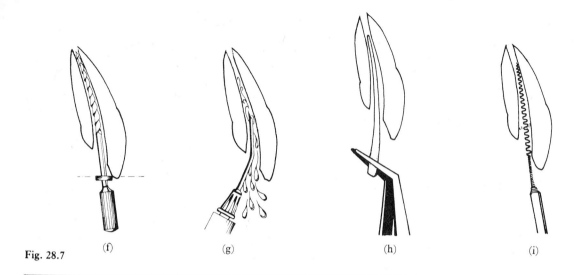

Fig. 28.7          (f)                    (g)                              (h)                              (i)

A gutta-percha 'plug' may first be made by warming points over a flame and rolling them together either with the fingers or between two glass slabs. When a 'plug' of the estimated diameter has been made, it is placed in the tooth to the known length of the canal, and a mark made on it with a hot instrument at the level of the incisal edge of the tooth (a radiograph may be taken to check its position). When the 'plug' is a satisfactory fit, it is coated with a proprietary root canal sealing cement and placed into position (a little of the cement may first be introduced into the canal with a rotary filling instrument or reamer, placing the cement at the apex and on the walls of the canal). Further small gutta percha points should be inserted if possible and condensed. The gutta percha is then cut at the base of the pulp chamber (using fine scissors or a heated dental instrument) and the palatal cavity is sealed.

## PARTIAL PULPECTOMY

Sometimes an immature tooth is assessed as being dead but, on proceeding with pulpectomy, vital pulp tissue is encountered at some point in the root canal. The alternative courses of action (after achieving local analgesia) are either to proceed with pulpectomy or to resect the pulp at the level of the vital tissue. The latter approach allows vital apical tissue to remain, in the hope that further root development may occur; this constitutes a partial pulpectomy, and is especially desirable when the walls of the root apex are divergent or parallel. The root canal up to the vital tissue is filled with calcium hydroxide paste.

## RETROGRADE ROOT CANAL FILLING

The recommended method of treating an immature, non-vital tooth is by pulpectomy and temporary root filling with calcium hydroxide, as described above. However, an alternative approach is retrograde root filling, which involves surgery to expose the root apex followed by sealing of the apex, usually with amalgam. The rest of the root canal should previously have been filled with a dental cement (e.g. zinc oxide-eugenol), either at the time of operation (using a quick-setting material) or at a previous occasion; the amalgam can then be packed down on to it, and the whole of the canal is effectively obturated.

The principal disadvantage of this approach is that it is much more unpleasant for the child than the conservative approach described previously. In addition, it is difficult to produce an effective apical seal in an immature tooth which has thin and divergent walls at its root apex.

Since conservative endodontic treatment usually

is effective, there seems to be no justification for preferring the surgical approach. However, when periapical infection persists despite repeated attempts to control it by conservative methods, surgery may be the only solution if the tooth is to be saved; retrograde root filling is then accompanied by curettage of the infected periapical bone.

## BLEACHING OF DISCOLOURED PULPLESS TEETH

Teeth that have received root canal treatment often become discoloured. This is usually caused by haemolysis of blood that diffused into dentinal tubules during pulpectomy, or by decomposition of pulp tissue that was not removed from the pulp chamber. Haemorrhage during pulpectomy of a vital pulp is inevitable, but every effort should be made to wash blood from the tooth. Incomplete removal of pulp usually results from making inadequate access to the pulp chamber.

There are several treatment alternatives for a discoloured root-filled tooth: covering the labial surface with a composite, acrylic or porcelain veneer (pp. 133–138); cutting off the crown and making a porcelain jacket crown on a post and core; and bleaching the crown.

The most commonly used bleaching techniques employ a 30 per cent (w/v) solution of hydrogen peroxide ($H_2O_2$). In the technique described below, sodium perborate is mixed with the solution to make a paste that is sealed into the pulp chamber (Nutting and Poe, 1967). More commonly, however, $H_2O_2$ solution is used alone on cotton pledgets, and heat and light are applied for periods of 20 to 30 minutes (Grossman, 1974; Nicholls, 1984). No studies have been conducted comparing the effectiveness of these methods, but the use of heat and light are certainly more time-consuming for the dentist and more unpleasant for the patient.

The $H_2O_2$ solution is available as Concentrated Hydrogen Peroxide Solution B.P. It must be handled with care because it is extremely irritant to soft tissues. A convenient source of sodium perborate is 'Bocasan' (Bocasan, Knox Laboratories).

## Technique: bleaching

1. Isolate the tooth with rubber dam.
2. Remove all filling materials from the pulp chamber.
   Remove also about 2 or 3 mm of root canal filling to expose dentine in the cervical region of the tooth (at least on the labial side).
3. Inspect the periphery of the palatal cavity. If it does not allow excellent access to all parts of the pulp chamber, extend the cavity.
4. Clean the walls of the pulp chamber with a large round bur, removing any obvious stains.
5. Check that the root canal is well sealed. If in doubt, apply a small amount of quick-setting cement.
6. Swab the walls of the pulp chamber with a cotton pledget soaked in chloroform; this dissolves fatty substances produced during pulp decomposition, which would interfere with the penetration of $H_2O_2$ solution.
7. Dehydrate the dentine by swabbing with 100 per cent ethyl alcohol, and dry thoroughly with compressed air; this aids the penetration of $H_2O_2$ solution.
8. Place 1–2 drops of $H_2O_2$ solution in a dappen dish and add powdered sodium perborate to make a thick paste.
9. Fill the pulp chamber with the paste. Alternatively, to facilitate removal, the paste may be incorporated into a cotton pledget.
10. Seal the pulp chamber with a quick-setting zinc oxide cement.
11. Assess in about 1 week. If necessary, repeat the treatment; it is desirable to overbleach slightly because some darkening usually follows.
12. When the bleaching treatment is completed, restore the tooth with composite resin.

## REFERENCES

Bhaskar S N, Rappaport H M 1973 Dental vitality tests and pulp status. Journal of the American Dental Association 86:409–411
Chambers I G 1982 The role and methods of pulp testing in oral diagnoisis: a review. International Endodontic Journal 15:1–5
Cvek M, Hollender I, Nord C E 1976 Treatment of non-vital permanent incisors with calcium hydroxide VI: a clinical, microbiological and radiological evaluation of treatment in

one sitting of teeth with mature or immature root. Odontologisk Revy 27:93–108

Grossman L I 1978 Endodontic practice, 9th edn. Lea & Febiger, Philadelphia, ch 18

Heithersay G S 1970 Study of root formation in incompletely developed pulpless teeth. Oral Surgery, Oral Medicine and Oral Pathology 29:620–630

Jordan R E, Suzuki M, Gwinnett A J, Hunter J K 1977 Restoration of fractured and hypoplastic incisors by the acid etch resin technique: a three-year report. Journal of the American Dental Association 95:795–803

Matthews B, Searle B N 1974 Some observations on pulp testers. British Dental Journal 137:307–312

Nicholls E 1984 Endodontics, 3rd edn. Wright, Bristol, ch 17

Nutting E B, Poe G S 1967 Chemical bleaching of discoloured endodontically treated teeth. Dental Clinics of North America (Nov.) 655–662

Watkins J J, Andlaw R J 1977 Restoration of fractured incisors with an ultraviolet light-polymerised composite resin. British Dental Journal 142:249–252

RECOMMENDED READING

Andreasen J O 1981 Traumatic injuries of the teeth, 2nd edn. Munksgaard, Copenhagen

Hargreaves J A, Craig J W, Needleman H L 1981 The Management of traumatised anterior teeth of children, 2nd edn. Churchill Livingstone, Edinburgh

# 29

# Injuries to primary teeth

About 8 per cent of 5-year-old children in England and Wales show signs of having suffered trauma to primary incisors (Todd, 1975). The most common results of trauma are loosening of the tooth (with or without tooth displacement), intrusion and avulsion; crown and root fractures are rare (Ravn, 1968).

Splinting of loosened teeth is difficult if not impossible in such young children; fortunately it is not required, because periodontal reattachment occurs rapidly. If the tooth is displaced it should be repositioned, and the parents advised to take obvious precautions regarding diet and general care. Similarly, an intruded tooth usually requires no treatment; it usually re-erupts within a few weeks and attains its original position within 6 months (Ravn, 1976). Although it is possible to replant an avulsed primary incisor (Mueller and Whitsett, 1978) this is rarely done because of inadequate patient cooperation and the difficulty of splinting satisfactorily. If, however, a primary incisor is replanted, it may be preferable to use a device designed to prevent the child placing fingers in his mouth and disturbing the tooth (Crabb and Crabb, 1971).

When crown fractures do occur, the same principles should be applied as in the treatment of permanent teeth. However, when the patient's cooperation is poor, a tooth fractured through dentine may be given no treatment and simply kept under observation. Many crown fractures, however, involve the pulp, and in these cases the tooth should be extracted if the patient does not allow appropriate pulp treatment to be given. The rare teeth with apical or middle third root fractures may be kept under observation, but those with coronal third fractures must be extracted.

Although traumatised primary incisors should be retained if possible, their loss is not as drastic as the loss of permanent incisors. The most serious aspect of trauma to primary incisors is the damage that may be caused to the permanent successors, which develop palatal to the roots of the deciduous teeth. The most common types of damage are hypoplasia and hypomineralisation of enamel (Ch. 13). In general, hypoplasia is caused by severe injuries sustained by infants under 3 or 4 years of age; hypomineralisation may be caused by milder injuries in this age group or by more severe injuries in older children. Less common types of damage are dilaceration (Ch. 14), odontome-like malformations, and the arrest of root development of the permanent tooth (Andreasen and Ravn, 1971).

The most severe types of injury to primary teeth are avulsion and intrusion. If avulsion occurs when the child is less than 2 years old, almost all (95 per cent) of permanent teeth are damaged; if it occurs between the ages of 2 and 4 years, about 80 per cent are affected, and if it occurs when the child is over 5 years of age, only 18 per cent are affected (Ravn, 1975). Intrusion of a primary tooth occurs mainly in children under 4 years of age and causes damage to 54 per cent of permanent successors (Ravn, 1976). These unfortunate possibilities should be explained to the parents, while attempting not to alarm them.

If a traumatised primary tooth subsequently dies, associated periapical infection may cause hypomineralisation or hypoplasia of the developing permanent tooth crown. Therefore, traumatised teeth should be kept under regular clinical and radiographic supervision. Pulp testing may not give reliable results with a young child, and the assessment of pulp death depends greatly on clinical signs: the appearance of a blue-grey discolouration of the tooth, or of a sinus on the gingiva, buccal to the root. Such a tooth, especially in a child below the age of 4 years, should either receive endodontic treatment (Ch. 9) or be extracted, to avoid the risk of causing damage to the permanent tooth. Sometimes a yellow discolouration occurs; this is a sign of calcification of the pulp, not of pulp death, and no treatment is necessary.

## REFERENCES

Andreasen J O, Ravn J J 1971 The effect of traumatic injuries to primary teeth on their permanent successors II: a clinical and radiographic follow-up study of 213 teeth. Scandinavian Journal of Dental Research 79:284–294

Crabb J J, Crabb V P 1971 Reimplantation of a primary central incisor: a case report. Dental Practitioner 21:353–354

Mueller B H, Whitsett B D 1978 Management of an avulsed deciduous incisor: report of a case. Oral Surgery, Oral Medicine and Oral Pathology 46:442–446

Ravn J J 1968 Sequelae of acute mechanical traumata in the primary dentition. Journal of Dentistry for Children 35:281–289

Ravn J J 1975 Developmental disturbances in permanent teeth after exarticulation of their primary predecessors. Scandinavian Journal of Dental Research 83:131–134

Ravn J J 1976 Development disturbances in permanent teeth after intrusion of their primary predecessors. Scandinavian Journal of Dental Research 84:137–141

# 30

# Non-accidental injuries to children

The term 'non-accidental injuries to children' (N.A.I.) is generally preferred to the more emotive 'battered child syndrome' which was introduced by Kempe *et al.* (1962) and later popularised by the media. The number of cases being reported is increasing; 5700 cases were reported in England during the last 9 months of 1974, of which 40 resulted in the death of the child (D.H.S.S., 1976). Most cases of N.A.I. involve children under the age of 3 years, and not many come to the attention of a dentist. However, 65 per cent of injuries involve the face or head (Becker, Needleman and Kotelchuck, 1978), and dentists are therefore able to assist others in diagnosis and management. A particularly distressing feature is the frequency of repeated attacks, with injuries tending to become more serious, and this emphasises the importance of early diagnosis (N.S.P.C.C., 1976). Many dentists are unaware of their legal and social responsibilities with respect to child abuse, and are reluctant to report suspected cases (Becker *et al.*, 1978).

## CLINICAL SIGNS

1. *Facial bruising*, especially if bilateral. Fingertip-sized bruises are found over bony prominences such as the forehead, zygoma and mandible. Bruises of different colours indicate injuries that have been inflicted on more than one occasion. Blows around the eyes may produce orbital haematomas ('black eyes').
2. *Damage to the lips*, especially tearing of the upper labial fraenum.
3. *Fractured or displaced teeth*, often associated with alveolar fracture.

4. *Severe head injuries.* Superficial scalp bruising may indicate more serious underlying damage. Intra-cranial bleeding may produce a subdural haematoma, which causes headache, drowsiness and vomiting. Injuries to the scalp must be investigated by radiography to exclude the possibility of skull fracture.
5. *Cigarette burns.* These are more common on the limbs and trunk, but may occasionally occur on the face. The typical circular outline of the injury is easily recognised. A recent burn will be a raw weeping wound; this is later covered by a scab, and further healing produces a depressed and puckered scar.
6. *Bite marks.* These are found most commonly on the limbs, but are sometimes found on the face. Careful study of the marks will usually reveal whether they were inflicted by a child or an adult (Sims, Grant and Cameron, 1973).

## MANAGEMENT

If clinical signs suggest the possibility of N.A.I., it is most important to obtain a detailed history from the parent or guardian and later, if possible, to question the child separately. Parents must not be challenged directly but questioned gently and tactfully to avoid antagonising them. It may be difficult not to appear critical but it must be borne in mind that the parents may themselves be in great need of care and attention. Most parents who injure their children are poor and socially deprived, and may also have been unloved and abused during childhood (Sims, 1985). Suspicion of N.A.I. is increased if there has been delay in bringing the child for treatment, if replies to questions are inadequate or evasive, if there is evidence that injuries have been suffered on more than one occasion, and if the child is dirty and appears generally neglected.

Health authorities have established guidelines for dealing with suspected cases of N.A.I. The recommended procedures include the following:

1. Perform emergency treatment of dental and soft tissue injuries, and prescribe antibiotic and antitetanus toxoid if necessary.
2. a *If there is only a suspicion of N.A.I.*: contact the family's doctor or a hospital paediatrician immediately by telephone, and arrange for the child to have a full medical examination. Explain the need for this examination to the parents in a careful and tactful manner, to avoid arousing their suspicion that child abuse is suspected.

   Check later that the parents took the child for examination. If they did not, suspicion of N.A.I. would be strengthened and the local Social Services Department should be informed immediately. The District Dental Officer would help, if required, in contacting the appropriate agency and in giving general advice. Every health authority maintains a Child Abuse Register; telephone to enquire whether the child is on the Register.

   b *If there is strong evidence of N.A.I.*: arrange for the child to be admitted immediately to a hospital. Ideally, arrange for an ambulance to take the child and the parents to the hospital. Alternatively, escort them personally or arrange for a colleague to do so. Hospital personnel will then be responsible for notifying the Social Services Department.

Admission to hospital is necessary to ensure the safety of the child while medical and social investigations are undertaken. When investigations and enquiries are complete, a case conference is convened for doctors, social workers, health visitors, and any other professional workers involved in the case, such as the dentist. It is therefore most important that the dentist keeps a detailed record of the child's injuries and of the history given by the parents. A decision is made either to return the child home and give the parents the support they need, or to place the child under local authority care.

Child abuse is most distressing and its causes are complex. Management of suspected cases requires tact and understanding by all professional staff, including the dentist. The most difficult cases to deal with are those in which there is only a suspicion of N.A.I., when investigation may be hampered by the scepticism of professional colleagues. However, it is better to risk being rebuffed and proved wrong than to risk exposing the child to further suffering.

## REFERENCES

Becker D B, Needleman H L, Kotelchuck M 1978 Child abuse and dentistry: orofacial trauma and its recognition by dentists. Journal of the American Dental Association 97:24–28

Department of Health and Social Security 1976 Non-accidental injury to children: Area Review Committees. Local Authority Social Services Letter 76:2

Jackson A D M 1976 Non-accidental injuries to children. Proceedings of the British Paedodontic Society 6:11–13

Kempe C H, Silverman F N, Steele B F, Droegmueller W, Silver H K 1962 The battered child syndrome. Journal of the American Medical Association 181:17–24

National Society for the Prevention of Cruelty to Children 1976 At Risk: An account of the work of the battered child research department. Routledge & Kegan Paul, London

Sims B G, Grant J H, Cameron J M 1973 Bite marks in the battered baby syndrome. Medicine, Science and the Law 13:207–210

Sims A P T 1985 Non-accidental injury in the child presenting as a suspected fracture of the zygomatic arch. British Dental Journal 158:292–293

# Appendix: Bur numbering systems

In this book the U.K. bur numbering system is used when referring to burs. The equivalent numbers by the International and U.S.A. systems are given below.

| | Maximum diameter of bur head (mm) | | | | | | | | | | | | | |
|---|---|---|---|---|---|---|---|---|---|---|---|---|---|---|
| | 0.60 | 0.80 | 0.90 | 1.00 | 1.20 | 1.40 | 1.60 | 1.80 | 2.10 | 2.30 | 2.50 | 2.70 | 2.90 | 3.10 |
| I.S.O.* | 006 | 008 | 009 | 010 | 012 | 014 | 016 | 018 | 021 | 023 | 025 | 027 | 029 | 031 |
| United Kingdom | | | | | | | | | | | | | | |
| round | ½ | 1 | | 2 | 3 | 4 | 5 | 6 | 7 | 8 | 9 | 10 | 11 | 12 |
| inverted cone | ½ | 1 | | 2 | 3 | 4 | 5 | 6 | 7 | 8 | 9 | 10 | | |
| flat fissure | | | | | | | | | | | | | | |
|   (plain & cross cut) | | ½ | 1 | 2 | 3 | 4 | 5 | 6 | 7 | 8 | 9 | 10 | 11 | 12 |
| tapered fissure (plain cut) | | | | 2 | 3 | | 5 | | | | | | | |
| tapered fissure (cross cut) | | | | 700 | 701 | | 702 | | 703 | | | | | |
| U.S.A. | | | | | | | | | | | | | | |
| round | ½ | 1 | | 2 | 3 | 4 | 5 | 6 | 7 | 8 | 9 | 10 | | |
| inverted cone | 33½ | 34 | | 35 | 36 | 37 | 38 | 39 | 40 | 41 | 42 | 43 | | |
| flat fissure (plain cut) | | 56 | | 57 | 58 | 59 | | | | | | | | |
| flat fissure (cross cut) | 555½ | 556 | | 557 | 558 | 559 | 560 | 561 | 562 | 563 | | | | |
| tapered fissure (plain cut) | | | | 170 | 171 | | 172 | | | | | | | |
| tapered fissure (cross cut) | | 699 | | 700 | 701 | | 702 | | 703 | | | | | |

* International Organisation for Standardisation

# Index

Note: entries in bold type refer to descriptions of techniques